Salt Wars

Salt Wars

The Battle Over the Biggest Killer in the American Diet

Michael F. Jacobson

foreword by Tom Frieden

The MIT Press
Cambridge, Massachusetts
London, England

This book was set in ITC Stone Serif Std and ITC Stone Sans Std by New Best-set Typesetters Ltd. Printed and bound in the United States of America.

Library of Congress Cataloging-in-Publication Data

Names: Jacobson, Michael F., author.
Title: Salt wars: the battle over the biggest killer in the American diet / Michael F. Jacobson.
Description: Cambridge, Massachusetts : The MIT Press, [2020] | Includes bibliographical references and index.
Identifiers: LCCN 2020002678 | ISBN 9780262044448 (hardcover)
Subjects: MESH: Sodium Chloride, Dietary—adverse effects | Diet—trends | Nutrition Policy | United States
Classification: LCC RM237.8 | NLM WA 712 | DDC 613.2/8522—dc23
LC record available at https://lccn.loc.gov/2020002678

10 9 8 7 6 5 4 3 2 1

To Donna and Sonya, with love

Contents

Foreword

Salt kills.

And that has led to a war—a life-and-death, but largely invisible, conflict. Between taste preferences formed when we were hunter-gatherers foraging for sustenance and our current environment of ultraprocessed, superabundant food. Between industrial profits and the public's health. Between misguided and sometimes corrupt scientists who have created a pseudo-controversy and rigorous researchers. Michael Jacobson has produced a thorough, clearly written, masterful analysis in *Salt Wars*.

It is a one-hundred-year war. Scientists first established evidence that salt kills a century ago, including a demonstration that a low-sodium diet could reverse hypertension. It is a war fought in the halls of Congress, the pages of scientific journals, and the aisles of supermarkets. It is a war with heroes, heroines, and villains—with millions of lives at stake. But, most importantly, it is a war that has not yet been won.

Excess salt intake kills an estimated 3 million people a year around the world and causes millions more strokes and heart attacks. And excess salt drives up health-care costs and undermines family, community, and national finances.

For more than fifty years, the US government has pledged to better protect Americans from heart attacks and strokes by reducing sodium in food. And, for fifty years, the US government has failed to do so. Why?

Three forces have blocked efforts to protect Americans from excess salt: scientific error, industry opposition, and the inherent difficulty of reducing sodium.

Scientific error is the most frustrating of the three. As Jacobson reviews, several scientific groups have purported to discover that at the lowest level of sodium intake, mortality increases. These groups claim to have found a so-called J- or U-shaped causal relationship, whereby both low and high levels of consumption increase health risk. Fortunately, there is now definitive proof that the salt skeptics are wrong. Reducing sodium lowers blood pressure and is associated with reduced risk of heart attacks and strokes. The J-shaped relationship described is the result of errors in study design: measurement of sodium intake has been inaccurate, the formula used to convert a single small urine sample into estimated consumption is fatally flawed, and, in some studies, subjects with the lowest sodium intakes died at a higher rate because they had worse health to begin with, unrelated to sodium intake. Recent analyses have demonstrated that the actual relationship that shows increasing mortality with increasing sodium appears, artifactually, to be J-shaped when these flawed methods are used.

The second force working for salt is easier to understand—money. Salt is cheap. It draws in water, which is even cheaper; foods in brine sold by weight have a higher profit margin. Salt encourages consumption, so industry is concerned, with reason, that if it reduces salt in the food it markets to people they will consume—and buy—less. And industry is inherently opposed to regulation. Like the infamous Tobacco Institute, which misled Congress and the public for decades by claiming that nicotine was not addictive and tobacco not harmful, the Salt Institute spread doubt and controversy for decades about the science of salt.

The third force—we like salt!—is essential to understand. One of my earliest memories is of pouring salt from a Morton box into my hand and licking it from my palm, feeling the tingling tartness on my tongue. We need salt—without it we would die, and some of our food would spoil sooner. Our tastes were created eons ago when salt was hard to come by, but it's cheap, plentiful, and deadly in the amounts we consume today. We need only a tiny fraction of what we consume. Salt is tricky: most of our salt intake doesn't come from salty foods but from foods we eat a lot of, such as bread. In higher-income countries, most salt is invisible to us in the food we buy in supermarkets and at restaurants. In lower-income countries, excess salt is added during cooking. If we steadily reduced the amount of salt we eat, our perception of what is salty will change steadily as well. If we do this, the food we eat now would taste unbearably salty, and our blood pressure and risk of heart attack would plummet.

For decades, Michael F. Jacobson and the Center for Science in the Public Interest have been strategic and persistent warriors against pro-salt forces.

They have sued the United States Food and Drug Administration—twice; lobbied Congress and successive administrations; and publicized shockingly high levels of salt in restaurant and other food. Jacobson's voice—methodical, passionate, plainspoken—comes through clearly in these pages.

Forces protecting people from excess salt have made progress on several fronts. Chile has shown that stark warning labels on the front of packages can cause industry to reformulate products quickly. Industry often claims that making change is impossible—until it is required to do so, after which it finds change surprisingly easy. Reducing sodium in most products by 20–30 percent can be done with virtually no one noticing. Further reductions are possible through both gradual changes in taste and, potentially, clever innovations in salt technology.

The United Kingdom set targets and held industry accountable for progress, saving lives and money in the process. This "health by stealth" approach worked: sodium intake gradually decreased, as did blood pressure and cardiovascular death rates. By encouraging all companies to reduce sodium, the UK showed that it is possible to overcome the "tragedy of the commons"—if one company reduces salt while others don't, that company may be at a competitive disadvantage. The importance of having an eyes-wide-open approach toward industry was confirmed when a new UK government reversed course and relied on voluntary efforts by industry. Progress stalled, resulting in thousands of preventable heart attacks and strokes.

Pro-health forces also have new weapons. Reformulated salt, including structural changes and replacement of some sodium with potassium, can cut sodium content by 20–50 percent with little or no impact on taste for many products.

The war on salt can be won—but only with a concerted and strategic effort that relies on leadership in government and in society. In the United States and other high-income countries, where most food consumed is packaged or restaurant food, strong and persistent policies such as those enacted in Chile and begun in the United Kingdom that create strong incentives for industry to reduce salt will be essential. For food made at home—the dominant source of excess sodium for people in lower-income countries—tools and information that empower people who cook will be needed.

Individuals can, with difficulty, reduce their own sodium intake somewhat, and *Salt Wars* has useful tools and information on how we can begin to make progress on that front. But victory in the United States and other high-income countries will come only when power is put into consumers' hands by removing much of the salt from packaged and restaurant food. It's not possible to remove sodium once it's in our food, but it is possible to add back only what's needed. In lower-income countries, steady progress will require a change in perceptions, government policies, and recipes, as well as evidence-driven innovation to find and spread effective interventions.

Contrary to the saying that there's no accounting for taste, in the case of salt, it's possible both to account for taste, and to return to a healthier world where our taste for salt isn't killing us. When we do this, we will have won the salt wars.

Tom Frieden

Prologue: An Overview of the Salt Battlefield

Salt? Yes, it is the most-used condiment in our food and present in every kitchen. Yes, it helps make foods taste good. Yes, it has been used for thousands of years. And yes, the US Food and Drug Administration (FDA) deems it "generally recognized as safe." So, you may wonder, why a whole book on salt? Why engage in salt wars when the public square is embattled with other controversies about diets high in calories, sugar, and fat, not to mention the political battles in Washington?

I confess that all through college and graduate school I had zero interest in nutrition—don't ask about my diet then! I only got interested in what Americans were eating, who was producing those foods, and how the government monitored their safety when I moved in 1970 from Cambridge, Massachusetts, and MIT to Washington, DC, to volunteer with consumer advocate Ralph Nader. His organization had just published a book about the FDA, and he suggested that I write a book that would take a close look at food additives and how the FDA regulates them.

Frankly, I knew nothing back then about food additives, let alone how to write a book. But I dove into the project and came out with *Eater's Digest*, in which I assessed the use and safety of more than a hundred additives. But— perhaps because familiarity can also breed disinterest—I said *nothing* about salt, even though I discussed in lavish detail the tiny amount of iodine added to it. Only a few years later, as my attention shifted from additives to nutrition, did I begin to learn about salt. And what I learned was deeply disturbing. Familiar as salt was to all of us, medical research had been discovering that consuming excess salt had serious, adverse health consequences. I ultimately concluded that salt is probably the single most harmful thing in our diet (perhaps with sugar a close second). *Salt Wars* follows naturally from the nearly 50 years of investigation into salt since the publication of my first book.

Salt has long been the focus of scientific and policy debates. But to put salt in context, let's focus for a minute on two other substances in our food—sugar and fat—that have received much more attention than salt. For many years sugar was vilified for causing tooth decay, but it was not linked by strong research to deadly diseases. Yet in the past decade or so, sugar has been increasingly studied and increasingly controversial. New research found that sugar and its kissing cousin high-fructose corn syrup promotes obesity, diabetes, and heart disease. That led to demands by health activists around the country for soft-drink taxes and warning labels. The soft-drink industry adamantly denied that its products were anything but safe sources of water and pleasure, and it hired a fleet of lobbyists and PR firms to influence legislators and the public. The new evidence on sugar has led to an 18 percent decline in sugar consumption, as well as improved Nutrition Facts labels that disclose the amount of added sugars.

Sugar is easy for people to understand (and target) because it is such a predominant ingredient in foods: a can of soda pop has about 10 teaspoons of sugar, and a breakfast cereal aimed at kids might be more than one-third sugar. That gets people's attention! In contrast, not many packaged foods have more than half a teaspoon of salt per serving.

Fatty foods and diets, too, have been perennially in the news. Countless stories have publicized the research on how polyunsaturated fatty acids (found mostly in vegetable oils) can reduce the risk of heart disease if they replace the saturated fatty acids (most abundant in meat, dairy products, and palm and coconut oils) in our diets. Other research has focused on whether fats contribute to obesity, a topic of great interest because two-thirds of Americans have overweight or obesity. Concerns about weight confront many of us every time we look in a mirror or step on a scale. In contrast, it is much easier to forget about the invisible signs of high blood pressure (hypertension) or heart disease caused by salty diets and other factors.

Trans fat, which generated a tsunami of attention beginning in the mid-1990s through the mid-2010s, was the perfect topic for journalists: it was a new threat, it was created in factories, it was a key ingredient in such iconic products as Crisco and Oreos—and most scientists and the FDA had considered it totally safe. The burst of reliable and unrebutted new research identifying trans fatty acids as a major cause of heart disease provided a practically open-and-shut case for action. In fact, the whole battle over trans fat was settled, by Washington standards, with astonishing speed. It took the FDA "only" 20 years to conclude that artificial trans fat was harmful and its source (partially hydrogenated vegetable oil, or PHO) was *not* "generally recognized as safe." In June 2018, the FDA banned the use of PHOs in all foods sold and served in grocery stores and restaurants, although it granted some extensions of the compliance date.

So, partly obscured by the supernova controversies surrounding sugars and fats, the salt wars being fought by researchers, health officials, health advocates, and industry have been waged largely under the radar. Most scientists who have studied the health effects of salt—aka sodium chloride—long ago concluded that eating too much salt (or sodium) increases blood pressure, which in turn increases the risk of strokes and heart attacks. And eating too much is easy, considering the ubiquity of salt in the food supply and the number of restaurant meals that contain well over a day's worth of sodium. Thus for many years, the American Heart Association, World Health Organization, and Centers for Disease Control and Prevention have urged food manufacturers and restaurants to sharply reduce sodium levels in their foods, which would automatically reduce sodium intakes by consumers.

But another group of researchers disagrees vehemently with the conventional wisdom. Their studies have indicated that Americans are eating a healthy amount of salt and that eating less would *increase* the risk of cardiovascular disease—a broad category that includes hypertension, coronary heart disease, heart failure, stroke, and other disorders. That was welcome news to food manufacturers and restaurants, which have long relied on salt as a cheap way to make and preserve delicious foods.

Medical journals were the initial battlefields of the salt wars, where opening shots were fired with the publication of controversial studies. Such studies have often elicited (and still do) fusillades of letters from opposing scientists. And that, in turn, spurred rebuttals from the original authors. Meanwhile, the usually restrained disagreements in journals turned into more spirited and candid arguments in newspapers and other popular media.

Quotable, outspoken warrior-professors have epitomized the two sides of the salt wars. For instance, Graham A. MacGregor, a British hypertension expert, is a leading advocate for consuming less sodium, whereas

Michael Alderman, an American hypertension expert and former editor of the *American Journal of Hypertension*, argues that current sodium levels are not only safe but also virtually unchangeable. Call them the yin and yang of salt researchers: MacGregor has authored hundreds of published papers, is quick with a barb aimed at the food industry and recalcitrant health officials, ardently defends the establishment view on the causes of hypertension, and seeks to influence consumers, governments, and companies. Alderman, who also has published hundreds of scientific papers, has been quoted in the *Wall Street Journal* and the *New York Times*, and has been a leader of the rebels (several Canadian and Danish scientists are in this camp, too) whose research counters the view that people should eat less salt. Alderman, MacGregor, and their colleagues in academe have helped catalyze a very public debate over a mineral that makes up less than 1 percent of our diet.

One reason that the debate has been so vigorous is that most journalists treat new reports supporting the conventional view on salt with a yawn. Dog bites man? Big deal. What does capture the interest of journalists and headline writers are the man-bites-dog reports—those suggesting that eating *less* salt would be harmful—especially when they are conducted by credentialed researchers at prominent universities and published in respected journals. More-mainstream researchers criticize the reliability of such pro-salt research. But their efforts usually materialize too late, after journalists have already pounded away at their keyboards to author cleverly titled articles suggesting—or stating bluntly—that everything we have been told about salt is wrong. The poor consumer, lacking an advanced degree in epidemiology or nutrition, can get dizzy trying to follow the arcane biomedical and statistical jousting.

Industry—including the late, benighted Salt Institute, the salt industry's PR and lobbying arm—then enlists studies that have found that cutting salt would be dangerous, and uses them to manufacture further doubt that high-sodium diets are as deadly as most experts say. Many companies do not want anyone mucking up their time-tested recipes (and profits), and so they contend that more research is needed before any conclusions are drawn or any government regulatory measures are deployed.

On the political battlefield in Washington, as in policy-making centers elsewhere in the world, industry and health advocates alike lobby their respective governments. They appear before Congress, or the FDA, or the White House to try to achieve their goals and to thwart their opponents' efforts, as each side seeks to obtain or repeal a regulation, or win or block funding for a program, or set or prevent limits on sodium in foods. Most of those skirmishes come to naught, swallowed up by more immediate concerns, such as health insurance, or global warming, or the federal budget. But occasionally a measure sneaks through for better (such as in 1990 when Congress required the labeling of sodium and other nutrients on most packaged foods) or for worse (when the US Department of Agriculture in 2018 postponed or dropped tighter sodium limits in school foods).

The key questions that I explore in *Salt Wars* include: What is a safe amount of sodium to consume? Should everyone cut back on salt or only people with high blood pressure? Would cutting back save or cost thousands of lives a year? What should government and companies do, if anything? And what should we consumers do when we sit down for our next meal?

Here's a chapter-by-chapter game plan for understanding the salt wars: I first describe how salt is used in food, how much we are consuming, and how much most nutrition experts say we should be consuming (chapter 1). In two key chapters, I investigate in some detail the health concerns connected to salt (chapter 2), focusing mostly on hypertension, heart attacks, and strokes, and move on to examine (in chapter 3) the contentions of the "sodium skeptics." Happily for readers, though, I focus on only a tiny—but key—fraction of the Niagara of studies, review articles, and letters to medical journals on the topic. Next comes a concise evaluation and summary of the research on salt's impact on cardiovascular disease (chapter 4). I follow that with revelations of the activities of the pugnacious Salt Institute (chapter 5), along with a brief discussion of the influence of money on scientists (chapter 6). I discuss what countries around the world, from Fiji to France, are doing to cut dietary salt (chapter 7), and recount the snail-like progress in the United States (chapter 8). There is good news to be had in chapter 9: the federal government, companies, and schools are finally beginning to address the salt problem. Continuing on a hopeful note, I present a plan for accelerating reductions of sodium in the food supply and in American diets (chapter 10), and discuss (in chapter 11) what *you* can do to protect your own and your family's health without waiting for government or industry to do anything. (Many of these chapters include illustrations, tables, and information boxes to supplement or summarize the material I present; in the appendixes I list their titles, and include as well the abbreviations for key agencies, studies, and terms that appear throughout the book.) Finally, the epilogue puts salt in the context of other health disputes in which industry has played a decidedly unhealthy role.

1 Salt: A Primer

Salt tastes good—and makes everything else taste good.
—Kimberly Y. Masibay, FineCooking.com[1]

Sodium chloride. Plain old salt: the condiment most used by consumers and the food industry alike. More than half of all packaged foods contain added salt. Practically every home has several loaded saltshakers, plus a canister of salt in the cupboard. We mostly use it to bring out the flavor of foods, either adding it when we're cooking a dish or sprinkling it on our food at the table. Its wide use is no surprise, because saltiness is one of the five basic tastes.

James Beard, the cookbook author who long advocated American cuisine, famously asked: *Where would we be without salt?* "Adrift in a sea of blandness," answered celebrity chef Samin Nosrat in her recent cookbook *Salt, Fat, Acid, Heat.*[2] Chef Rick Bayless, owner of Frontera Grill, a Chicago institution, declared that home chefs make one of their biggest mistakes when "they don't salt enough."[3]

Chefs in restaurants or homes—and food manufacturers as well—love salt because it is so flavorful and so cheap. That's a major reason we find salt in 52 percent of all packaged foods—a higher percentage than any other ingredient (sugar and high-fructose corn syrup are found in "only" 40 percent of foods).[4] Even a pinch of salt injects a desirable taste, at almost no cost, into an otherwise bland dish or masks the unpleasant taste of one with bitter ingredients. Companies invest heavily in taste testing to identify the "bliss point" at which flavor, whether from salt, fat, sugar, or other ingredients, is optimized.

In addition to adding flavor, salt performs a multitude of other functions, not least as a preservative. In cured meats and seafood, it retards bacterial growth. In bread, it strengthens gluten and inhibits the growth of acid-producing bacteria. In cheesemaking, it helps separate the curds from the whey, facilitates melting, provides flavor, and inhibits the growth of some microorganisms. Salt also adds a sense of thickness ("mouthfeel," as food technologists say) to soups and beverages.[5] Pickle makers know that using the right amount of salt encourages the growth of "good" lactic acid–producing bacteria and discourages the growth of spoilage bacteria.[6] Salt brings out the flavor of other seasonings, and it reduces bitterness or sourness in some foods, allowing sweetness or other flavors to pop out.

Add to the versatility of salt the fact that the body absolutely needs small amounts of it to function. Without salt, or with inadequate amounts of it, our bodies would simply break down: it is present throughout the body and involved in countless physiologic processes, from ensuring healthy blood volume to maintaining the optimal potassium levels in cells, from transmitting nerve impulses to contracting and relaxing muscle fibers. Fortunately, our bodies do not need much salt, so virtually no one needs to worry about consuming too little. Even endurance athletes, such as ultra-marathoners who sweat profusely, do not seem to need salt supplements.[7] In the rare cases of people who have too little sodium in their blood (hyponatremia), symptoms might include fatigue, nausea, and confusion, among others.[8]

Aside from possible harms to health when people consume too much, salt serves at least two dubious, often-unrecognized commercial functions. First, food manufacturers add it to mask the off-flavors created when the ingredients they use are low quality or cooked for excessive times or at high temperatures or extruded at high pressures. Richard Horton, the longtime editor of the *Lancet* medical journal, minced no words when he said (perhaps with a dash of hyperbole) that food manufacturers "desperately need salt to persuade us to swallow the otherwise inedible rubbish they serve up to us daily."[9]

Second, as Thomas G. Pickering, a professor of medicine at New York City's College of Physicians and Surgeons, Columbia University Medical Center, once explained:

> In the 19th century, cattle drivers who were taking their cattle to market in Poughkeepsie, NY, used to stop at a place called Salt Lick on the day before they reached the market, where the cattle would take on salt and water, thereby increasing their weight and market value.[10]

Today, implicitly admitting to a modern-day version of that chicanery, many meat and poultry processors inject or otherwise add water (and flavor) to their product along with a disclaimer on labels: "__% solution of chicken broth and salt added." I've seen "meat" containing as much as 30 percent added water. The ham shown in figure 1.1 had 23 percent added water, sugar, salt, and other ingredients, for which a consumer paid almost five dollars. Companies called such meat "enhanced" until the US Department of Agriculture (USDA) outlawed that euphemism in 2015.[11] I call it adulterated, which it surely is. At a press conference I once held up a seven-and-a-half pound package of chicken and deplored that consumers were paying chicken prices for the water added to it, which amounted to 15 percent of its weight, or slightly more than a pound![12]

Sodium chloride and sodium phosphates make it possible for meat to hold on to that much extra water. According to the USDA, 21 percent of beef, 78 percent of chicken, and 57 percent of pork is bulked out this way.[13]

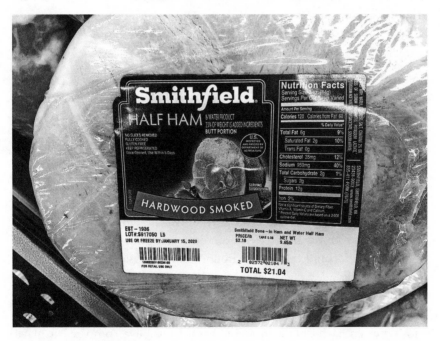

Figure 1.1
Water-added ham. This Smithfield ham contains 23 percent of mostly water, sugar, and salt. *Source*: Photo by the author.

Such products are far higher in sodium than plain, natural meat. Judging from a 2006 study of poultry conducted by California state officials, consumers nationwide were paying $2.6 billion (adjusted for inflation to 2020 dollars) annually for the added solution.[14] Add in the beef and pork products that are watered down, and it appears that consumers are now being cheated out of at least $4 billion annually and possibly much more.

Pickering also noted that because salt stimulates thirst, the bars that offer free salted peanuts, pretzels, and potato chips may do so not out of generosity but because people will order more drinks. (Incidentally, Pickering coined the term "white-coat hypertension," whereby patients experience higher blood pressure in a doctor's office than elsewhere.[15])

Salt itself provides about 90 percent of the sodium added to food, with a host of additives providing the rest.[16] Sodium is integral to baking soda (bicarbonate of soda), baking powder (often containing sodium aluminum phosphate), sodium ascorbate (vitamin C added as a nutrient or preservative), monosodium glutamate (MSG, a flavor enhancer), sodium propionate (a mold inhibitor), sodium stearoyl lactylate (an emulsifier that increases bread volume), sodium nitrite (another preservative), and dozens of other ingredients.

How Much Sodium Do We Need?

In the days before people preserved fish, sausages, and other foods with salt, salty foods were rare or nonexistent. People living back then did well with far less sodium—and still do so today in a few communities—than even the strictest, most current advice recommends.

More than 12,000 years ago our Paleolithic ancestors foraged savannas and forests for their food. Their diets are thought to have consisted of roughly two-thirds fruits, legumes, roots, and nuts and one-third wild game. They probably consumed around 3,000 calories a day, somewhat more than the average American consumes today.[17] But those calories were accompanied by less than 800 milligrams (mg) of sodium (see figure 1.2). Those modest quantities of sodium were accompanied by potassium, another essential nutrient, in amounts that are huge compared to what processed-food-eating people now consume.

Jeremiah Stamler of the Northwestern University Feinberg School of Medicine observed:

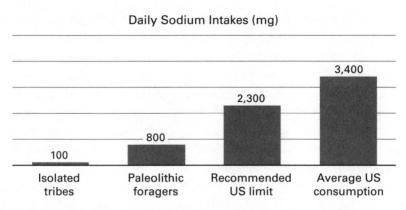

Figure 1.2
Daily sodium intakes of different populations.

> During the 4–15 million years of hominoid and hominid evolution leading to *Homo sapiens sapiens,* our hunter-gatherer nomadic predecessors had no exposures to the several components of contemporary lifestyles now known to be related present-day to population BP patterns—no exposures to: habitual high salt intake due daily to addition of salt to foods, or to a fare with a high ratio of [sodium to potassium]. . . . On the contrary, having evolved in the warm climate of Africa, a salt-poor continent, on a fare low in salt by present-day practices, the human species became—and remains—exquisitely adapted for the physiological conservation of the limited salt in the food supply, i.e., for salt retention, not for excretion of a chronically excessive intake, 10–20+ times physiological need.[18]

Stamler, a legendary epidemiologist who has been doing research since 1948, has been called the Father of Preventive Cardiology; he celebrated his one hundredth birthday in 2019.[19]

Finnish researchers have calculated that because unprocessed, natural foods are so low in sodium, it is almost impossible to consume a totally natural-foods diet that contains more than 1,200 mg of sodium per day.[20] Those scientists concluded that "our genetic mechanisms are programmed" to work best with that level of sodium. We are now witnessing what happens when our intake of sodium gets out of kilter with what our bodies evolved to expect.

The hunter-gatherers of today are a throwback to cave dwellers of yore. Let's travel to South America and meet the Yanomami Indians, an isolated tribe living in the rainforest straddling Venezuela and Brazil. (That isolation is eroding, thanks in part to the illegal entry of miners into tribal lands since the 1970s; the problem worsened since 2018 with an invasion by upwards of 20,000 more miners.)[21] Researchers first visited the Yanomamis in the early 1970s and found that they were physically active, short, and rarely obese.[22] They ate mostly plantains, cassava, along with some game, fish, and wild vegetables. Using the gold standard for determining sodium intake—the amount excreted in urine over 24 hours—the researchers found that the Yanomamis excreted only about 20 mg of sodium per day, though they consumed somewhat more. They were healthy and presumably had lived with little sodium for millennia.

A 2005 committee of the Institute of Medicine, now the National Academy of Medicine (NAM), said that the minimum sodium requirement for adults is 180 mg per day, but it set the Adequate Intake at 1,500 mg to ensure that people could consume necessary levels of other nutrients and to account for different patterns of physical activity and climate.[23] The generous 1,500-mg level, which the NAM still considers adequate, is far above what the isolated tribes consume, but less than what almost every American consumes.

At the other extreme, some people in the northern part of Japan may consume as much as 10,000 mg per day. In the 1600s, aristocrats in northern Europe flaunted their affluence by consuming an estimated 20,000 mg per day—at least five times as much as today's average American.[24]

Why do people now find such pleasure in diets that contain 50 or 100 times more sodium than those of our prehistoric ancestors? Probably our taste buds and brains evolved in that salt-scarce era to make us love the taste of salt, and so our ancestors ate salt or salty foods whenever they could. Unfortunately, once people began consuming thousands of milligrams of sodium per day, evolution did not put a brake on our innate love of salty foods or cause us to reject very salty foods or diets. Although we do find extremely salty foods unpalatable, the "distaste level" is too high to be helpful when it comes to limiting ourselves to reasonable, healthful amounts of sodium.

How Much Sodium *Should* We Consume?

If hunter-gatherers consume well under 1,000 mg of sodium per day and the average American consumes around 3,000 (women) or 4,000 (men) mg per day, you might wonder how much sodium *you* should consume to protect your health. The federal government's official recommendation for healthy adults—2,300 milligrams per day—is provided in its "Dietary Guidelines for Americans 2015–2020." The NAM reiterated that figure in 2019, though the committee did not provide different recommended intakes for those at high risk of, or with, hypertension (high blood pressure).[25] But the "Dietary Guidelines," as well as the American Heart Association, recognize that adults with elevated blood pressure—both prehypertension and hypertension— would especially benefit from consuming closer to 1,500 mg per day.[26]

The World Health Organization (WHO), which advises governments throughout the world, sets a somewhat stricter standard than the "Dietary Guidelines" by recommending that adults consume less than 2,000 mg per day.[27] Perhaps the most restrictive (and protective) advice comes from the United Kingdom government's National Institute for Health and Care Excellence. In 2010 it set extremely ambitious goals (which are not being met) of having adults consume no more than 2,400 mg per day by 2015 and just 1,200 mg of sodium per day by 2025.[28] To be candid, if the average American reduced consumption to 2,300 mg by 2030 that would be a miracle. Currently, only 2 percent of adult men and 20 percent of adult women consume less than 2,300 mg per day.[29] (It's probably not that women are watching their sodium intake more closely than men, it's that women consume less food.) The percentage of people consuming less than 1,500 mg is microscopic. Getting the average daily intake down to or below 2,300 or 2,000 mg is challenging, especially considering that about 600 mg of the sodium we consume occurs naturally in dairy products, fruit, seafood, and other foods. That doesn't leave much room for the added sodium in processed and restaurant foods.

Food manufacturers use the number 2,300 to calculate the "% Daily Value" on food labels. Because salt is 40 percent sodium, 2,300 mg of sodium is equivalent to 5,750 mg of salt—just shy of 6 grams (roughly one teaspoonful) of table salt. Note that the 2,300 mg benchmark is an average for men and women, so men (who consume more food) could consume a couple of hundred milligrams more and women should consume a couple of hundred milligrams less.

Young children, being smaller, should consume less sodium than adults. The recommended daily limit for children 1 to 3 years old is 1,200 mg; for children 4 to 8 that limit is 1,500 mg; for children 9 to 13 it is 1,800 mg.[30] Health officials hope that when children raised on less-salty foods grow older, they will be satisfied with similar salt levels.

Table 1.1

Calorie and sodium (mg) intakes for people with a sedentary lifestyle*

Age	2–3	4–8	9–13	14–18	19–30	31–50	51–70	71+
Males	1,000	1,400	1,800	2,300	2,400	2,300	2,100	2,000
Females	1,000	1,200	1,500	1,800	2,000	1,800	1,600	1,600

*Sedentary lifestyle includes only the physical activity associated with independent living. Calorie intakes will be higher at greater physical activity levels.

Adapted from data in US Department of Agriculture, US Department of Health and Human Services. "Dietary Guidelines for Americans 2015–2020," tables A2-1, A7-1; Center for Nutrition Policy and Promotion, US Department of Agriculture. Nutrients in healthy US-style food pattern at each calorie level. https://www.cnpp.usda.gov/sites/default/files/usda_food_patterns/NutrientsInHealthyUS-StyleFoodPattern.pdf (accessed November 17, 2018).

A more refined way of estimating *your* maximum recommended sodium intake is to tie it to your calorie intake. Young adult women and men around 30 or 40 years old with a sedentary lifestyle consume an average of about 2,100 calories per day. That 2,100 number representing calorie intake is just a little under the 2,300 mg recommendation for daily sodium intake. Hence, you could aim to consume no more than about 1 milligram of sodium per calorie, a 1:1 ratio. Someone consuming 1,600 calories per day should aim for no more than about 1,600 mg of sodium, but someone consuming 2,400 calories would have a looser target of about 2,400 mg. Table 1.1 shows how that translates into recommendations for males and females of different ages whose activity level is described as sedentary (that means most of us).

You could also use that 1:1 ratio of sodium to calories as a guide when you're reading food labels or recipes. If a food contains much more than 1 mg of sodium per calorie, or 100 mg per 100 calories, that is probably too much. But finding those "1:1 or less" foods may not be easy. A study conducted by the USDA and the Centers for Disease Control and Prevention (CDC) found that only 13 out of 125 different kinds of food (ranging from breakfast cereals to beef hot dogs to barbecue sauce) averaged under 110 mg per 100 calories. Moreover, most of the 13 were not low in sodium but high in calories, such as sugary baked goods and high-fat French fries and peanut butter.[31]

There are a couple of exceptions to the 1:1 rule. A cup of packaged soup typically provides only about a hundred calories, but its large volume needs anywhere from several hundred to a thousand milligrams of sodium to taste good. Another exception is canned or frozen vegetables, which are also low in calories, so modest amounts of salt could easily exceed the guideline.

How Much Sodium *Do* We Consume?

Determining exactly how much salt, or sodium, people consume turns out to be a far more challenging task than just conducting a survey to find out what foods they ate. Most people could estimate pretty accurately how many eggs they had for breakfast. But salt is different. Salt is added to countless packaged foods. Natural or processed, organically grown or not, homemade or restaurant-made, almost everything contains sodium. Moreover, levels may vary widely from brand to brand of the same food. You cannot even count on food labels to provide accurate information. Nutrition Facts labels often overstate by 10 percent or so the amount of sodium in a serving, because companies don't want to be caught illegally understating the amount. The sodium content of meals at chain restaurants is disclosed on websites (calories must be disclosed on menus), but the sodium content of foods served at non-chain restaurants is essentially unknowable.

A 2017 survey of people leaving fast-food restaurants underscored consumers' ignorance of sodium levels.[32] Their average meal contained 1,292 mg of sodium. But they estimated—or, more accurately, guessed—that the meals contained only 279 mg.

For the past several decades, sodium consumption and many other measures of health have been assessed in the National Health and Nutrition Examination Survey (NHANES) conducted by the CDC. The surveyors interview several thousand people from around the country each year, asking them detailed questions about, among other topics, their medical history, what they ate the previous day or about other food-related concerns, and then weighing them and measuring their blood pressure. The dietary responses are then translated into milligrams of sodium by using USDA food composition databases (see USDA's FoodData Central).[33]

NHANES found that Americans consume much more than the recommended intake: the average person consumes about 3,400 mg of sodium per day (about 500 mg less for women and 500 mg more for men); that 3,400 mg figure has not budged much in 30 years despite the many recommendations to cut back.[34] People in many other countries consume about the same amount, making humans the only animal species that consumes large quantities of salt.

In fact, the CDC found that 88 percent of people consume more than the recommended 2,300 mg, and 98.6 percent of people who met the "Dietary Guidelines" criteria to limit their sodium intake to 1,500 mg per day consume more than that amount.[35] Eric Decker, the head of the Department of Food Science at the University of Massachusetts, Amherst, commented on the obvious: "We keep making recommendations and making recommendations and the needle doesn't move at all."[36]

Children, who love salty foods, such as canned soup, hot dogs with mustard on white buns, French fries, and Oscar Mayer Lunchables, also consume much more sodium than is ideal. Three out of four children 1 to 4 years old consume more than the recommended amounts of sodium.[37] Children 8 to 17 consume an average of 1,000 mg more than is recommended. But in one promising change, for reasons unknown, in the years 2015 and 2016 combined, children were consuming about 5 percent less sodium than they were a dozen years earlier. Perhaps related, they were experiencing slightly lower rates of elevated and high blood pressure.[38]

One limitation of dietary surveys is that they tend to understate food intakes. NHANES relies on people's memories to accurately report the foods and portion sizes they have eaten. Not surprisingly, many people tend to underestimate how much they consume, especially when it comes to unhealthy foods. People may "forget" to tell researchers about that second serving of soup, or they won't mention they ate the whole 3-ounce bag of pretzels instead of calling it quits after 1 ounce. Researchers believe that the underreporting of foods and serving sizes probably results in a 10 percent underestimate of calorie and sodium intakes. Also, USDA databases may not have accurate data or even any data for certain items. For instance, it is impossible for the databases to know just how much sodium was in that meal you ate at the Thai restaurant last night.

Another problem is that NHANES does not ask people how much salt they use in cooking or add at the table. As I show later in the chapter with figure 1.3, those uses of salt would add another 10 percent to sodium intake. Thus, correcting for the two limitations would boost the actual sodium-intake average by 800 mg to 4,000 mg per day.

To overcome the problems with dietary-recall estimates, in 2014 the CDC began using a more accurate method to measure sodium consumption.

They asked some NHANES participants to collect their urine for 24 hours. The amount of sodium in the urine pretty accurately reflects the amount of sodium consumed in a day. But even that approach fails to reflect the 10 percent or so that is lost in sweat and stool. Also, not every participant scrupulously collects every drop of urine. Notwithstanding those limitations, 24-hour urinary excretion is the best way to measure sodium consumption. Based on 24-hour urine samples, Mary Cogswell and others at the CDC found that men between the ages of 20 and 69 excreted 4,205 mg of sodium per day, and women excreted 3,039 mg per day.[39] When those numbers were adjusted for the missing 10 percent from sweat and urine, the average actual intake of sodium was found to be 4,008 mg.

Thus, the actual average sodium intake of American adults, as determined by two different methods, is about 4,000 mg per day, not 3,400. (If that figure were incorporated in recommendations, to be consistent the 2,300 mg goal would be raised proportionately to 2,700 mg.) But because most scientists, health officials, and journalists use the uncorrected number—3,400 mg—as the average intake, *Salt Wars* will generally use that number.

Sodium consumption has remained about the same during the past several decades, even though some manufacturers have reduced sodium moderately in some of their products (see chapter 9). It appears that those decreases were balanced by our consumption of more food, by some companies increasing sodium, or by our eating out more often, where the sky is the limit when it comes to sodium.

It would be interesting to compare how much sodium Americans are consuming now to what our forebearers consumed a hundred years ago. Back then most people ate home-cooked meals in which the sodium came from the salt used in cooking or while eating, the small naturally occurring amounts in foods, or the relatively few packaged foods. But, lacking refrigeration, they were also eating hefty amounts of cured meats and fish (ham, bacon, salted cod, and the like), which were loaded with salt and the preservatives sodium nitrate and sodium nitrite. Furthermore, many more people engaged in physical labor, leading them to consume more food—and, hence, more sodium. Unfortunately, though USDA has tracked food consumption since 1909, it didn't track nutrient intakes until recent decades. Thus we can only speculate on whether our ancestors consumed more or less sodium than we do today.

Nutrition Facts labels are a starting point for figuring out how much sodium we consume now. Most packaged foods do not have shockingly large amounts of sodium, partly because the portions listed on many labels are unrealistically small, but the milligrams do add up. While 1 ounce of those potato chips contains about 160 mg of sodium, eat an entire 3-ounce bag and you've consumed about one-fifth of your recommended daily sodium limit. A typical Campbell condensed soup contains around 800 mg per cup, but many people eat the entire can and consume 2,000 mg. Foods that contain half a day's sodium or more (see examples in table 1.2, "Salt Bombs at Grocery Stores") simply can't fit into a healthy diet.

In contrast to individual servings of packaged foods, countless meals eaten outside the home are loaded with salt. That's an increasingly important problem because we are increasingly reliant on restaurant meals. In the late 1970s, away-from-home meals and snacks—from restaurants, cafeterias, food trucks, and vending machines—accounted for 18 percent of Americans' calories.[40] In the early 2010s, that figure almost doubled to 34 percent. USDA found that foods served at table-service restaurants had 35 percent more sodium per 1,000 calories than foods prepared at home.[41] Fast foods had "only" 22 percent more sodium than home-prepared meals.

But those are averages. Many restaurant meals are huge and contain a whole day's worth of sodium, with some meals providing two or occasionally even three times as much sodium as a person should consume in an entire day. (The calorie, saturated fat, and sugar contents are equally startling.) In the 1990s, my organization, the Center for Science in the Public Interest (CSPI), conducted widely publicized analyses of the nutrient content of popular foods served at table-service restaurants, ranging from Chinese and Italian to seafood and steak houses.[42] We dubbed Fettuccine Alfredo a "heart attack on a plate" and shocked people when we publicized the calorie, fat, and sodium content of movie-theater popcorn (sales of which immediately plummeted). While the fat or saturated fat content varied widely from one type of restaurant to another, the meals were uniformly high in sodium and calories. We found, for instance, that an order of Beef with Broccoli at a Chinese restaurant had 3,150 mg of sodium and a Fried Seafood Combo with tartar sauce, fries, coleslaw, and buttered biscuits at a seafood restaurant had 4,390 mg. Those amounts are way over the recommended daily target of 2,300 mg and, if anything, may have become even saltier since then.[43]

Table 1.2

Salt bombs at grocery stores

Company	Food	Sodium content per serving (mg)	Days' worth of sodium*
Campbell	Chicken Noodle Soup, condensed (whole can)	2,120	1
Kohinoor Foods	Mughlai Kofta Curry with Peas Pulao	2,120	1
ConAgra Brands	Banquet Mega Bowls Buffalo-Style Chicken Mac 'N Cheese	2,100	1
The Original Soupman	Crab & Corn Chowder (whole box, 17 oz.)	2,080	1
Pinnacle Foods	Hungry-Man Selects Mesquite Classic Fried Chicken (16 oz.)	2,060	1
La Choy	Chicken Chow Mein (½ can)	2,055	1
Maruchan	Ramen Noodle Soup Soy Sauce Flavor (whole package)	1,760	¾
Walmart	Great Value Meatlovers Calzone	1,600	⅔
Hormel	Dinty Moore Beef Stew (XL) (12.5 oz.)	1,570	⅔
Campbell	Chili with Beans Chunky Soup (15¼ oz. microwaveable bowl)	1,540	⅔
Bob Evans	Sausage & Potatoes Bowl	1,470	⅔
Campbell	Slow Kettle Style Creamy Broccoli Cheddar Bisque (15.5 oz.)	1,420	⅗
Tabasco	Bloody Mary Mix (8 oz.)	1,380	⅗
Tyson	Fully Cooked Chicken Pomodoro Dinner Kit (½ package)	1,350	⅗
Libby's	Spaghetti & Meatballs (14.5 oz.)	1,280	½
Hormel	Macaroni and Cheese Pasta (10 oz.)	1,250	½

*Based on the recommended limit of 2,300 mg per day; serving sizes not all labeled servings.

Today, by restaurants' own admission, many meals have far more than 2,300 mg of sodium (see table 1.3, "Salt Bombs at Restaurants"). Because of their larger portion sizes and additional components (salads, bread, etc.), meals at table-service restaurants generally have more salt than those at fast-food restaurants. According to company websites, IHOP's Bacon Temptation Omelette with a side of three Buttermilk Pancakes has 3,790 mg of sodium, two-thirds more than someone should consume in an entire day. Applebee's three-course dinner of Chipotle Lime Chicken Quesadilla appetizer, House Salad with Mexi-Ranch Dressing, and the Fiesta Lime Chicken entrée delivers a whopping 7,150 mg of sodium. Chili's gigantic Ultimate Smokehouse Combo, with its three meats and side dishes, may contain as much as an astonishing 8,050 mg![44] Those last two meals provide three days' worth of sodium. With meals like that on restaurant menus, it is no surprise that the New York City health department found that the average meal ordered by diners at IHOP and TGI Fridays had more than 2,800 mg and more than 3,400 mg, respectively.[45]

Restaurants try to explain away those huge amounts of sodium by claiming that people treat eating out as an occasional indulgence and put their health concerns aside. Or they say that the lower-sodium (and lower-calorie) meals also on the menu provide a choice for people who want to avoid the heart attack that many of their other meals might cause. Justifications aside, restaurants need to do a better job of lowering the calorie and sodium content of what they sell to a nation of people who have overweight, obesity, or hypertension.

While almost everyone is consuming too much sodium, a recent national survey found that only about half of all consumers try to limit sodium.[46] Another survey found that only 29 percent of people were trying to limit sodium, though 38 percent were trying to limit sugar and 44 percent were trying to avoid artificial sweeteners (which pose a small health risk).[47] Still, the percentages of people concerned about salt and trying to reduce their intake are twice as large as in the 1990s.[48]

If we wanted to consume less salt, it would be helpful to know which foods contribute the most sodium. According to the CDC, 71 percent of all the sodium we consume is added to food by manufacturers and restaurants, not by consumers using a saltshaker (see figure 1.3).[49] About 14 percent of our sodium intake is unavoidable because it occurs naturally in everything from spinach to meat; 6 percent comes from salt (and soy sauce,

Table 1.3

Salt bombs at restaurants

Company	Food	Sodium content (mg)	Days' worth of sodium*
Chili's	Ultimate Smokehouse Combo (with Cheesy Bacon BBQ Chicken, Honey Chipotle Crispers w/Ranch, and Dry Rub Ribs)	8,050 mg	3½
Jimmy John's	Gargantuan on French bread (16-inch)	7,830	3½
AMC (movie theaters)	Bavarian Legend Soft Pretzel	7,600	3⅓
Applebee's	Chipotle Lime Chicken Quesadilla, House Salad with Mexi-Ranch Dressing, Fiesta Lime Chicken	7,150	3
Outback Steakhouse	Baked Potato Soup (bowl), Blue Cheese Side Salad with dressing, Grilled Pork Chop	6,990	3
Red Lobster	Admiral's Feast	5,000	2⅓
Jersey Mike's Subs	Chipotle Chicken Cheese Steak (giant), Fries (5 oz.)	4,950	2
Chili's	Honey-Chipotle Crispers & Waffles	4,730	2
Uno Pizzeria & Grill	Deep Dish Buffalo Chicken Mac & Cheese	4,310	1¾
Jason's Deli	Roasted Turkey Breast Muffaletta (½)	4,240	1¾
Shake Shack	Double SmokeShack (cheeseburger), Fries, Black & White Shake	4,230	1¾
P. F. Chang's	Long Life Noodles and Prawns	4,120	1¾
Denny's	The Grand Slamwich with bacon, Bacon Cheddar Tots	3,920	1¾
Chick-fil-A	Spicy Chicken Sandwich, Waffle Potato Fries (medium), Chicken Soup (large)	3,820	1⅔
IHOP	Bacon Temptation Omelette with three Buttermilk Pancakes	3,790	1⅔
The Cheesecake Factory	Breakfast Burrito	3,640	1⅔
Sbarro	Chicken Vesuvio with Spaghetti, Breadstick	3,130	1⅓
KFC	Popcorn (chicken) Nuggets (large)	1,890	⅘

*Based on the recommended limit of 2,300 mg per day. Data obtained from restaurants' websites.

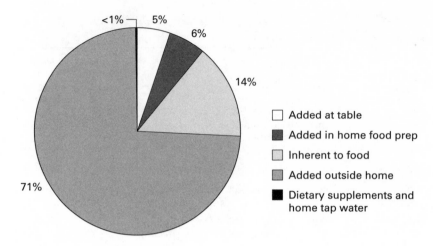

Figure 1.3
Most sodium comes from processed and restaurant foods. *Source*: Illustration by J. Bach, CSPI, based on L. J. Harnack, M. E. Cogswell, J. M. Shikany et al., "Sources of Sodium in US Adults from 3 Geographic Regions," *Circulation* 135 (2017): 1775–1783.

baking powder, MSG, and other ingredients) used when we cook; and just 5 percent comes from what we add at the table. Tap water, drugs, and other sources provide the rest. In other words, except for people who use them with abandon, saltshakers are not a big part of the problem—yet nearly half of all adults believe that table salt is the biggest source of sodium.[50]

The sodium content of most natural foods is quite low. One estimate has put the average sodium content of natural foods from plants at only 14 mg per 3.5 ounces (100g), and foods from animals at 59 mg per 3.5 ounces. But processing typically sends those numbers soaring. For instance, a 3.5-ounce boiled potato has 4 mg of sodium (adding a tablespoon of margarine might bring that up to 75 mg),[51] while a 1-ounce serving of Lay's Classic Potato Chips has 170 mg. Four ounces of natural chicken has about 87 mg of sodium. In contrast, a Washington, DC, supermarket was selling a roaster chicken plumped up with so much water, salt, and sodium phosphate that it had 610 mg of sodium in a 4-ounce (raw) portion.[52] Even worse, a 3.5-ounce KFC Original Recipe Thigh has 910 mg.[53]

Tap water is usually not a concern with regard to sodium. In Chicago, New York, and most other cities, water has less than 20 mg per liter (a bit more than four 8-ounce glasses). The EPA considers levels between 30 and

60 mg per liter best for taste. But in some cities, especially in the southwestern United States, tap water can supply a fair amount of sodium. The water in El Paso, Texas, for instance, has about 35 mg of sodium per 8-ounce glass.[54] So the five cups of water someone drinks in a day has as much as an ounce of potato chips. (People can ask their city water provider for sodium information.)

Well water, too, may contain excessive sodium. The University of Maryland Extension recommends that people on a sodium-restricted diet get their well water tested.[55] The extension service has an online calculator for estimating how much sodium well water might contribute to a diet.

Water softeners can add to the problem. They exchange the minerals that make water hard (calcium, magnesium, and iron) for sodium. The result is a decrease in hardness but an increase in sodium; the harder the water, the more sodium is added. Healthier water softeners exchange the hardness minerals for potassium.

Most drugs and dietary supplements have little or no sodium. An exception is over-the-counter drugs for heartburn or acid indigestion. Alka-Seltzer has about 535 mg of sodium per tablet, averaging the Original and Extra Strength versions. Taking the recommended limit of seven tablets a day for people 12 to 59 years old would provide a whopping 3,750 mg—far more than the daily sodium recommendation.[56] (The label advises older adults not to take more than three tablets a day, or 1,630 mg.)

Another way to slice the data on where we get our sodium is to see which individual foods provide the largest amount of sodium. In reality, consumers have no idea where their sodium is coming from. An industry survey asked consumers to name the three biggest sources of sodium in their diet. About half of consumers named snacks like chips and crackers (52 percent), while about one-third named luncheon meats and hot dogs (36 percent) and canned soup (32 percent). Only 24 percent of people rated pizza as one of their three biggest sources of sodium, and only 7 percent thought that bread was one of their biggest sources.[57]

In fact, the No. 1 source of sodium in the average diet is bread and rolls (see table 1.4). It's not that bread itself is so high in sodium, but rather that we tend to eat a lot of it. Only 6.2 percent of sodium comes from bread and rolls, though the percentage would be much higher if the bread in sandwiches and the crust of pizza were included in that figure. That is half again more than the sodium from soups and snack foods. The second-biggest

Table 1.4

Top 10 sources of sodium

Food	Percent of sodium intake
1. Bread, Rolls, Bagels	6.2
2. Pizza	5.9
3. Sandwiches (burgers, hot dogs, egg/breakfast, chicken, etc.)	5.7
4. Cold Cuts, Cured Meats	5.4
5. Soups	3.8
6. Burritos, Tacos	3.8
7. Savory Snacks (chips, popcorn, pretzels, etc.)	3.7
8. Chicken (whole pieces)	3.7
9. Cheese	3.5
10. Eggs and Omelets	2.6

Source: Z. S. Quader, L. Zhao, C. Gillespie, et al., "Sodium Intake among Persons Aged ≥2 Years—United States, 2013–2014," *Morbidity and Mortality Weekly Report* 66 (2017): 324–328. https://www.cdc.gov/mmwr/volumes/66/wr/pdfs/mm6612a3.pdf.

source of sodium is pizza, which provides 5.9 percent of the average person's intake. Salt and other sodium-containing additives are integral ingredients in the crust, sauce, cheese, pepperoni, olives, bacon, and other toppings.

Still, those Top 10 categories account for only 44 percent of the sodium we eat. The rest is split among scores of other foods.

Bonnie Liebman, the nutrition director and my long-time colleague at CSPI, warns that at fast-food restaurants "the fries, which people typically identify as salty, aren't the problem; it's the large amounts of salt hidden in the burgers, the nuggets, the McMuffins, the chicken and fish sandwiches, the biscuits, and more."[58] The same can be said for packaged foods. Yes, some soups and snacks may be pretty salty, but they don't make up a large part of the average diet. The problem, Liebman says, is that there's a lot of salt in a lot of foods, and many of them don't even taste salty.

Eating less of any one or two foods probably would not have a great impact on a person's total sodium intake. In contrast, average Americans get fully half of their added sugars from soft drinks and other sugar-sweetened beverages, so just cutting out sugar drinks would likely make a big difference in their sugar consumption.[59]

If we are going to reduce sodium intake, the way to start is by eating more natural foods and less processed and restaurant foods. But, inevitably and realistically, almost all of us are going to continue buying some processed foods (including bread), and we're not going to stop eating out. That means that we need the food industry to help us by manufacturing and marketing foods with far less added salt. In chapter 9, I explain what some companies have been doing. But first, we need to dig deep into the evidence for and against consuming less sodium. In the next two chapters I describe a great deal of scientific research, so let's get ready to meet some experts and discover what they have learned from it.

2 The Case *for* Eating Less Salt

Population-wide reductions in sodium intake could prevent more than 100,000 deaths annually.

—Institute of Medicine, 2010[1]

The stakes could not be greater.

Every year almost 800,000 people in the United States suffer a heart attack, and 365,000 die as a result of coronary heart disease.[2] Heart attacks typically occur when a blood clot blocks one of the arteries that supply blood to the heart muscle. The lack of blood can kill muscle cells quickly, so it is critical to get to the hospital as quickly as possible after experiencing symptoms suggestive of a heart attack.

I recall well a beautiful July day at the Delaware shore when my wife felt unusual discomfort in her chest while riding a bike. We quickly rode back to a friend's home and read some articles that described what heart attacks might feel like to women. Then, resisting the lure of the beach, we rushed to the hospital. Tests showed that Donna had suffered a mild heart attack, doctors installed two stents, and she has been fine ever since. If we had delayed, the outcome might have been very different.

A stroke is like a heart attack of the brain, but the stakes can be higher. The heart is just a dumb muscle—whereas the brain controls virtually every aspect of our life. Every year about 800,000 Americans suffer a stroke; 140,000 of them die as a result, while many of the rest suffer long-term debilitating effects.[3]

A stroke occurs because either an artery bursts (hemorrhagic stroke) or, in 87 percent of cases, gets clogged by a blood clot (ischemic stroke).[4]

When the blood supply is interrupted, brain cells start dying within minutes. Where in the brain a stroke occurs (and how severe it is) determines what the symptoms are. Symptoms vary greatly, but strokes may totally alter a person's (and family's) life. Victims can experience loss of balance, difficulty talking or breathing, incontinence, emotional changes, impaired thinking, memory loss, blurred vision, partial paralysis, inability to eat or get dressed, and numerous other problems.

Read how Jill Bolte Taylor, a brain scientist, explained in a TED talk what it feels like to have a stroke—based on her own experience when she was just 37:

> I woke up to a pounding pain behind my left eye. . . . In the course of four hours, I watched my brain completely deteriorate in its ability to process all information. On the morning of the hemorrhage, I could not walk, talk, read, write, or recall any of my life.[5]

It turned out that the cause of Taylor's stroke was a clot the size of a golf ball.

A ministroke, or transient ischemic attack (TIA) may sound less ominous, but the future consequences can be deadly. While a TIA only temporarily interrupts the blood flow and does not cause permanent damage, it signals a greater chance of having a major stroke: one out of three people suffering a ministroke go on to have major one within a year.[6]

Fortunately, medical advances and healthier lifestyles have led to a remarkable 75 percent reduction in the incidence of stroke deaths since 1968 despite the soaring rate of obesity, a major risk factor; between 2013 and 2015, however, stroke incidence inexplicably ticked up.[7] Perhaps the influence of obesity is finally making the impact that some researchers have been predicting for years.

Early Research on Salt and Blood Pressure

More than a hundred years ago, two French researchers—based on their study of a handful of patients—were among the first to contend that high salt intake was a major cause of hypertension, though they blamed the chloride half of sodium chloride, not the sodium.[8] The *Journal of the American Medical Association* acknowledged that research, but opined, notwithstanding the meager amount of evidence at the time:

> We can not dispense with the use of salt. . . . Its usefulness to the average individual in health and to the population generally can not be questioned. It would be an interesting calculation how much the world's progress is due to salt and how our present civilization could really exist without this important food preservative.[9]

(Note that *JAMA* conflates using less salt with eliminating it entirely.)

Though the French research was greeted with skepticism, around 1920 Frederick M. Allen and James W. Sherrill at the Psychiatric Institute in Morristown, New Jersey, tested salt-restricted diets anew. Those diets, made as palatable as possible, contained as little as 200 mg of sodium per day, far less than the 3,400 mg in today's average American diet.[10] Allen and Sherrill confirmed that patients with hypertension could tolerate those extremely low-sodium diets even over several years. The diets lowered blood pressure in 70 percent of the patients, including to normal levels in one out of five. Box 2.1 provides recent numbers on sodium, blood pressure, and cardiovascular disease, which includes hypertension, coronary heart disease, heart failure, stroke, and other disorders.[11]

The concept of using a low-sodium diet to treat hypertension—which was called "malignant hypertension" because it was as deadly as the most untreatable cancers—did not really capture the attention of doctors or the public until 1939.[12] That's when Walter Kempner, a German physician and refugee working at Duke University, started testing a diet containing nothing but rice, fruit (or juice), and sugar plus some vitamins and iron to treat potentially fatal kidney disease and hypertension. The diet was extremely low in sodium, fat, and protein—as well as in taste and variety. Those were the days before antihypertensive medicines, and the Kempner Rice Diet, as it became known, was virtually the only treatment for hypertension. It simultaneously reduced heart size, cleared up damage to the retina, and improved electrocardiograms. The *New England Journal of Medicine* editorialized that "Kempner's own therapeutic results are little short of miraculous."[13] Sixty-five years later, a review in the *Journal of Electrocardiology* concluded that the diet was effective "simply beyond belief."[14]

Unfortunately, not all physicians embraced Kempner's dietary treatment. When Kempner spoke at a 1946 meeting of cardiologists at the New York Academy of Medicine, some doctors doubted his findings and even accused him of exaggerating and falsifying his findings.[15] Another problem was that not all of his patients enjoyed dining on the boring, austere diet. The Rice Diet was so restricted and unpalatable that Kempner—whose personal

---

Box 2.1
Sodium, hypertension, and cardiovascular disease by the numbers

- Among adults, 54% of African Americans have hypertension (blood pressure over 130/80) compared to 46% of non-Hispanic whites, 39% of non-Hispanic Asians, and 36% of Hispanics. Those percentages account for 108 million people. Millions more have pre-hypertension.

- 80 to 90 percent of adults will develop hypertension over their lifetime.

- Hypertension is responsible for over $131 billion in annual healthcare costs.

- Together, coronary heart disease and stroke kill about 500,000 people annually (more than one in six deaths).

- High blood pressure is a primary or contributing cause of 472,000 deaths per year, about 1 out of 6 deaths.

- About 7 of every 10 people suffering a first heart attack have high blood pressure. About 8 of every 10 people suffering their first stroke have high blood pressure. About 7 of every 10 people with chronic heart failure have high blood pressure.

- The average adult should consume no more than 2,300 mg of sodium per day; people with prehypertension and hypertension should aim for no more than 1,500 mg per day.

- Average sodium intake of sodium for everyone 2 and older is 3,400 mg per day,* or about 50 percent more than the recommended 2,300 mg. About 71 percent of the sodium comes from salt (and other additives) added to foods by manufacturers and restaurants.

- 3,400 mg of sodium is equivalent to about 1½ teaspoonfuls of salt. One teaspoon of salt has 2,325 mg of sodium.

- For children, the recommended sodium limits are 1,200 mg for ages 1 to 3; 1,500 mg for ages 4 to 8; 1,800 mg per day for ages 9 to 13; and 2,300 (same as adults) for ages 14 to 18. However, children 6 to 10 years old actually consume 2,900 mg of sodium per day; teens 14 to 18 consume 3,700 mg per day.

- Worldwide, reducing sodium intakes to an average of 2,000 mg per day could prevent about 2.5 million deaths per year, mostly among older adults.

---

*As I discussed in chapter 1, after appropriate adjustments, actual sodium intake is closer to 4,000 mg per day. See note 11 for box 2.1 sources.

predilection for questionable behavior-modification methods might have distracted from his scientific achievements—actually beat some of his patients to get them to stick with it. (Kempner said in a court deposition, "I have whipped people in order to help them and because they say they want to be whipped.")[16] To increase compliance, Kempner allowed a more varied diet as his patients' blood pressure declined.

The Rice Diet, or more palatable versions of it, reduced blood pressure by a remarkable 25 percent or so in about half the patients.[17] Adding salt to that diet, as researchers at Columbia University's College of Physicians and Surgeons discovered, generally negated its effect, confirming that salt was the culprit. But as one physician said, and Kempner acknowledged, the diet "imposes such hardship upon the patient and so much difficulty in control as to make it virtually impracticable for general use."[18] By the late 1950s and 1960s, however, the availability of antihypertensive drugs relieved the need for the Rice Diet.

Animal research in the early 1950s shed more light on the effect of sodium and potassium on hypertension. With humor in medical journals being rarer than a two-headed giraffe in the wild or a zoo, it was amusing to read an article written by two hypertension experts, George R. Meneely and Con O. T. Ball of the Vanderbilt University School of Medicine:

> For reasons probably not even known to himself, one of us developed at that time a curiosity about the long-term effect of added sodium chloride in the diet. . . . We had in mind the possibility that excess salt might manifest itself as a source of degenerative disease, nature unspecified. Our minds were open, even perhaps blank.[19]

Those researchers put large numbers of laboratory rats on "diets" that contained sodium chloride in levels ranging from toxically low to toxically high, with or without potassium chloride. They found, now unsurprisingly, that higher-sodium diets raised the rodents' blood pressure. Potassium negated some of the effect of the sodium. Their important findings helped pave the way for similar research in humans.

Animal research also shed light on why some people are more susceptible to developing high blood pressure than others. In the 1970s, Lewis K. Dahl and Martha Heine, at the Brookhaven National Laboratory in Upton, New York, transplanted kidneys from rats that did not develop high blood pressure into rats that did.[20] The result? The previously sensitive rats did not develop high blood pressure. Likewise, when the kidneys from susceptible rats were transplanted into resistant rats, those rats did develop high blood pressure. Clearly, assuming that the kidneys in rats and humans behaved similarly, our genes could have a dramatic effect on our chance of developing hypertension.

Animal research like Dahl and Heine's, which used highly inbred laboratory rats, led many researchers to think that people were either sensitive to or resistant to salt's effects on blood pressure. In fact, though, unlike those specially bred rats, people display wide variation in sensitivity.[21] Some people—such as African Americans, those with hypertension, and elders— are especially sensitive. And some lucky people go through life with normal or even low blood pressure, with a high-sodium diet and other factors posing little problem. Most other people have intermediate sensitivities. In one striking example, in the prefecture of Akita in northern Japan, several decades ago average sodium consumption was a sky-high 10,000 mg per day.[22] Thirty-nine percent of people (average age 45) were hypertensive— but the majority was not. Researchers are currently trying to understand the genetic determinants of salt sensitivity in order to identify people at high risk of hypertension and strongly encourage them to lower their sodium intake as soon as possible.[23]

Humans are much more closely related to apes than rats, which suggested studying the effect of salt on blood pressure in chimpanzees. In one failed experiment in the United States, the chimps involved were accustomed to consuming high-sodium biscuits providing 2,400 to 4,800 mg of sodium per day. When researchers tried giving the chimps low-sodium replacements, the animals refused to eat the biscuits and lost weight. The chimps ultimately won the battle and resumed enjoying their customary high-sodium diet.[24]

The researchers went back to the drawing board and found a colony of chimpanzees eating a natural, low-sodium diet at a research center in Gabon.[25] They gradually increased the sodium content (up to 6,000 mg per day) in the animals' diet for 20 months. As expected, the animals' average blood pressure soared. As earlier studies had shown for humans and rats, some chimpanzees experienced large increases in blood pressure, some had smaller or even no increase, but on average their blood pressure rose steadily and dramatically. When the chimps were returned to their original low-sodium diet, their blood pressure gradually decreased to the original level.

Small, but interesting, studies on hunter-gatherer tribes added to the case that a high sodium intake boosts blood pressure and the risk of cardiovascular disease. Many thousands of years ago most humans consumed very little sodium, and that was the case for our primate and earlier ancestors going back millions of years. Today, most humans consume a high-sodium diet. But a few communities, such as the Yanomami Indians I mentioned in chapter 1, have barely been touched by our style of civilization and still consume ultra-low-sodium diets. The Yanomami consume less than one-tenth as much sodium as Americans.[26]

Strikingly, the Yanomami have much lower blood pressure, averaging only around 95/63 mm Hg, than young and middle-aged Americans, who average over 120 mm Hg systolic.[27] (See box 2.2 for more about blood pressure: how our bodies react when our sodium intake changes, how our blood pressure responds, and how blood pressure is measured and monitored.)[28] Equally striking, unlike in most Americans, the tribe members' blood pressure does not rise with age. That phenomenon has also been observed in other isolated indigenous populations from South Pacific islands to the Kalahari bush in southern Africa.[29] In one such community in New Guinea, sodium consumption was about 400 mg per day. Judging from blood pressure measurements and electrocardiograms, "only 3 per cent of males over the age of 40 . . . were hypertensive in contrast to 20 per cent of middle-aged American men. . . . Heart disease was rare if not absent."[30] That doesn't mean salt was the only factor—more physical activity and dietary fiber, little obesity, less animal fat, and other lifestyle differences also were at play. But judging from the medical evidence—and the fact that those populations are not tempted by nearby McDonald's and IHOP restaurants or canned soups and bags of chips—the lack of salt likely was a significant factor.

Also consider the Tsimane tribe in the Bolivian Amazon. It was more acculturated than the Yanomami and probably consumed more sodium.[31] Nevertheless, their blood pressure rose much less with age compared to people in industrialized countries. Moreover, the prevalence of hypertension in people over 70 was only 8 percent in men and 27 percent in women compared to about 70 percent or more among older Americans.[32]

One basic question is whether hunter-gatherers are simply genetically resistant to the effects of salt on blood pressure. We can glean answers from instances in which they consume more salt or move to urban

Box 2.2
What high blood pressure is and does

Over millions of years, our prehistoric animal and human ancestors evolved in areas away from the sea and other sources of salt. Because a bit of sodium is so essential to life, prehistoric animals developed powerful physiological processes, not only to retain sodium that might otherwise be lost in urine and sweat, but also to develop a strong appetite for salt that would provide the urge to seek it out. Those animals (including humans) were thus able to thrive on diets that contained precious little sodium, as well as an abundance of potassium.

But what happens when diets change and people consume far more sodium and far less potassium than the body was designed for? The result for all too many people is elevated blood pressure. But, thanks to genetic variations, individuals may be more or less susceptible to the ill effects of excessive salt in their diets (and other lifestyle characteristics).

The body's organs, with kidneys playing a key role, are part of a complex system (including hormones, nerves, and blood vessels) that works to maintain healthy levels of sodium and other nutrients in blood, and healthy blood pressure. But eating too much salt increases the amount of sodium in the bloodstream and may wreck that delicate balance. The increased sodium tends to increase blood volume, thicken and stiffen blood vessels, and boost blood pressure. The stiffer blood vessels force the heart to work harder to circulate blood, and that can lead to an enlarged heart and heart failure. They also are more susceptible to rupturing, which, if in the brain, can lead to a stroke, and to clogging, which can lead to a stroke or heart attack. The kidneys need to excrete the extra water and sodium, but high blood pressure not only interferes with that process but also can lead to kidney failure, heart attacks, and strokes. Aging worsens the problem because excreting unnaturally large amounts of sodium for many years impairs the kidney's ability to excrete sodium.

Fortunately, in contrast to sodium, potassium helps relax blood vessels and reduce blood pressure. Unfortunately, thanks to the ubiquity of processed foods, almost everyone consumes less potassium than they should and far less than what Paleolithic humans likely consumed. Potassium is one important reason why we should be eating plenty of fruits and vegetables, which have 5, 10, or even 100 times more potassium than sodium.

The "pressure" in blood pressure refers to the force of blood pushing against the walls of the arteries. That pressure, measured using a blood pressure cuff or digital device, is denoted by two numbers, such as 140/95 mm Hg ("140 over 95"). The "mm Hg" refers to how many millimeters ("mm") high a column of mercury ("Hg") rose in an old-fashioned sphygmomanometer, the

Box 2.2 (continued)

device long used to measure blood pressure. The higher number is the *systolic* pressure, the pressure when the heart has just pumped blood to the rest of the body. (Systolic is derived from the Greek word for contract.) The lower number is the *diastolic* blood pressure, the pressure when the heart is resting between beats. (Diastolic comes from the Greek word for expand.)

Blood pressure (BP) is considered to be normal when the systolic pressure is under 120 mm Hg and the diastolic pressure is under 80 mm Hg. But as Japanese researchers observed, "When compared with the BP of wild animals or of primitive man, BP levels considered to be 'normal' in civilized countries may actually be hypertensive, with high salt intake making a great contribution." Figure 2.1 describes what different blood pressure categories mean.

President Franklin Delano Roosevelt long had a blood pressure problem. In the first years of his presidency, between 1933 and 1938, his blood pressure climbed gradually to 175/90. That blood pressure would be considered high-risk today. By the end of 1944 it was about 225/125—a "crisis" level. On April 12, 1945, the day he had a massive fatal cerebral hemorrhage, it was thought to be 350/195. Roosevelt was only 63 years old when he died. Sadly, few physicians knew at the time, long before effective blood pressure–lowering medications became available, that a low-sodium diet could effectively treat hypertension. Had the president switched to such a diet a year or two before his fatal stroke, he might well have lived long after World War II ended, changing the course of history.

A trio of hypertension experts, led by Stephen Havas of the University of Maryland School of Medicine, has expressed the consensus view today: "The relationship between blood pressure level and risk of developing cardiovascular disease is strong, continuous, graded, consistent, independent, and etiologically significant. The risks of heart attack, congestive heart failure, stroke, and end-stage renal disease increase progressively as blood pressure rises above optimal levels."

That means a person need not have sky-high blood pressure before beginning to worry—and making lifestyle changes. As medical research advanced, scientists discovered that health risks occurred at lower and lower blood pressures than previously thought. In the 1970s, the threshold for hypertension was 160/95. By 1990, the definition was reduced to 140/90. And then in 2017 the threshold for stage 1 hypertension was lowered again to 130 mm Hg systolic *or* 80 mm Hg diastolic blood pressure. That lower threshold for concern meant that the percentage of adults who are considered to have high blood pressure jumped from 32 percent to 46 percent. It also meant that many more people would probably be prescribed medications.

Box 2.2 (continued)

African Americans suffer comparatively high rates of high blood pressure, or hypertension. Moreover, rises in blood pressure strike blacks earlier, hypertension is often more severe, and some medications are less effective. According to the American Heart Association, African Americans may carry a gene that makes them more salt sensitive, increasing the risk of high blood pressure. Besides genes, the average African American lives with more poverty, less healthcare, and poorer diets (though blacks consume slightly less sodium than whites), exacerbating the problem.

While obesity, alcohol, and other factors boost blood pressure, lowering sodium in foods is a factor particularly amenable to public health action. Consuming 1,000 mg less sodium should lower systolic blood pressure by about 5 mm Hg in people with hypertension and about 2 mm Hg in people with normal blood pressure. That's roughly the same benefit one might get from losing 11 pounds or consuming a diet rich in potassium.

Blood Pressure Categories

BLOOD PRESSURE CATEGORY	SYSTOLIC mm Hg (upper number)		DIASTOLIC mm Hg (lower number)
NORMAL	LESS THAN 120	and	LESS THAN 80
ELEVATED	120 – 129	and	LESS THAN 80
HIGH BLOOD PRESSURE (HYPERTENSION) STAGE 1	130 – 139	or	80 – 89
HIGH BLOOD PRESSURE (HYPERTENSION) STAGE 2	140 OR HIGHER	or	90 OR HIGHER
HYPERTENSIVE CRISIS (consult your doctor immediately)	HIGHER THAN 180	and/or	HIGHER THAN 120

©American Heart Association

heart.org/bplevels

Figure 2.1
Blood pressure categories. *Source*: Reprinted with permission (https://www.heart.org/-/media/files/health-topics/high-blood-pressure/hbp-rainbow-chart-english-pdf-ucm_499220.pdf). © American Heart Association.

areas rife with processed foods, motor vehicles, cigarettes, and other accou-trements of modern life. In some cases, such as Easter Islanders who moved to South America and rural Zulus who migrated to African cities, the migrants had more opportunities to consume processed foods. Their blood pressure rose.[33]

Scientists also have compared communities that had access to salt or used saltwater in cooking to nearly identical communities that did not.[34] One study focused on two rural communities in Nigeria that had similar diets and lifestyles. But the community that had access to salt from a salt lake had a higher sodium intake and higher blood pressure than the other.

Another study examined six isolated tribes with similar lifestyles in the Solomon Islands, a thousand miles northeast of Australia. In five of those tribes sodium consumption was under 700 mg per day, one-fifth what Americans ingest. People in those tribes were healthy overall and had "an almost total lack of coronary heart disease."[35] The one exception was a tribe that cooked vegetables in seawater. They had higher blood pressure than the other groups. Such studies provide strong evidence that the tribes' health status is due more to the scarcity of salt than to genetics.

Of course, all of that ethnographic research does not *prove* that salt causes high blood pressure and heart disease, but the findings are certainly consistent with that hypothesis.

As those early clinical, animal, and ethnographic studies fostered con-cerns about the healthfulness of salty diets, more and more scientists and public health officials began calling for lower-salt foods. That spurred a counteroffensive from a few scientists and food industry officials who called for more evidence that lowering salt would be safe before any pub-lic health advice was issued or any regulatory actions taken. Public health action was delayed while a wide variety of increasingly sophisticated stud-ies have been conducted to investigate the benefits and safety of lowering sodium consumption.

Key Research Supporting Lower-Sodium Diets

Controlled, human studies were one type of research needed to establish the relationship between sodium and blood pressure. Scores of studies have now been conducted in which blood pressure was monitored in people who were given different amounts of sodium for several weeks or months.

One of the early, well-designed experiments was done in England in 1989 with 20 patients who had mild high blood pressure.[36] Graham A. MacGregor, a hypertension expert (more about him later), and his colleagues then at the St. George's Hospital Medical School in London trained their patients how to eat a diet very low in sodium; to help achieve those low intakes, the researchers gave the patients salt-free bread, margarine, and certain other foods. After one month on the diet, the participants entered a new three-part phase during which researchers gave them pills to bring their sodium intakes to 1,150, 2,300, or 4,600 mg per day. Then, after one month at a particular intake level, the participants were switched to one of the other two levels; and after another month they were switched to the third level.

The initial results of the London study showed that going from a low-sodium intake to a mid-sodium intake boosted blood pressure by 5 percent. The high-sodium intake boosted their blood pressure another 5 percent. After one year, most of the participants pretty much stuck to the low-sodium diet, averaging 1,240 mg daily, and continued to have the same reduced blood pressure. The researchers said that patients found that "after 3–4 weeks of the diet, high-salt foods taste unpleasant and for many patients become unpalatable." Blood pressure in 16 of the 20 patients was low enough for them to stop taking antihypertension drugs, though more recent, stricter guidelines would recommend that some of them take drugs on top of the low-sodium diet.

The DASH–Sodium Intervention Diet

The best and most influential of all the clinical studies on salt and blood pressure is the DASH–sodium intervention trial, which was conducted by researchers at Harvard Medical School, Johns Hopkins, and other institutions.[37] DASH (short for Dietary Approaches to Stop Hypertension) was a randomized placebo-controlled trial (RCT), the "gold standard" of biomedical research. Such studies can determine cause-and-effect relationships, whereas most other research, such as observational studies that follow large groups of people over many years, can only identify associations.

DASH's primary developer was Frank M. Sacks, now a professor of cardiac disease prevention at the Harvard T.H. Chan School of Public Health. It grew out of two studies he conducted in the early 1970s, before entering and during medical school, on blood pressure and cholesterol levels in young adherents to a macrobiotic, largely vegan diet (a diet that Sacks himself then ate). Both studies found the vegetarians to be in far better health than the control groups of typical Americans. For instance, the vegetarians' average blood pressure of just 106/60 mm Hg was much lower than in most young people in the United States.[38] Sacks said, "That gave me the dietary-patterns concept that I used a couple decades later to design the DASH diet and study." Having confirmed the benefits of eating a healthy, mostly vegetarian diet, he led the DASH–sodium trial, in which healthy and ordinary non-vegetarian diets were tested at three levels of sodium.[39]

A key strength of the DASH–sodium trial is that the researchers provided the 412 participants—who had either slightly elevated blood pressure or hypertension—all of their meals and snacks. People were randomly assigned to eat either a control diet similar to what the average American eats or the DASH diet, which is higher in potassium-rich fruit and vegetables, calcium-rich, low-fat dairy products, fiber-rich whole grains, fish, lean poultry, and nuts. Versions of those two diets were prepared with low, medium, or high (typical of the American diet) levels of sodium: 1,500 mg, 2,500 mg, and 3,300 mg for people eating a 2,100-calorie diet. Sodium was increased or decreased proportionally for people who ate more or fewer calories. Participants ate their specified meals with each sodium level for 30 days, long enough for their blood pressure to largely adjust to the diets. The researchers measured the participants' sodium intakes using the most accurate method available—24-hour urinary excretion—and their blood pressure.

Figure 2.2 summarizes the exciting DASH–sodium results. The broken vertical arrows show that when people switched from the control diet to the DASH diet their blood pressure declined by 2 to 6 mm Hg, depending on the sodium level. That indicates one benefit of eating an overall healthy diet, rich in dietary fiber, potassium, and other nutrients and low in saturated fat, cholesterol, and sugar.

Furthermore, the solid arrows show that when people reduced their sodium intake from the high to the low level their systolic blood pressure dropped by 6.7 mm Hg (control diet) or 3 mm Hg (DASH diet). Lowering sodium from 2,500 mg to 1,500 mg (1,000 mg drop) provided a disproportionately greater benefit, especially for people on the control diet, than lowering sodium from 3,300 mg to 2,500 mg (800 mg drop).

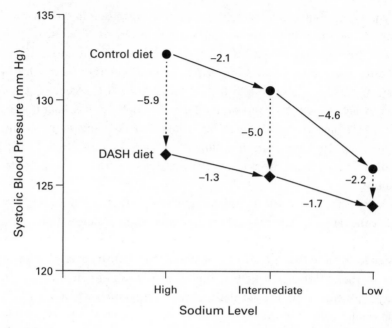

Figure 2.2

Changes in systolic blood pressure on the DASH and DASH–Sodium diets at three sodium levels. The "High" sodium level is 3,300 mg per day, "Intermediate" is 2,500 mg, and "Low" is 1,500 mg based on a 2,100-calorie diet. The numbers show the reductions in systolic blood pressure (mm Hg) that occurred when going from one sodium level (solid horizontal arrows) or diet (broken vertical arrows) to another. (Diastolic blood pressures showed a similar pattern.) *Source*: Illustration by J. Bach, CSPI. Adapted from Sodium Collaborative Research Group, "Effects on Blood Pressure of Reduced Dietary Sodium and the Dietary Approaches to Stop Hypertension (DASH) Diet," *New England Journal of Medicine*, 344 (2001): 3–10.

The DASH researchers also reported the following results (not shown in the figure):

- Blood pressure declined more in African Americans than in whites.
- Blood pressure declined more in people with than without hypertension.
- In participants with hypertension, the low-sodium version of the DASH diet was as potent as treatment using one or two blood pressure–lowering drugs (doctors often prescribe multiple drugs).
- The biggest benefit—a whopping 15.1 mm Hg average decrease in systolic blood pressure—was seen in hypertensive African American women older than 45 who switched to the healthy, low-salt diet.

- The decrease in people over 45 without hypertension, and who were eating a typical American diet or a DASH diet, was twice as great as in younger adults.[40]

DASH–sodium was a landmark study that demonstrated decisively that consuming less sodium lowers blood pressure. Richard Cooper, a cardiovascular researcher at the Loyola University Parkinson School of Health Sciences and Public Health in Chicago later called DASH "the most beautiful piece of data I've seen in my whole life."[41]

The DASH authors stated that their study "should settle the controversy over whether the reduction of sodium has a worthwhile effect on blood pressure in persons *without* hypertension" (emphasis added). The study was so persuasive that the National Heart, Lung, and Blood Institute has publicized the DASH diet widely, including with a free booklet that is available on its website.[42] Numerous privately published books, including cookbooks, based on the DASH diet are available at bookstores or online.

Fortuitously, the DASH–sodium trial provided a real-life opportunity to gauge what people thought of the taste of lower-sodium foods. Were they as off-putting as some people believe? Surprisingly, the participants liked the intermediate-sodium foods *more than* the foods with smaller or larger amounts of sodium.[43] And the low-sodium diet tasted just as good as the high-sodium diet typical of how Americans now eat. So much for the argument that people would never stick to a lower-sodium diet!

More Trials and Meta-Analyses

Further strengthening the evidence that higher sodium intakes increase blood pressure, in 2002, a year after DASH–sodium was published, Feng J. He and MacGregor in London performed two "meta-analyses" of well-done RCTs.[44] A meta-analysis combines the results of several similar studies to increase the ability to detect health effects of a diet, chemical, or drug. But the devil is in the details: results can vary widely depending on the studies included.

One of the He–MacGregor meta-analyses included 17 trials involving people with hypertension; the second included 11 trials of people with normal blood pressure. In people with hypertension, a 1,800 mg per day decrease in sodium led to a 5 mm Hg decrease in systolic blood pressure. Among people with normal blood pressure, a similar drop in sodium consumption led to a 2 mm Hg decline in systolic blood pressure. The researchers estimated that a long-term 1,800 mg reduction in a population's sodium intake[45] (more than a 50 percent reduction for Americans) reduced blood pressure in people with hypertension enough to prevent 14 percent of stroke deaths and 9 percent of deaths from coronary heart disease. Among people with normal blood pressure, they estimated that a sodium reduction of that magnitude would reduce stroke and coronary deaths by about 6 percent and 4 percent, respectively.

The most finely detailed and recent meta-analysis was undertaken by researchers in Australia, the United Kingdom, the United States, Canada, and Japan.[46] They incorporated the results of 133 previous studies with more than 12,000 participants. The results were just as expected. They found a strong dose–response relationship: the larger the reduction in sodium the larger the fall in blood pressure. The effects of a major reduction in sodium were strongest in people with high blood pressure (a decline of almost 3 mm Hg systolic), but trivial in those with normal blood pressure (under 120/80). Almost every segment of the population benefited from consuming less sodium, with the blood pressure of women, blacks, and older adults dropping more than men, whites, and younger adults. For example, the effect of lowering sodium by about 1,150 mg was about 10 times as great in adults between 56 and 65 years old (–3.88 mm Hg systolic) as in those 35 and younger (–0.39 mm Hg). Also, the effect of that same reduction in sodium intake in blacks (–4.07 mm Hg) was two-and-a-half times greater than in whites (–1.60 mm Hg). And showing that it takes a bit of time for blood pressure to adjust to lower sodium levels, larger decreases were seen in tests lasting two to four weeks than in shorter ones.

Those single-digit reductions in blood pressure may seem small—and for a given individual they would be modest—but they would yield a huge health benefit for the population at large. Nancy Cook, a biostatistician and epidemiologist at Brigham and Women's Hospital and Harvard Medical School in Boston, and her co-workers estimated that an average decrease of just 2 mm Hg in diastolic blood pressure in the entire American population would lead to a 17 percent decrease in the prevalence of hypertension, a 6 percent decrease in the risk of coronary heart disease, and a 15 percent decrease in the risk of stroke. That "small" decrease would prevent an estimated 67,000 heart attacks and 34,000 strokes and TIAs every year.[47]

Another illuminating trial looked at the sodium issue from a different perspective. It compared whether treating mild hypertension with lower sodium consumption or drugs was more effective. Lawrence J. Appel, a professor of medicine at the Johns Hopkins School of Medicine and a long-time adviser to the American Heart Association, led the Trial of Nonpharmacologic Interventions in the Elderly, or TONE.[48] As the name suggests, TONE was done in people 60 to 80 years old. The participants who were counseled to consume low-sodium meals and then taken off their blood pressure medication succeeded in dramatically lowering their sodium intake from 3,300 to 2,300 mg per day. After more than two years, not only did their average blood pressure decline (in the absence of drugs), but also many participants were able to stay off their meds. They also experienced fewer headaches and cases of angina (chest pain that might indicate heart disease), though the latter was not statistically significant.

Salt and Blood Pressure in Children

Many parents wonder whether diets high in sodium pose a problem for their young children, even though the risk of heart attacks and strokes may be decades away. That is a good question, considering that most kids' diets are as bad as their parents' and are certain to promote heart attacks and strokes when they grow up. Almost half a century ago, Edward D. Freis, a prominent hypertension expert at the Veterans Administration Hospital in Washington and Georgetown University School of Medicine, urged parents not to accustom their infants and older children to salty foods.[49]

In 1983 MacGregor wrote, "It may be that . . . hypertension becomes established in childhood rather than in early adulthood as thought previously."[50] Twenty-seven years later, with salty diets still no less a problem, Jane Henney, a former commissioner of the US Food and Drug Administration (FDA) who chaired an Institute of Medicine committee on lowering sodium intakes, said, "High blood pressure is a progressive condition that can begin to increase the risk of cardiovascular disease even in childhood."[51]

The CDC found that about 4 percent of children 12 to 19 years old (1.3 million of them!) already have hypertension.[52] Another 10 percent had higher-than-desirable blood pressure, but not rising to the level of hypertension. Children with higher blood pressure tend to have higher blood pressure as adults.[53] (It's a mystery why the percentage of adolescents with hypertension dropped by almost half between 2001 and 2016, a time of rising obesity and constant sodium intake.)[54]

Several interesting studies shed light on the impact of sodium on blood pressure in infants and children; one of the most revealing was begun in Holland in the 1980s.[55] Its design was simple: Researchers randomly divided a group of 476 newborn babies into two groups. They gave 245 babies a normal-sodium diet including both formula and solid foods, while 231 babies ate a similar diet but with one-third as much sodium. After six months the low-sodium diet led to a 2.1 mm Hg lower systolic blood pressure.

Fifteen years later, the Dutch researchers were able to track down about one-third of the children. They found that all those years later the difference in blood pressure persisted. The infants who consumed a low-sodium diet grew into teenagers who presumably also consumed a lower-sodium diet and whose systolic blood pressure was 3.6 mm Hg lower than the children in the control group.[56] That indicates the value of protecting children with a low-sodium diet from infancy. Fortunately, companies stopped adding salt to infant foods in the 1980s. But after children graduate to regular foods, their sodium intake soars. A study led by CDC scientists found that in 2015 a shocking 84 percent of 43 toddler dinners or meals were high in sodium.[57] The average dinner or meal contained 2,233 mg of sodium per 1,000 calories—far in excess of our suggested limit of 1,000 mg per 1,000 calories.

Students at two private schools, Exeter and Andover, served as guinea pigs in another classic experiment.[58] The students, who were about 15 years old, were taught to record what they ate in food diaries and to measure their blood pressure. Chefs in both schools were trained to cook lower-sodium meals. The intervention alternated during a two-year period: the chefs at Exeter served the lower-sodium meals one year; the Andover chefs served them the next year. The students in the intervention schools consumed about 15 to 20 percent less sodium—and their systolic blood pressure was an average of 1.7 mm Hg lower than the students eating a regular diet. Girls, who reduced their sodium more than the boys, had greater reductions in blood pressure. The study also demonstrated the power of the food environment. Even though all the students had access to saltshakers, cooking with less salt led to lower sodium intakes. "It is believed that such food preparation practices among young people, if maintained over many years," the researchers observed, "could have a profound effect on their future risk of . . . hypertension."

As every parent has heard, it is never too early to get kids off to a healthy start, including keeping them away from most salty packaged foods and restaurant meals. As every parent knows, that is easier said than done, but it starts by having plenty of fresh fruits, vegetables, and other low-sodium foods in the house and then cooking irresistibly delicious low-sodium meals for the whole family. Eating out does not help.

Final Pieces of the Sodium Puzzle

Health experts have long agreed on two critical and uncontested facts based on massive evidence: (1) sodium boosts blood pressure and (2) the higher the blood pressure, the greater the risk of heart attacks and strokes.[59] Based on those findings, most hypertension experts have concluded that diets higher in sodium cause cardiovascular disease. But the sodium skeptics have demanded proof that lowering sodium lowers disease risk, not just blood pressure. A small, but important, body of research shows just that.

One piece of evidence comes from observational studies, which follow hundreds or thousands of people over several years. The researchers then correlate how much sodium people consumed at the beginning of the studies with disease rates at the end. This kind of research is informative, but it cannot prove cause and effect.

European Union scientists combined the results of more than a dozen observational studies into one meta-analysis.[60] Each of the studies had limitations, but the meta-analysis technique, by greatly increasing the number of people studied, can oftentimes increase the ability to detect associations between different lifestyles and various diseases. In this case, the researchers found a consistent relationship between sodium and cardiovascular disease. Higher sodium intake was associated with a 23 percent higher risk of stroke and, when one low-quality report was excluded, a 17 percent higher risk of total cardiovascular disease. However—and all too often there is a "however" or "but" when discussing nutrition research!—observational studies and meta-analyses of them (as I discuss in chapter 3) have serious weaknesses, especially regarding the accuracy of measuring sodium intake and the possibility that people consuming less sodium may have overall healthier diets and lifestyles, which can undermine their reliability.

The biggest observational "study" involved the entire British population. In 2003, the British government began a serious campaign, which I describe more fully in chapter 7, to encourage consumers to choose lower-sodium foods and encourage industry to lower sodium levels in their products. The goal was to cut sodium consumption by more than one-third, from 3,800 to 2,400 mg per day. By 2008, daily sodium intake fell by 360 mg per person, or about 9 percent.

The British National Institute for Health and Care Excellence estimated that the campaign, "which cost just £15 million [$30 million at the time[61]], led to approximately 6,000 fewer [cardiovascular disease] deaths per year, saving the UK economy approximately £1.5 billion [$3 billion] per annum."[62] By 2011, the Department of Health reported a 15 percent reduction in sodium, from 3,800 to 3,240 mg per day[63] (the government later revised the reduction down to 11 percent[64]). A 15 percent reduction was estimated to have contributed to an 11 percent reduction in stroke mortality and a 6 percent reduction in fatal heart attacks, preventing 9,000 non-fatal cardiovascular events and 9,000 deaths per year.[65] The health department estimated that getting sodium down to 2,400 mg per day would lead to 14,000 to 20,000 fewer deaths annually.[66] Note that those were computer-based estimates of health benefits, not direct observations of actual deaths.

Impressive as the British experience and the meta-analysis of observational studies might appear—along with the undisputed fact that higher sodium intakes raise blood pressure—they still did not prove in a single controlled trial that higher sodium levels cause disease, or that lowering intakes to the recommended 2,300 mg per day (let alone to the 1,500 mg that some authorities recommend for many people) would prevent disease. Sodium skeptics, including those who argue that lowering sodium intakes could be harmful, continued to insist that RCTs must be conducted before consumers should sharply reduce their sodium intakes and before governments should force industry to produce lower-sodium foods. But that's easier said than done. RCTs sensitive enough to detect differences in rates of stroke and heart disease are tough to do and expensive. They necessitate following large groups of people consuming similar diets except for sodium content over a long period of time. No perfect study has been done, but several controlled trials that lowered sodium intake *did* demonstrate a lower risk of cardiovascular disease.

In one of the best-known experiments, researchers in Taiwan used as their "laboratory" a large retirement facility for veterans, where the men's diets could be carefully controlled.[67] In two of the facility's five kitchens, they replaced half the regular salt with potassium chloride, which is somewhat salty and lowers blood pressure. But they were not able to replace soy sauce and the flavor enhancer monosodium glutamate (MSG), both big sources of sodium, with potassium-containing versions. The change in salt lowered sodium consumption by about one-third and almost doubled potassium intake. The sodium and potassium intakes of veterans who ate meals from the three other kitchens remained the same. After two and a half years, deaths due to cardiovascular disease dropped a remarkable 41 percent among the veterans who ate the lower-sodium, higher-potassium meals. The study also demonstrated reduced medical costs. Those are remarkable effects that resulted from simply replacing less than half the salt in the men's diets with potassium chloride.

Notwithstanding its clear-cut results, the Taiwan trial still does not settle the dispute about whether lowering sodium intake to the recommended 2,300 mg decreases disease rates. That is because the "low" level of sodium in the Taiwan study was actually pretty high—about 3,800 mg per day, far more than what elderly American men consume.[68] (The control group consumed about 5,200 mg of sodium per day.) So the study could not establish the effects on health of consuming the recommended intake, nor could it determine whether the veterans' improved health was due to consuming less sodium, or more potassium, or (probably) both. (I have more to say about potassium later in this chapter and in chapter 9.)

Other key research on sodium and cardiovascular disease was done in the United States. Appel and his colleagues conducted two Trials of Hypertension Prevention (TOHP I and the much larger and longer TOHP II).[69] The 3,000 participants were 30 to 54 years old and had prehypertension. The researchers trained about half the participants in the first trial to lower their sodium intake for 18 months and in the second trial for three to four years. The other half served as a control group in each trial. The intervention groups lowered their average sodium intake by about 1,200 mg per day, or one-third. As expected, the lower intakes were associated with slightly lower blood pressure. The declines were small (systolic blood pressure was reduced by less than 2 mm Hg) though not a surprise, considering that the participants were only 30 to 54 years old and did not have hypertension. Still, in TOHP II the incidence of hypertension was 18 percent lower in the sodium-reduction group; no change was seen in the briefer, smaller TOHP I.

(Another part of the studies found that weight loss led to somewhat greater reductions in blood pressure than consuming less salt.)

The TOHP researchers continued to track the participants for 15 years after the controlled part of TOHP I ended and 10 years after the controlled part of TOHP II ended. Their major finding was impressive. The participants who had cut their sodium intake enjoyed a 25 to 30 percent lower risk of cardiovascular events compared to the control group: the researchers emphasized that TOHP "provides some of the strongest objective evidence to date that lowering sodium intake, even among those without hypertension, reduces the risk of future cardiovascular disease."[70] The follow-up was an uncontrolled extension of the controlled parts of the studies. If anything, participants in the lower-sodium group probably gradually increased their sodium intake, which would have lessened the reduction in cardiovascular events.

The authors recognized that the substantial reduction in cardiovascular disease might seem unrealistically large considering that blood pressure was just a bit lower in the people who reduced their sodium intake. But they speculated that in addition to boosting blood pressure, consuming more sodium might be causing harm in other ways, such as stiffening tiny arteries or thickening the heart muscle. They said that such "mechanisms may explain the sizeable reduction in cardiovascular disease, despite the relatively modest effects on blood pressure seen during the TOHP trials."[71]

Fiona Godlee, the editor of the *BMJ* (formerly the *British Medical Journal*), where the paper was published, applauded the TOHP follow-up study, saying it "may be the final bugle call in the battle of the evidence."[72] But alas, bugles kept calling, as we'll see in chapter 3.

To add some statistical muscle to the TOHP and TONE trials, a committee of the NAM combined them into a meta-analysis. It found that people eating the lower-sodium diets had a 26 percent reduction in the incidence of any form of cardiovascular disease (including angina, strokes, heart attacks, and others).[73] A somewhat broader meta-analysis published in 2020 found a statistically significant 20 percent decrease in disease for every 1,000-mg decrease in sodium.[74]

A British group that conducted a similar meta-analysis found a similar result with borderline statistical significance. It emphasized the need for more effective ways than just cajoling people—the approach that has failed for several decades—to lower sodium consumption.

In any case, while the meta-analyses included just a handful of studies with modest numbers of participants, the positive findings were certainly supportive of the conclusion that lowering sodium intakes reduces the risk of heart disease and strokes, but were not decisive enough to end the controversy.

Health and Economic Benefits from Lowering Blood Pressure

Many studies have quantified the decreases in blood pressure when sodium consumption is lowered. Many others have quantified the reduction in cardiovascular disease when blood pressure is lowered. Based on those two bodies of information, health economists have used computer-based methods to estimate the population-wide benefits—in terms of illnesses, deaths, and dollars—of lower sodium consumption. Their findings are eye opening:

- The first estimate I am aware of was made in 2004: Stephen Havas (from University of Maryland School of Medicine), with Edward Roccella and Claude Lenfant (both from National Heart, Lung, and Blood Institute [NHLBI], which researches cardiovascular disease) estimated that cutting sodium by 50 percent in packaged and restaurant foods would save 150,000 lives per year.[75]

- Kartika Palar and Roland Sturm at the RAND Corporation in Santa Monica, California, using more sophisticated methods, estimated that reducing sodium intake from 3,400 mg per day to 2,300 mg would reduce the prevalence of hypertension by 11 million people and save $18 billion in healthcare costs each year.[76]

- Researchers at Harvard and elsewhere estimated that sodium consumption in excess of 500 mg per day, which they considered the theoretical minimum intake (but impossible for Americans to attain), was causing about 100,000 premature deaths annually.[77] Reducing sodium less would have proportionately smaller benefits.

- In 2010 a team led by Stanford University researchers estimated the effects of a small, 9.5 percent reduction (only about 350 mg per day) in sodium.[78] Reducing sodium by that amount would translate into a seemingly tiny 1.25 mm Hg decrease in the systolic blood pressure of people aged 40 to 85. But the researchers estimated that the small decrease would avert about a million strokes and heart attacks, as well as save more than 1.3 million years of life and an estimated $32 billion in direct medical costs, over the people's lifetimes.

- Kirsten Bibbins-Domingo of the University of California, San Francisco, and her co-authors calculated that reducing sodium intake by 1,200 mg per day (about one-third) would prevent 44,000 to 92,000 deaths per year.[79] They also estimated that a reduction of 1,200 mg per day would save $10 billion to $24 billion in healthcare costs annually—similar to Palar and Sturm's estimate. The researchers said that such an intervention would be more cost-effective than using medications to lower blood pressure in everyone with hypertension.

- Subsequently, Bibbins-Domingo and fellow researchers estimated that current sodium intakes were causing 110,000 more deaths per year than if average intake was 1,500 mg per day.[80] They also estimated that gradually decreasing intakes by 4 percent (145 mg) a year for 10 years, or from 3,600 mg to about 2,160 mg per day, would save an average of 28,000 to 50,000 deaths per year over 10 years (many more in the tenth year than the first year). In the understated lingo of medical journals, the authors concluded that the "magnitude of health benefit for the US population will be substantial."

- Researchers led by Dariush Mozaffarian, the dean of the Gerald J. and Dorothy R. Friedman School of Nutrition Science and Policy at Tufts University, estimated that lowering sodium to 2,000 mg per day would save more than 50,000 lives per year.[81]

- European and American scientists estimated that gradually lowering sodium in food over 10 years until diets included only 2,300 mg of sodium per day would save 83,000 lives and $57 billion in health-related costs over 20 years (and even more over lifetimes).[82] Differences in methodology led to lower estimates than in the other studies, but the scientists found that even much smaller reductions in sodium still would be highly cost-effective.

- Analysts at the US Department of Health and Human Services (FDA's parent agency) calculated that a one-third reduction in sodium consumption (1,264 mg per day) would save $10 billion a year in medical expenses and $142 billion over 20 years.[83] Unlike the other studies, they estimated the value of having longer, healthier lives: $239 billion in one year and $3.556 trillion over 20 years. "A total value of about $3,699

billion over 20 years." (Because sodium would not be reduced instan-
taneously, the actual benefits would be less. Also, based on previous
research they valued a healthy year of life at $400,000, higher than what
other government agencies have assumed. On the other hand, they only
considered benefits flowing from lower blood pressures and not other
possible benefits of reduced sodium intakes.)

Because the health economists used different statistical methods, different reductions in sodium, and different estimates of the effects of lowering
sodium on blood pressure, their estimates of benefits are not directly com-
parable. Some of the projected cost-savings may be exaggerated, because
the people who lived longer would have additional medical expenses and
greater Social Security costs. Also, some critics question whether lower
sodium intakes always translate proportionally into lower blood pressure
and whether lower blood pressure always means lower death rates.[84] On the
other hand, the benefits might be underestimated, because they did not
include any of sodium's possible detrimental effects other than the contribution of blood pressure to heart attacks and strokes (as I discuss later
in this chapter). Finally, when researchers refer to deaths prevented, they
really mean deaths postponed.

The CDC director Tom Frieden and his colleague Peter Briss were certainly emphatic when they told physicians in 2010 that about 100,000
deaths a year could be attributed to excess sodium. After all, that is more
deaths than are caused by alcohol consumption[85] and two-and-a-half times
as many as are caused by motor vehicle crashes.[86] "After tobacco control,"
Frieden and Briss wrote, "the most cost-effective intervention to control
chronic diseases might be reduction of sodium intake."[87]

The bottom line is that America is suffering an astounding *tens of thousands of unnecessary deaths and wasting many billions of dollars annually* simply because we are consuming too much sodium. That kind of toll would
cause a national furor if the deaths were immediately obvious after eating
a salty meal. But the harm from overly salted foods accumulates quietly
and invisibly over the decades. No one writing obituaries or filling out
death certificates attributes premature deaths to "salty diet." So, instead
of being outraged and taking action, people continue to dine obliviously
on high-sodium foods, most food manufacturers and restaurants do little to slash sodium levels in their products, and the federal government,

largely because of industry pressure, has not made lowering sodium a high priority.

Giving Drugs Their Due

While it is far better to avoid high blood pressure in the first place than to get it and then try to treat it, we need to give drugs their due. After all, most people with high blood pressure would much rather just take a few daily pills than undertake the chore of improving their diets, losing weight, and exercising more. And taking drugs is certainly the fastest, most convenient, most effective way to reduce blood pressure quickly. Antihypertensive medications, such as diuretics and ACE inhibitors, deserve much of the credit for the plummeting incidence of stroke since the 1960s.[88] (The reduced need for salt-preserved foods, thanks to greater use of refrigerators and freezers, might also have played a significant role in the decline in stroke rates since 1925.)[89]

As extraordinary as drugs are, though, they have their limitations. A Canadian study found that half of newly diagnosed patients stopped taking their hypertension medications within three years.[90] European investigators found that about half of the patients stopped taking the drugs within one year.[91] People stop taking the drugs because of cost, or because hypertension has no symptoms and is easy to ignore, or because taking drugs every day is an easily forgotten nuisance. Drugs may cause side effects, such as disturbed sleep, headache, muscle cramps, a cough, and an increased need to urinate. Another concern emerged in 2018 and 2019 when companies had to recall from the marketplace some widely used hypertension drugs containing valsartan, irbesartan, and losartan, because they were contaminated with cancer-causing chemicals.[92]

But let's look again at cost. With hypertension being the single most commonly treated health condition, antihypertensive drugs cost Americans upwards of $20 billion per year.[93] That is about six times the entire annual budget of the NHLBI.[94] Beyond drugs, Americans spend an additional $27 billion for doctor visits, emergency room costs, and other care related to hypertension. That is about eight times the annual budget of NHLBI.

About 1 out of 10 people with hypertension experience "resistant hypertension" that cannot be sufficiently reduced even by taking as many as three antihypertensive medications.[95] A healthier diet can be lifesaving for them. In one tightly controlled study of a dozen such patients, switching from a high-sodium (5,750 mg/day) to a low-sodium (1,150 mg/day) diet dramatically reduced blood pressure within one week from 152/85 mm Hg to a much safer 131/75 mm Hg.[96] Those results suggest that many people with resistant hypertension are "exquisitely salt sensitive." The American Heart Association called that study "compelling."[97]

While consuming less salt is important, it is not the only way to reduce blood pressure and its deadly consequences. Maintaining a healthy weight is a top priority. And, as DASH demonstrated, so is consuming plenty of foods rich in potassium—such as bananas, sweet potatoes, salmon, lentils, peas, cooked spinach, and many more, as shown in chapter 11 (table 11.2)—to counteract the blood pressure–raising effect of sodium. It is equally important to refrain from smoking cigarettes and to limit alcohol consumption to no more than two drinks per day. Last but not least, remember that getting plenty of physical activity is associated with healthier blood pressure and many other benefits. But in theory—and without requiring each individual to make lifestyle choices many times a day—perhaps the easiest, most efficient way to improve blood pressure would be for companies to lower sodium levels substantially throughout the food supply.

More Damage Due to Hypertension

High blood pressure takes its toll on the kidneys and the eyes; it challenges some of our normal bodily functions and exacerbates the role that aging plays in others. In the sections below I offer several more reasons to switch to a low-sodium diet.

Cut the Salt . . . for Your Kidneys

High blood pressure is a major risk factor for chronic kidney disease (CKD). The CDC estimates that some 30 million adults have CKD, and most are undiagnosed. Kidney disease is the ninth leading cause of death and enormously expensive. Medicare paid $114 billion in 2016 to treat chronic and end-stage kidney disease (in which patients need dialysis or a kidney transplant),[98] with private insurance and patients paying tens of billions more. Across the globe, kidney disease kills as many as 5 to 10 million people every year.[99] Because most people who have chronic kidney disease do not even know it, the National Kidney Foundation calls kidney disease *"the under-recognized public health crisis."*[100]

Kidneys are key workhorses in the human body. To keep the body functioning optimally, kidneys maintain healthy levels of calcium, sodium, potassium, and other minerals that circulate in the blood. To filter extra water and wastes (including sodium) out of the blood, they make urine. The kidneys also release hormones that help make red blood cells, regulate blood pressure, and keep bones strong.

But elevated blood pressure makes it harder for kidneys to excrete water. That leads to fluid build-up and even higher blood pressure—and the cycle continues, possibly leading to kidney failure (also called end-stage renal disease), the often-deadly end result of CKD. Diets high in sodium, potassium, phosphorus, and water can be especially harmful to the kidneys of elderly, obese, diabetic, or black patients with kidney failure.[101]

Numerous experiments have tested diets high or low in sodium in patients with various stages of chronic kidney disease. A meta-analysis of good studies (all used 24-hour urine collections to measure sodium excretion) found that a low-sodium diet not only reduced blood pressure, but also the amount of protein in urine, a hallmark of kidney disease.[102] The researchers, based at the University of Campania in Naples, Italy, said that the big challenge is overcoming the food environment and making it easier for patients to eat a lower-sodium diet over the long term.

The Chronic Renal Insufficiency Cohort (CRIC), a major, seven-year-long study involving more than 3,700 people with kidney disease, explored the effect of sodium, not just on blood pressure and markers for kidney disease, but on rates of heart disease. It found that patients consuming a high-sodium diet—more than about 4,500 mg of sodium per day—had a 50 percent greater risk of cardiovascular disease than those who consumed under 2,900 mg.[103] The high sodium levels (based on multiple 24-hour urine collections) seemed to be harmful in ways in addition to boosting blood pressure, possibly by interfering with blood vessels' ability to expand and contract. CRIC should inspire people suffering from kidney disease to stick to a lower-sodium diet.

. . . for Your Eyesight

High blood pressure can affect the eye in several ways. A stroke (or even a TIA) can damage the part of the brain that processes visual images. It can also damage the optic nerve, which carries information from the retina—the light-sensitive part of the eye—to the brain.[104] Those effects cause partial loss of vision, blurred vision, or droopy eyelids. Such symptoms should trigger an immediate trip to the emergency room.

High blood pressure also can thicken or stiffen tiny blood vessels in the retina, a condition called retinopathy. The retina is the light-sensitive part of the eye that receives light and sends the information to the brain. An "eye stroke" occurs when the flow of oxygen-rich blood to the retina is blocked.[105] That could lead to permanent blurred vision or even blindness. Diet and drugs need to be used to prevent or reverse the damage.

. . . to Fight Cognitive Decline and Dementia

A landmark trial funded by the National Institutes of Health (NIH) found that reducing systolic blood pressure by means of pharmaceuticals from 140 mm Hg down to normal levels—120 mm Hg—led to an almost 20 percent decrease in mild cognitive impairment (MCI). MCI is characterized by a decline in memory and thinking skills.[106] The risk of dementia itself also appeared to decline by almost as much, but the decrease was not quite statistically significant. Those results, from the SPRINT MIND study, are certainly promising but need to be replicated before they will be widely accepted. Presumably, reducing blood pressure by means of a low-sodium diet, as well as losing weight and other lifestyle changes, would also improve cognition.

Kristine Yaffe, a professor at the University of California, San Francisco, wrote about SPRINT MIND in the *Journal of the American Medical Association*, saying that it "offers great hope."[107] Maria C. Carrillo, the chief science officer of the Alzheimer's Association, was a bit more exuberant, exclaiming, "to reduce new cases of MCI and dementia globally we must do everything we can—as professionals and individuals—to reduce blood pressure to the levels indicated in this study, which we know is beneficial to cardiovascular risk."[108]

Research on mice supports the link between salt and mental performance. Scientists at Weill Cornell Medicine in New York City and Washington University in St. Louis found that consuming a diet several times saltier than what Americans consume for just eight weeks impaired the mice's normal nest-building activities—they spent less time and used less nesting material than normal mice—and their memory.[109] Costantino Iadecola, one of those researchers and the director of the Feil Family Brain and Mind Research Institute (BMRI) at Weill Cornell, said, "mice fed a high-salt diet developed dementia even when blood pressure did not rise."[110] Digging deeper, the scientists found that the high-salt diet reduced the production of nitric oxide, which in turn altered proteins in the brain in the same way that the proteins are altered in patients suffering from Alzheimer's disease. Interestingly, the salty diet acted on cells in the gut to produce the molecules (interleukin-17) that reduced nitric oxide production in the brain.

. . . to Prevent Headaches

Two high-quality RCTs—DASH–sodium (involving people with normal or high blood pressure) and TONE (involving people with hypertension)—found that people who reduced their sodium intake had fewer headaches.[111] The researchers speculated that the headaches might be caused either by increased blood pressure or by a direct effect of sodium.

. . . to Relieve Erectile Dysfunction

The link between high blood pressure and erectile dysfunction (ED) is so well known that doctors use the occurrence of ED as an indication that a man might have previously undetected high blood pressure or heart disease.[112] High blood pressure causes ED because it stiffens and narrows arteries, reducing blood flow to the penis and making it difficult for men to have an erection. The problem becomes increasingly prevalent as men age, with the rate of complete impotence tripling from 5 percent in 40-year-olds to 15 percent in 70-year-olds.[113] Exacerbating the risk of ED for men with high blood pressure are the medications used to treat hypertension: some of them, including diuretics and beta blockers, may themselves cause ED and contribute to the popularity of Viagra and similar drugs among seniors.

According to the Mayo Clinic, high blood pressure may also affect a woman's sex life. It does so by reducing blood flow to the vagina, possibly leading to a decrease in sexual desire, vaginal dryness, or difficulty achieving orgasm.[114]

Potassium: Salt's "Friendly Co-conspirator"

Potassium is an essential nutrient that helps maintain fluid and electrolyte balances and normal cell function. According to Emory University researchers, our Stone Age ancestors, with their largely plant-based diets, consumed 10,000 mg or more of potassium per day (and under 1,000 mg of sodium), a level that is unheard of in the United States.[115] That was the high-potassium dietary environment in which early humans and their primate predecessors evolved. In fact, the Emory researchers observed, "Americans, like nearly all people living today, consume more sodium than potassium. Humans are the only free-living, non-marine mammals to do so." Our bodies are not designed to function optimally when we are consuming so little potassium and so much sodium.

Higher potassium intakes reduce blood pressure.[116] For example, researchers at the World Health Organization (WHO) and elsewhere conducted meta-analyses of clinical trials that looked at potassium's effect on both blood pressure and cardiovascular disease. The meta-analyses found that people with hypertension who consumed 3,500 to 4,700 mg of potassium per day ended up with a 7 mm Hg lower systolic and a 4 mm Hg lower diastolic blood pressure than those in control groups who consumed less.[117] The scientists also combined observational studies into another meta-analysis that found about a 25 percent reduced risk of stroke in people who were consuming at least the recommended amount of potassium. But they did not see a decrease in heart attacks. And neither did they (nor did others) detect much, if any, benefit for people without hypertension.[118]

Another meta-analysis of observational studies, this one performed by Italian scientists, found similar results. Consuming more potassium (1,500 mg more per day) was associated with a 20 percent reduced risk of stroke in the general population.[119] In addition, they saw smaller reductions in coronary heart disease and total cardiovascular disease, but those were not statistically significant. The researchers estimated that increasing potassium intake by 1,500 mg per day throughout the world could prevent a million stroke deaths per year.

Because consuming less sodium and more potassium both reduce blood pressure, the ratio of sodium to potassium in the diet appears to be a better indicator of the risk of hypertension than the amounts of sodium and potassium looked at individually.[120] According to the American College of Cardiology and other health groups, "A lower sodium–potassium ratio [is] associated with a lower level of [blood pressure] than that noted for corresponding levels of sodium or potassium on their own." A high potassium intake could help lower the risks related to a high sodium intake.[121]

Likewise, a low sodium intake could reduce the need for potassium. But the bulk of research suggests that lowering sodium has more impact than raising potassium.[122] My advice is to both reduce sodium *and* increase potassium to maximize your health benefit.

The NAM recommends that women should consume at least 2,600 mg of potassium per day and men 3,400 mg per day, with no concerns about consuming more.[123] The WHO recommends an intake of at least 3,500 mg per day.[124] The American College of Cardiology, the American Heart Association, and other health groups consider higher potassium intakes to be one of the best non-pharmaceutical means of lowering blood pressure.[125] They recommend that people with hypertension, whether they are taking medications or not, should consume 3,500 to 5,000 mg per day. While the average person may consume an adequate amount of potassium,[126] it could only be helpful—particularly for people with high blood pressure—to consume more, especially from healthy diets. Potassium supplements are not a great option because they rarely contain more than 99 mg of potassium per pill, which is only about 3 percent of a day's recommended intake. (The FDA requires a warning label on pills with more potassium out of fear that the higher dose might cause ulcerative lesions in the small intestine.)[127] To get more potassium, consumers should eat more potassium-rich foods (see chapter 11, table 11.2); they could also use a potassium-containing salt substitute when they cook or at the table (see chapter 9).

Beyond Blood Pressure: Other Potential High-Salt Risks

Higher blood pressure and the ensuing higher risk of cardiovascular disease are the most serious and common harmful effects of salty diets. But salty diets also may undermine health in other ways. Measured in terms of lives and dollars, the harm caused by high-sodium diets may be much greater than the estimates discussed earlier, because those estimates were based only on salt's effect on blood pressure and blood pressure's effect on cardiovascular disease. Let's explore briefly some of the other ways that high-sodium diets appear to affect health.

Stones and bones   "Kidney stone pain is not subtle," says Dr. Gary Curhan, a professor of epidemiology at the Harvard T.H. Chan School of Public Health.[128] It is often described as being worse than childbirth. High intakes of sodium stimulate the body to excrete calcium, while potassium has the opposite effect.[129] The extra calcium in the kidney can crystallize into stones, which range in size from a grain of sand to a ping-pong ball. The evidence on sodium and calcium excretion led He and MacGregor to conclude that salt intake is an important cause of kidney stones.[130] Almost everyone who has had a kidney stone would urge people to do everything imaginable—including lowering sodium intakes, drinking plenty of fluids, and eating a DASH diet—to avoid them.

Whether salty diets not only increase calcium excretion but also lead to osteoporosis is still an open question.[131] One trial found that high sodium intakes were not detrimental to older women's bones.[132] But those women were given calcium supplements to boost their average intake to about 1,400 mg per day, roughly 50 percent higher than women in the general public. Similar trials need to be conducted with women who have marginal calcium intakes, as is the case for all too many people.

In the absence of conclusive evidence regarding bone health, Bess Dawson-Hughes, director of the Bone Metabolism Laboratory at Tufts University's Jean Mayer USDA Human Nutrition Research Center on Aging, offers some sensible bottom-line advice:

> Higher salt intake triggers greater calcium excretion. People with a low calcium intake would be most vulnerable to the adverse effect of sodium intake on bone. While offsetting the adverse effect of excess sodium intake by increasing calcium intake would be one strategy, the general recommendation to reduce salt intake for bone health is sound, especially since salt intake is far above recommended levels in most diets.[133]

Obesity   The global epidemic of overweight and obesity has many causes. Surprisingly, salt, which has no calories, may be one of them. When Feng J. He and her colleagues analyzed the diets of British children, they found that increased sodium intake correlated with both overall fluid intake and soft drink intake.[134] The scientists then calculated that by cutting salt intake in half, the children would consume an average of 2.3 fewer eight-ounce servings of sugar drinks—a definite cause of obesity—per week. They further calculated that drinking that many fewer sugar drinks could reduce the number of overweight and obese children by more than 15 percent. Richard Horton, the plainspoken editor of the *Lancet*, offers an explanation: "Salt makes you thirsty. Without salt, our need to guzzle endless soft drinks would evaporate."[135]

But there might be salt-related mechanisms other than through increased consumption of sugar drinks that promote obesity. In a study that collected 24-hour urine samples to measure sodium intake, scientists at the CDC, the National Center for Health Statistics, and NIH found a strong association between sodium consumption and overweight and obesity.[136] That association remained even after they accounted for different soft drink and calorie intakes, suggesting that sodium might act directly on hormone levels or other factors. The authors concluded, "Our findings, together with others, provide important evidence suggesting that high sodium intake may play a role in obesity."

Another recent study done by an international group of researchers looked at possible links between sodium intake and obesity in China, Japan, the United Kingdom, and the United States.[137] It found significant associations in all four countries (after controlling for calorie intake, physical activity, and other factors). In the United States, every 400 mg increase in sodium consumption was associated with a 24 percent increased incidence of overweight and obesity.

That (or other) research does not prove that salty diets are a cause of obesity. But there certainly is some smoke, and further research may find a fire.

Bloating, edema Salty foods may lead to bloating or edema. That issue is discussed more on women-oriented websites than in medical journals, but millions of women and men alike would swear to it. Edema might show up as swollen fingers, feet, or ankles. When people increase their sodium intake, their bodies retain more water to dilute out the sodium, and that may lead to feeling bloated.[138] The ever-informative DASH–sodium trial provided scientific evidence that a higher-sodium diet increases bloating.[139]

Stomach cancer The World Cancer Research Fund found "strong evidence" that consuming foods preserved by salt increases the risk of stomach cancer.[140] The main culprits appeared to be foods like pickled vegetables and salted or dried fish as traditionally prepared in East Asia. Those foods may irritate the delicate lining of the stomach, inviting infections from *Helicobacter pylori* bacteria, the underlying cause of many cases of stomach cancer (and stomach ulcers). But few Americans eat that kind of diet. In addition, when researchers looked at total salt intake, not just salt-preserved fish and pickled vegetables, they did not find an association with stomach cancer.[141] Cancer should be near the bottom of your list of salt-related worries.

Summarizing the Science

Copious evidence from numerous kinds of studies proves that consuming less sodium reduces blood pressure and that lower blood pressure reduces the risks of heart attacks and strokes, as well as kidney disease. In addition, some of the research indicates that lowering sodium reduces the risk of cardiovascular disease via mechanisms other than lowering blood pressure. Meanwhile, computer models based on the relationships between sodium, blood pressure, and disease have estimated that reducing sodium intakes to healthy levels would prevent tens of thousands of deaths and save many billions of healthcare dollars each year. Consuming more potassium would increase those benefits.

Notwithstanding that research, some well-credentialed critics at major universities contend that "there is not a shred of evidence whatsoever" to prove that a lower-sodium diet is healthier than the current American diet, but rather argue that lowering sodium would actually be harmful.[142] In this chapter I have sought to explain that there is much more than "a shred of evidence" that lower-sodium diets would save many lives. In the next chapter let's examine the evidence that consuming less sodium would be harmful.

3 The Case *against* Eating Less Salt

The vast majority of Americans can take comfort in knowing their chosen dietary sodium intake is not a health hazard.
—Michael H. Alderman, MD,[1] Albert Einstein College of Medicine

Most health authorities have concluded that as people increase their sodium intake their risk of heart attacks and strokes also increases. That's what has led governments and health organizations around the world to urge people to eat—and companies to make—less-salty foods. The recommendations vary, depending on the organization, but they generally advise that people limit their sodium intake to less than 2,000 or 2,300 mg per day. In contrast, Americans' current intake is around 3,400 mg. To most hypertension and cardiovascular disease experts, the case against salt was closed decades ago.

But there's an alternative universe of thinking. As long ago as 1980, a minority of researchers opposed reducing sodium consumption. Citing conflicting evidence on the effects on health of moderate sodium reductions, John D. Swales, a medical professor at England's University of Leicester, warned against "such massive public health measures as reducing the sodium content of food."[2] (It was later revealed that Swales was secretly working with the British salt industry.)[3] A few years later, an international group of researchers wrote: "There is no scientific evidence" that reducing sodium intake would benefit the general public. The group further claimed that population-wide reductions were "unjustified and irresponsible."[4] That was more than a decade after the White House Conference on Food, Nutrition, and Health recommended that sodium consumption be reduced.[5] Still, research then was not as fully developed as now, and delving more deeply into sodium's effect on blood pressure and health made sense.

Similar criticisms have continued to this day, with some newer studies suggesting that current sodium intakes are *optimal* and that cutting back would be useless or even harmful. But even critics of reducing sodium across the population agree that people with enormous intakes of sodium, such as more than 5,000 mg per day, should cut back.

Andrew Mente, a nutritional epidemiologist and sodium-reduction critic at McMaster University in Hamilton, Ontario, said, "The bottom line is that there is not a shred of evidence whatsoever that low sodium, 2,500 mg per day or lower, is better than average sodium, around 3,500 mg per day, in reducing cardiovascular events or mortality."[6]

In 2016, David A. McCarron and Michael H. Alderman, both long-time opponents of lowering sodium intakes, wrote in the *Journal of the American Medical Association*: "The general population's greatest risk is at intakes below 2800 to 3000 mg/d. . . . The proposed FDA target of 2300 mg/d is significantly below that lower limit and thus unsafe."[7]

I asked Alderman, now an emeritus professor at the Albert Einstein College of Medicine, for his current views on the salt debate. When he was starting to do research in the early 1970s, he told me, "I, like everybody else in the world, knew that a low-salt diet would lower blood pressure [and] was really a good thing to do."

> But [now] I think the issue . . . is really silly. There is not any evidence that reducing sodium to less than 2,300 milligrams per day is a benefit. . . . Why should we ask millions of people to change their diet when there is no evidence? I mean, it seems to me you need strong evidence to do something. Our evidence isn't perfect, but I'm not asking anybody to change anything.[8]

Alderman also told me he's convinced that people can't change their sodium-intake habits, even if it were beneficial to consume less sodium.

Scientists have long debated the health effects of salt at countless conferences, at government advisory committee meetings, and in the pages of scientific journals. But in recent years, journalists at prominent news outlets—with their voices augmented by social media and bloggers—have broadcast those debates to the public in the form of "man bites dog" stories. Those articles have fueled confusion, leaving people buffeted by seemingly endless arguments between two camps of credentialed scientists:

Wall Street Journal (June 3, 2019): "Are You Getting Too Much Salt in Your Diet? Probably Not."[9]

Forbes (August 9, 2018): "A new . . . study offers additional and more powerful evidence that dramatic reductions in salt consumption may not be beneficial and might even prove harmful."[10]

New York Times (May 25, 2016): "A Low-Salt Diet May Be Bad for the Heart."[11]

Washington Post (May 26, 2015): "Some scientists are questioning the wisdom of the public health campaigns pushing people to alter their salty diets. 'I cannot see why the society should spend billions on sodium reduction,' Graudal [a prominent Danish researcher] said."[12]

Washington Post (May 4, 2015): "Pass the salt, please. It's good for you. . . . And, in fact, salt is good for us."[13]

Washington Post (April 6, 2014): "Is the American diet too salty? Scientists challenge the longstanding government warning."[14]

New York Times editorial (May 15, 2013): "After years of warnings to cut sodium consumption to reduce heart attacks and strokes, it is disturbing to learn how little evidence exists that such reductions would actually be beneficial to health. There is even emerging evidence that some groups in the population could suffer harm from levels that are too low."[15]

New York Times (June 2, 2012): "The evidence from studies published over the past two years actually suggests that restricting how much salt we eat can increase our likelihood of dying prematurely. Put simply, the possibility has been raised that if we were to eat as little salt as the USDA and the CDC recommend, we'd be harming rather than helping ourselves."[16]

Daily Express (July 6, 2011; UK): "Now salt is safe to eat: Health fascists proved wrong after lecturing us all for years. . . . Cutting our daily intake does nothing to lower the risk of suffering from heart disease, research shows."[17]

And those articles have "legs." Jeremiah Stamler, the Northwestern University epidemiologist, complained to the publisher and top editors of the *New York Times* about a *Times* article that was syndicated nationally and headlined "Hypertension Research Challenges Role of Salt." In 1992, long before the internet and social media turbo-charged the art of propagandizing, Stamler observed that whenever an article questioning salt's harmfulness was published, within a short time it [was] sent, under the aegis and at the expense of private commercial and trade associations, all over the country, to doctors, researchers, nutritionists, etc. Press conferences are held, exhibits that misrepresent research findings are prepared and circulated. In short, efforts are made to make the health questions take a back seat, in favor of commercial interests.[18]

Even some medical journals publish papers that are more attention getting than reliable. Maybe that attracts readers, "clicks" on the web, and more advertisers, but it certainly does not serve the public interest.

What had seemed to be well-settled science became controversial, at least in the United States, though not much elsewhere in the world. It happened with climate change, it happened with cigarettes, it happened with lead. Is it now happening with salt? Or have the sodium skeptics truly proven that Americans are eating an optimal level of sodium, that lower-sodium diets would be harmful, and that government should not press companies to lower sodium levels?

Way back in 1989, a committee of the National Academy of Sciences, in its report titled *Diet and Health: Implications for Reducing Chronic Disease Risk*, recognized that diets high in sodium and low in potassium increase the risk of hypertension. But the committee also stated:

By far the greatest difference of opinion, and the most strongly held opinions, relate to the desirability of recommending to the general public that dietary sodium intake should be restricted. . . . There is little likelihood that these controversies will be entirely resolved in the foreseeable future.[19]

How right they were! Let's now examine some of the pivotal studies that defenders of salt have cited when they proclaim that eating a lower-sodium diet would be worthless and even dangerous.

People with Normal Blood Pressure Need Not Consume Less Sodium

A linchpin of the plea by public health experts to lower sodium throughout the population is that doing so would lower blood pressure and prevent heart attacks and strokes. But what if lowering sodium had no effect on blood pressure in most people?

In 2019, Niels Graudal of the Copenhagen University Hospital in Denmark and several colleagues conducted a large meta-analysis of controlled clinical trials on sodium and blood pressure.[20] Coincidentally, it included 133 studies, the same number as were included in a 2020 meta-analysis that

I described in chapter 2.[21] Like the subsequent study, this one found that a major decrease in sodium intake decreased systolic blood pressure only slightly (–1.46 mm Hg) in the majority of people whose blood pressure was normal, under 132 mm Hg. (The change in people with higher blood pressures was far higher: 7.7 mg Hg.) The authors used the smallness of the increase to argue that sodium reduction "should probably not be a target for the general population but only for hypertensives with a high sodium intake."

The conclusion that most people need not reduce their sodium intake was seriously misguided. First, as I also noted in chapter 2, even small reductions in blood pressure averaged over the millions of people with normal or high-normal blood pressure would prevent a modest number of heart attacks and strokes in the coming decades. Second, people who have hypertension cannot lower their sodium intake significantly over the long term unless sodium is decreased in the overall food supply. Third, reducing sodium would recalibrate Americans' taste buds, starting in childhood, and help reduce the taste for salt and the risk or severity of hypertension. Finally, the authors ignored the likelihood that salt may well be harmful by mechanisms other than boosting blood pressure and that elevated blood pressure causes problems other than cardiovascular disease.

The "Earth-Shattering" Institute of Medicine Report

The heart of sodium skeptics' argument, though, does not rely on the effects of sodium on blood pressure, but rather on disease. In 2013, the Institute of Medicine (IOM; now the National Academy of Medicine or NAM) published a major, attention-getting report on how low-sodium diets might affect health.[22] The journalist who wrote about the report in the *New York Times*—under the sensationalized headline "No Benefit Seen in Sharp Limits on Salt in Diet"—said it "undercuts years of public health warnings" and stated that Alderman called the report's findings "earth-shattering."[23]

The IOM committee was established to consider whether diets in the range of 1,500 to 2,300 mg of sodium per day affected health outcomes, such as strokes, instead of just risk factors such as blood pressure. The committee supported lowering sodium consumption from today's high levels to 2,300 mg per day, yielding a substantial benefit and causing no harm.[24] But it also concluded that the evidence was inconsistent and insufficient because of the paucity of evidence on whether intakes below 2,300 mg of sodium were beneficial or risky to the general population. Recall that the government's then-current "Dietary Guidelines for Americans 2010" had recommended that older people, African Americans, and people with pre-hypertension and hypertension should shoot for 1,500 mg per day, something the makers of salt and salty foods did not appreciate.

Importantly, the committee did not evaluate the voluminous research showing that low-sodium diets, including ones with well under 2,300 mg per day, reduce blood pressure and that lower blood pressure reduces the risk of cardiovascular disease. According to the committee, that was not within the scope of the charge it was given by the government sponsors.

But here is the "earth-shattering" part of the evaluation, which led to huge publicity: the IOM committee stated that lowering sodium intake to 1,840 mg per day "may lead to greater risk of adverse events" in patients with heart failure. The word "risk" exerted its magnetic pull on journalists who discussed the IOM assessment.

The alleged risk was based largely on six studies done in Italy, where many patients with congestive heart failure (CHF) who were put on a low-sodium diet had died.[25] It was not widely publicized that the doctors followed an unwise therapeutic regimen that was rarely used (and probably not at all in the United States). The IOM qualified its statement by noting that the patients whose sodium intakes were restricted had severe heart failure, had been subject to "aggressive" treatment with high doses of a powerful diuretic, and were on fluid-restricted diets. The American Heart Association (AHA) dismissed the Italian research entirely—and the committee's reference to it—by emphasizing that "experience in such a sick and highly medicated group has no relevance for the general population or even for most patients with heart failure."[26]

Putting a nail in the Italian research's coffin, the journal *Heart* retracted (that is, it disavowed) a meta-analysis it had previously published of those six studies. The journal's ethics committee stated that two of the studies contained duplicate data as well as raw data that could not be substantiated because, the researchers claimed, it had been "lost as a result of computer failure."[27] That's either a good example of "the dog ate my homework" or an inexcusable failure to properly store data, which is further evidence that the study was poorly conducted. Before the meta-analysis had been retracted, the pro-salt health journalist Gary Taubes published "Salt We

Misjudged You," a prominently placed opinion piece in the *New York Times* that gave national publicity to the Italian research. Taubes wrote: "Italian researchers began publishing the results from a series of clinical trials, all of which reported that, among patients with heart failure, reducing salt consumption increased the risk of death."[28] Actually, it wasn't the lack of salt that killed the patients; it was the doctors' risky therapeutic regimen.

The IOM committee also found "some evidence suggesting risk" from consuming less than 2,300 mg of sodium per day for people with diabetes, chronic kidney disease, or preexisting cardiovascular disease. The evidence of risk to those various groups of patients was skimpy, but in any case patients with serious illnesses are ordinarily under their doctors' care and are very different from healthy consumers, at whom public-health dietary advice is directed.

Dariush Mozaffarian, the dean of the Friedman School of Nutrition Science and Policy at Tufts University, later sharply criticized the 2013 IOM committee, saying that it

> was not tasked with reviewing all available evidence nor with setting a target level. Rather, they were instructed to limit their focus to studies of clinical endpoints, and only to studies published from 2003 to 2012 . . . and only to the question of comparing a target level of 2,300 to 1,500 mg/day. Their task, in other words, was *not* to determine the best evidence base for a dietary target, but to evaluate *one* type of the evidence and over a specified period and only for the question of lowering the target from 2,300 to 1,500 mg/day.[29]

Controversy aside, the 2013 IOM report endorsed long-standing advice to cut sodium to 2,300 mg per day, but it did not support going below that amount. Truth be told, debating whether people should consume 1,500 or 2,300 mg is currently a bit academic considering that the average American consumes so much more—3,400 mg. It's going to be a long, long time before the country gets down to an average of 2,300, let alone 1,500. But *you*, of course, don't have to wait to consume less salt. I'll have tips for doing that in chapter 11.

Similar to the IOM committee, in 2017 a joint committee of the World Heart Federation, European Society of Hypertension, and European Public Health Association pointed to the absence of controlled trials on the health effects of diets in the range of 2,300 mg per day. They advised remedial actions only when a population's average sodium consumption exceeds 5,000 mg per day.[30] That would give the green light to almost everyone in almost every nation to eat just about all the salt they want—with disastrous consequences for public health. In light of the mountain of research on sodium and disease, their advice should be ignored!

Observational Studies Suggest That Low-Sodium Diets Promote Cardiovascular Disease

Perhaps the most widely publicized evidence that low-sodium diets could be harmful was based on studies of sodium intakes of large groups of people over a number of years. In such observational studies the participants are not asked to change their diets, they are just observed. In contrast, people in trials are put on diets (or urged to adhere to certain diets) with different amounts of sodium and then followed for months or years to identify any differences in blood pressure or rates of disease or deaths. Observational studies probably (and unfortunately) have muddied the waters and confused the salt debate rather than clarified it. Because this issue is at the heart of the debate over how much sodium we should consume, I am going to delve deeply into it.

Observational studies have been highly controversial: although some found a lower risk of cardiovascular disease at lower sodium intakes (see chapter 2), others linked a higher risk of cardiovascular disease to sodium intakes at both higher- *and* lower-than-typical intakes.

Some major observational studies are based on dietary intakes measured by the federal government's National Health and Nutrition Examination Survey (NHANES). Researchers mine those data for all sorts of relationships between diet and disease. Hillel W. Cohen and Michael H. Alderman of the Albert Einstein College of Medicine and their co-authors have published several papers based on NHANES surveys conducted in different years. They consistently found that the lowest sodium intakes were associated with a higher risk of deaths from cardiovascular disease. For instance, a 2006 article concluded that consuming less than 2,300 mg of sodium per day was associated with a 37 percent greater risk of cardiovascular disease and a 28 percent greater risk of dying from any cause compared to people who consumed more than 2,300 mg per day.[31]

Stated plainly, those investigators found that the people consuming the *least* sodium and the *most* sodium had a *greater* risk of cardiovascular disease than those consuming middling levels. The authors acknowledged certain inherent weaknesses in their and other observational studies, but the unexpected results, published in major medical journals, lent credence—and publicity—to the notion that people need not lower their sodium intake. To overcome those weaknesses, Alderman and others have urged that controlled trials be done in which large numbers of people would be asked to eat, or be provided with, diets with different levels of sodium. Then they would be followed for years to determine the rates of heart disease, strokes, and overall deaths. I write more about that later in this chapter.

Feng J. He and her fellow researchers in London blasted the Cohen-Alderman study. They decried that "the method used to assess salt intake (one 24-hour dietary recall at the beginning) is notoriously unreliable, particularly because no account is taken of discretionary [table] salt." And, because Cohen's group had conducted earlier studies using the same flawed methods, they added, "It is quite extraordinary that Cohen et al. choose to ignore the scientific criticisms that followed their [previous] article."[32]

Alderman is not totally doctrinaire about the harmfulness of lowering sodium. He has acknowledged that salt restriction, though "relatively weak and costly," does lower the blood pressure of some patients.[33] And he agrees that it would be sensible for people with enormous intakes or who have hypertension to reduce their intake. I asked him if he ever has doubts about his position that current salt intake is generally fine, especially when health organizations with the stature of the World Health Organization (WHO) and Centers for Disease Control and Prevention (CDC) strongly favor public health measures to lower their sodium intake population-wide. He said "of course."[34]

But Alderman questions whether it is even possible for people to consume less salt—because, he says, decades' worth of advice to the public to cut the salt has had no effect. That argument is weak at best. Official policy is to cut the salt, but the US government has never mounted a well-funded, persuasive, persistent education campaign. Relying on a standard low-budget and perfunctory education program to lower sodium is like using scissors to cut the greens on a golf course. Living in a world of salty packaged and restaurant foods makes it very challenging for average consumers, who have many more immediate worries on their minds, to opt for a lower-salt diet.

Critics charge that many observational studies do not just have weaknesses, but are so flawed as to be misleading. Finnish researchers said about earlier (1978) research, "Rather than shed new light on sodium intake and mortality, Alderman and colleagues' report brings unnecessary confusion into the discussion on the relation between dietary sodium and mortality."[35] They pointed out that the people who had supposedly consumed low levels of sodium had "a calorie intake that should have resulted in death from starvation." People in the lowest one-fourth of sodium consumption reported that they consumed only about half the recommended calorie intake. Clearly, those people were underestimating how much food (and, hence, sodium) they had eaten.

Fatal and PURE Flaws

In a systematic critique of the research indicating that low sodium intakes were harmful—with most of that assessment coming from observational studies—CDC researchers, including CDC's then-director Tom Frieden, emphasized the studies' often-poor estimates of sodium intake.[36] They noted that basing sodium intakes on participants' recollections of what they ate on just one day at the beginning of a long study is unreliable and might well lead to inaccurate results. People's diets vary radically from one day to another (just think of your own diet). Moreover, people tend to under-report the soups, restaurant meals, and other unhealthy foods they ate and over-report the broccoli, spinach, peaches, and other healthy foods. Even Alderman and two colleagues acknowledged that measuring sodium intakes just once in a multiyear study, as is done in much observational research, might not be adequate.[37]

The CDC scientists also noticed that a disproportionate number of participants consuming a low-sodium diet had diabetes, hypertension, heart disease, or other chronic illness when the studies started. But sick people eat less food and therefore less sodium, and some of those people likely had consumed less salt to help treat their illness. It makes no sense to assume that low sodium intake caused them to be sick. That kind of "reverse causality," also called "reverse causation," confuses cause and effect and is an inherent defect of a great deal of observational research.

To get beyond individual observational studies, Graudal, Alderman, and two other researchers conducted a meta-analysis based on some two dozen observational studies on sodium consumption and the risk of cardiovascular disease.[38] They found that the lowest intakes of sodium (under about

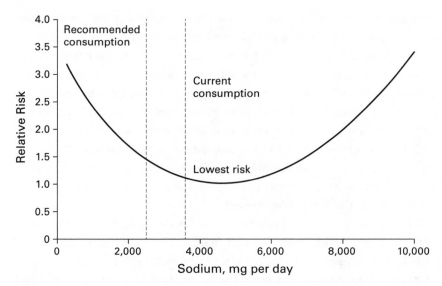

Figure 3.1
Both high- and low-sodium intakes appear to be harmful. Several observational studies found a J- or U-shaped relationship between sodium intake (along the horizontal
axis) and the risk of cardiovascular disease. In this hypothetical example, the lowest
risk of disease was with a daily sodium intake of 4,500 mg. *Source*: Illustration by J.
Bach, CSPI.

2,600 mg per day) and highest (above 4,900 mg per day) were associated
with a higher risk of cardiovascular disease than intakes between those levels. That is, they observed a J- or U-shaped relationship between sodium
intake and the incidence of disease, as depicted in figure 3.1.

Findings that are so contrary to the larger body of research on salt and
disease must be scrutinized carefully. In fact, meta-analyses, which are
sometimes considered especially reliable because of their increased statistical power, may distract from weaknesses in the underlying individual studies and, hence, in the meta-analysis itself. When the indefatigable British
researchers Feng J. He and Graham A. MacGregor put the Graudal meta-
analysis under their microscope, they stated that its "conclusion is invalid
because of the severe methodological flaws of the studies [it] included."[39]
They pointed especially to inaccurate measurements of sodium consumption ("it varies hugely day to day"), as well as the likelihood of reverse
causality. More recently He and her colleagues wrote: "These J- or U-shaped

findings should not have been used to challenge the current public health policies due to their severe methodological limitations."[40]

By coincidence, the Graudal meta-analysis of observational studies was published in 2014 just after the American Heart Association (AHA) had released a detailed "science advisory" that explained why many such studies are unreliable.[41] The advisory emphasized, like He and MacGregor, erroneous measurements of sodium intakes and reverse causality. The AHA advisory concluded, "It remains appropriate to base [sodium] guidelines on the robust body of evidence linking [sodium] with elevated blood pressure and the few existing general population trials of the effects of [sodium] reduction on [cardiovascular disease]."

The giant among observational studies is the Prospective Urban Rural Epidemiology (PURE) study—actually a series of studies begun in 2001 and led by Salim Yusuf of McMaster University Medical School in Hamilton, Ontario. PURE is frequently portrayed as being exceptionally powerful and reliable because of its enormous size. For example, for a 2014 study, the researchers collected urine samples from 101,945 persons in 17 countries to determine sodium intake, and then followed individuals for three-and-a-half years.[42] They found that consuming between 3,000 and 6,000 mg of sodium per day was associated with a lower risk of death and fewer heart attacks and strokes than consuming a higher or lower intake.

In a subsequent and even larger analysis involving 133,000 individuals, PURE researchers found the same J-shaped relationship between sodium consumption and the risk of cardiovascular disease.[43] (Other PURE studies found that saturated fat was not harmful and perhaps even beneficial, and that polyunsaturated oils and vegetables were not beneficial; both findings are contrary to most medical research.)[44]

Martin O'Donnell, a colleague of Yusuf, told one journalist that PURE undermines much of the advice that health officials have been telling the public for years:

> This study . . . questions the appropriateness of current guidelines that recommend low sodium intake in the entire population. An approach that recommends salt in moderation, particularly focused on those with hypertension, appears more in line with current evidence.[45]

Graudal, who was not an author but also opposes lowering sodium intakes below about 3,000 mg per day, said flatly that PURE "is based on genuine scientific data" and "confirms that low sodium intake is an independent risk factor for increased mortality."[46] In other words, he implied, everything you've heard about the importance of cutting sodium well below the current 3,400-mg average diet is wrong. And journalists, impressed by PURE's size, quickly pounded out prominent and favorable stories that spread the message. Unfortunately, such media coverage amplifies and gives credence to unreliable studies, and that can lead consumers to think that cutting back on salt is dangerous.

PURE's conclusions were immediately challenged. Francesco Cappuccio, professor of Cardiovascular Medicine & Epidemiology at the Warwick Medical School in England and head of the WHO's Collaborating Center for Nutrition, slammed both the PURE paper and the *Lancet* medical journal for publishing it. He told the *Independent* newspaper, "It is with disbelief that we should read such bad science published in *The Lancet*. . . . The flaws that were extensively noted in [the researchers'] previous accounts are maintained and criticisms ignored."[47]

Nancy Cook, the biostatistician at Brigham and Women's Hospital and Harvard Medical School, took on the issue of study size:

> The fact that the PURE study is the largest to date should not influence its interpretation. A large study size does not eliminate bias resulting from selection, reverse causation, or confounding [i.e., interference by a third variable] but could lead to spurious results.[48]

The observations of the heart association's science advisory are particularly applicable to PURE: "It is difficult to conduct rigorous, high-quality investigations of the relationship between [sodium] intake and [cardiovascular disease]." The advisory included a further comment: "For the foreseeable future, the high-quality body of evidence linking [sodium] intake to [blood pressure] should remain the basis for setting recommended levels of [sodium] intake."[49]

The PURE authors themselves acknowledged some "limitations" in their methodology, and many critics heartily agreed. The "limitations," though, were disqualifying flaws. One of the biggest was the reliability of participants' sodium intakes. I touched on the problem earlier when discussing the Graudal study, and it's worth exploring here in more detail.

Instead of obtaining multiple 24-hour urine samples to estimate usual sodium intakes, PURE used just one "spot" urine sample—peeing into a container once—at the beginning of the studies. That method saves money, but it does not accurately reflect a person's average sodium intake both at the beginning of a study and over time. (Intakes based on what participants said they ate on the previous day or based on which foods they reported consuming over the course of months—Food Frequency Questionnaires—are similarly flawed.) To correct for the measurement problem, the PURE investigators used a formula—the Kawasaki formula—to try to convert the sodium content of the spot urine samples to what would have been excreted over 24 hours. But the Kawasaki formula has been dubbed a "poor performer" because it overestimates sodium at lower levels and underestimates it at higher levels.[50] Statistical alchemy simply cannot turn bad data into good data.

In addition, two reports demonstrated the perils of using spot urines and the Kawasaki formula. In one, Dutch researchers took advantage of their previous project in which people provided several 24-hour urine samples over 15 years.[51] That study found that the average sodium content of multiple urine samples was often markedly different from the initial sample. When they used only the initial 24-hour urine sample to correlate sodium intake with cardiovascular risk—note that even a single 24-hour sample is more reliable than the spot urines in PURE—the notorious J-shaped relationship emerged. But they then included urine samples obtained after one year and five years to get a truer estimate of a subject's typical sodium intake. Like magic, the J-shaped curve indicating a greater risk at the low end of sodium consumption vanished. Instead, the relationship between sodium and cardiovascular disease became the expected linear one, with the lowest sodium intakes being associated with the lowest risk of disease. The Dutch scientists warned against relying on a "wobbly parameter" (a single urine sample) and took a direct poke at PURE's basic methodology: "Future [observational] studies should therefore focus on accurate assessment of sodium intake rather than the inclusion of many subjects."[52]

In a second rebuttal, a team of British, Canadian, and American experts also disputed the reliability of PURE. They did a reanalysis based on the two TOHP studies that I discussed in chapter 2, which found that the participants with a lower sodium intake had a lower mortality rate. Similar to the Dutch study, when the team reanalyzed their data using the Kawasaki formula to estimate sodium intake, the J-shaped curve appeared. That finding, like the Dutch one, demonstrated that the curve was an artifact of

PURE's methodology and not a true indication that low salt intakes are harmful. The researchers' stinging conclusion was that "paradoxical results from methodologically flawed studies should not be used to derail critical public health policy, nor divert action."[53]

Most damning, the TOHP researchers investigated whether participants in their control group who consumed the least sodium, under 2,300 mg per day, had higher rates of cardiovascular disease than people who consumed middling levels.[54] In fact, they found the opposite: people who consumed less than 2,300 mg had a 32 percent *lower* risk than people who consumed 3,600 to 4,800 mg. That finding was shy of statistical significance, but that might have been due to the small number of participants who consumed so little sodium. As the researchers concluded, "estimates from spot urine are unreliable, not reproducible and systematically biased."

Cook highlighted yet another limitation of PURE and other observational studies: "residual confounding." That is the term researchers use for unaccounted-for factors that can distort the apparent relationship between an exposure and a health outcome. Because they are unknown, researchers cannot compensate for them by making statistical adjustments. Residual confounding is an especially important problem, Cook said, in a study that includes "people from a host of countries, ranging from low to high income, with very different background health status, nutritional standards, and health care systems." Cook further explained:

> [The PURE researchers] only control for a few variables and don't capture the heterogeneity in the data. For example, some of the participants could even be malnourished or have other uncontrolled health conditions including infectious diseases, and that could easily account for the effects seen.[55]

Yusuf, the lead PURE researcher, has acknowledged the problem: "Even the best work has limitations, including ours. So, I worry how much of our work is potentially confounded. I truly worry."[56] In a presentation to the National Academy of Medicine, he said, "That's our data. Would I like better data, yes."[57]

Still, the PURE researchers continue to campaign against sodium reductions. Their persistence has driven some leading hypertension experts to frustration. In a detailed, scholarly rebuttal to the sodium skeptics, Norm R. C. Campbell, a professor at the University of Calgary's O'Brien Institute of Public Health and Libin Cardiovascular Institute of Alberta, charged:

> Several dissenting scientists have conducted low-quality research, taken research
> out of context, made factual errors or misinterpreted results, altered scientific for-
> mulae/protocols in a fashion that makes their controversial research appear more
> robust, and used low-quality evidence to trump higher quality.[58]

More colloquially, a quip favored by software engineers comes to mind.
When you combine data from rich and poor countries and healthy and
sick people into one big study, you end up with "garbage in, garbage out."

No matter how big the studies and how hard the researchers worked on
them, the PURE studies (and others conducted like them) are red herrings,
especially in the context of the vast body of reliable research on sodium
and health.[59] The AHA told consumers bluntly, "The findings in this [PURE]
study are not valid, and you shouldn't use it to inform yourself about how
you're going to eat."[60]

The "Set-Point" Theory of Sodium Consumption

In 2013, based on their reviews of sodium consumption in 45 countries,
several widely published researchers have asserted that the "'normal' range
of human sodium intake [is] defined by physiology and biological needs
and not by the food supply."[61] Those researchers—McCarron, a consultant
who previously headed the nephrology division at Oregon Health & Science University, Niels A. Graudal in Copenhagen, and others—found that
average sodium consumption in almost all countries ranged from 2,600 to
4,800 mg per day. They also noted that in the Trials of Hypertension Prevention (TOHP) II trial (see chapter 2) participants were vigorously counseled
to consume about 1,800 mg of sodium per day, but they actually consumed
closer to 2,600 mg.

Based on such observations, the researchers suggested that humans have
a safe and natural "set point" for sodium consumption that is determined
by hormones that regulate the excretion of water and sodium and not by
what people try to consume or what the food industry is marketing. They
also raised the specter of harm if consumption dipped below 2,300 mg per
day, saying, "to attempt to use public policy to abrogate human physiology
would be futile and possibly harmful to human health."[62]

The true situation is more complicated. It may sound reasonable to say
that people around the world are consuming the optimum level of sodium,

but it is misleading.[63] For starters, McCarron and his colleagues excluded from their study populations that consume very salty diets, as well as groups that consume very little sodium, such as hunter-gatherer tribes with intakes amounting to just a few hundred milligrams per day. Also, because salt is such an integral ingredient of packaged and restaurant foods throughout most of the world, consuming at least 3,000 mg of sodium per day is not a conscious choice or a physiological requirement, but an almost inevitable consequence of our salty food environment.

What really puts the lie to the set-point theory of sodium consumption is that people *can* consume less sodium. In Finland, average sodium consumption was cut by one-third. In a controlled experiment in two small Portuguese communities, people in the intervention community reduced their sodium intake by 43 percent after two years.[64] Average consumption in the United Kingdom was cut by 10 to 15 percent over a decade. The participants in the TOHP and TONE trials reduced their intake by one-third, with those in TOHP I consuming 2,300 mg per day. Admittedly, though, no entire country has cut sodium consumption all the way down to 2,300 mg per day or less. That's impossible to do when packaged and prepared foods are suffused with salt and other sources of sodium.

Yet More Criticisms of Low-Sodium Diets

Might choosing a low-sodium diet somehow lead to nutrient deficiencies? Two University of Washington nutrition researchers were curious to see how practical it would be for Americans to reduce sodium intakes substantially and still consume adequate amounts of protein, vitamins, and other nutrients. Matthieu Maillot and Adam Drewnowski used a mathematical model to estimate the dietary changes that would be needed to consume a diet with 2,300 or 1,500 mg of sodium per day accompanied by 100 percent of the recommended intakes of two-dozen other nutrients. They concluded that eating a nutritionally adequate diet with as little as 2,300 mg of sodium was feasible for most men and women. Yet to get down to between 1,500 and 2,000 mg, they said, would require "wrenching" changes in food choices and the American food supply. To get to 1,500 mg or less would necessitate totally omitting meats and grains. Maillot and Drewnowski stated: "No combination of food categories satisfied the model requirements of a nutrient-adequate food pattern. . . . In other words, at this low level of sodium, the requirements for multiple other nutrients could not be met."[65]

But the situation is not as dire as the University of Washington researchers suggest. The 2010 Dietary Guidelines Advisory Committee described food patterns with 2,300 mg of sodium and 100 percent of the recommended intakes for almost all nutrients (exceptions were vitamins D and E).[66] To adhere to those dietary patterns, however, most people indeed would have to eat more natural, whole foods and less (and less-salty) packaged and restaurant foods—changes that would be salubrious for many reasons. Getting down to 1,500 mg a day would certainly require greater changes in food composition and choices, but for now let's be satisfied getting down to 2,300 mg in the next decade or so.

In another line of attack, some researchers have suggested mechanisms by which low sodium intakes could be harmful. One possibility, they contend, is that lowering sodium consumption could upset hormonal balances. They focus on the body's renin-angiotensin-aldosterone system (RAAS), a group of critically important hormones that regulate sodium and fluid balances in the body. Alderman wrote that at sodium intakes under 2,500 mg per day, plasma renin activity increases and mortality increases.[67]

Indeed, major, sudden reductions in sodium consumption sharply increase levels of renin and aldosterone, which could be harmful. But over the longer term and with more modest (and realistic) reductions in sodium, renin and aldosterone levels stay about the same.[68]

Cappuccio, the head of the WHO's Collaborating Center for Nutrition, told National Public Radio that elevated renin-angiotensin activity is the body's normal physiologic response to decreased sodium, and is not worrisome.[69] The Yanomami Indians, as a result of their extremely low sodium intakes, have renin levels 10 times higher than Americans' levels without any apparent problem.[70] It is likely that those are historically normal levels, and that our *low* levels of renin and aldosterone are aberrant. Also, taking diuretics to treat hypertension stimulates the renin-angiotensin system, but diuretics are known to reduce cardiovascular mortality.[71] Finally, in 2010 the IOM said, "in contrast to the well-accepted benefits of blood pressure reduction, the clinical relevance of modest rises in plasma renin activity as a result of sodium reduction is uncertain."[72] So let's not worry that gradually declining sodium intakes might lead to dangerously high levels of those hormones.

The Dangers of Waiting for the Perfect Trial

Sodium skeptics have opposed lowering sodium consumption by the general population until definitive research has shown that reductions would be safe and effective in reducing disease rates. Alderman urges that before health officials take actions to lower sodium, "all researchers should press for well-designed, rigorous, and robust [randomized controlled trials, or RCTs] to determine the health consequences of universal salt restriction."[73] Alderman and several others have been saying that for at least 30 years.

In theory, definitive RCTs to determine whether sodium intakes under 1,500, 2,300, or 3,000 mg per day decrease or increase the risk of disease would be the ultimate test of the "sodium hypothesis." The ideal trial would enlist a large number of healthy volunteers, split them into two groups, and for many years give them all their meals and snacks, which would be identical except for differences in sodium content. Then the researchers would compare the numbers of strokes, heart attacks, and other health problems that people in each group suffered.

Partly because of the huge cost of that kind of trial, almost two decades ago two prominent experts predicted flatly, "it will never be done."[74] Many researchers, who almost reflexively support doing more research, are not supportive here. According to Lawrence J. Appel, a professor at the Johns Hopkins School of Medicine and one of the lead researchers in the DASH trials, "it would not be worth the considerable time and expense because of the overwhelming evidence for salt's adverse effects on blood pressure."[75] I suspect that because the National Institutes of Health and other agencies around the world have not provided funding, they have apparently come to the same conclusion.

MacGregor emphasizes that nutrition research is often not like drug research where randomized trials are generally feasible. He likened the situation to that of tobacco, where we have no trials showing the benefits of smoking cessation. Instead, he said, "We need to rely on all the other types of evidence, and for salt we are fortunate to have over 10 different types of evidence, all of which indicates that salt is important in increasing blood pressure."[76]

Pasquale Strazzullo, a professor at the University of Naples Medical School in Italy, echoed that sentiment, asking, "Should we refrain from this life-saving measure and let people die of hypertension and its cardiovascular complications while waiting for the 'mother of all trials'?"[77] Health officials should not be paralyzed by the paucity of trials.

Despite the obstacles to conducting a definitive trial, in 2018, eight well-known researchers, including both advocates and opponents of reducing sodium intakes—such as Paul Whelton of the Tulane University School of Public Health on the pro side and McCarron and Alderman representing the cons—explored options for conducting an RCT with prisoners.[78] They wanted to work with prisons to provide some inmates a diet with the usual amount of sodium and to give other prisoners, in the same or different prisons, the exact same diet but with less sodium. Because the Federal Bureau of Prisons does not allow research other than that which advances knowledge about corrections, such a study would probably have to be conducted in state or private prisons.[79]

Some public health experts, however, were leery. They contended that an RCT involving prisoners was (a) unnecessary (because of the strong and consistent animal, clinical, and epidemiologic research, the several existing trials, and the experience in the United Kingdom and Finland showing the benefits of lowering sodium intakes); (b) too expensive (and potentially siphoning funding from higher-priority research); (c) possibly unethical; and (d) almost certainly inconclusive, leading to calls for additional costly and lengthy trials.

Sonia Y. Angell, then a deputy commissioner of health in New York City and now the director of the California Department of Public Health, pointed out that "prison conditions are unique," and prisoners not only have higher rates of mental illness, cardiovascular disease, and other problems, but they also experience stress levels that the general population does not endure. Angell said, "Modifying a single nutrient in a diet of a population in prison won't produce a study with answers relevant to our population at large."[80]

Ethical considerations raised additional concerns: Would the inmates truly be giving their informed consent to participate in the study? Should some of the participants be forced to eat a low-sodium diet that they would rather not eat? Should others be required to eat a standard, unhealthy, high-sodium diet?

Finally, and importantly, postponing public health action pending the results from an RCT could undermine public health because, according to Appel, planning, conducting, analyzing, and publishing a study might delay policies to lower sodium in the food supply for 15 years.[81] During that time companies and supportive politicians would likely argue that the government should not encourage consumers or require companies to reduce sodium until the results were available. (My organization, the Center for Science in the Public Interest, did not oppose the study, but pointed to the ethical, practical, and financial obstacles to conducting it. We also said that any such research should not be permitted to delay government action on salt.)

Ultimately, according to two members of the committee who spoke to me confidentially, the notion of a prison study fizzled when the advocates could not develop a design that would pass scientific and ethical muster, let alone be financially feasible. Even Alderman, who was on the committee and has called for trials for 30 years, stated in August 2019: "I don't think it's possible" to conduct an RCT.[82] One insoluble problem he pointed to was the prisoners' uncontrolled access to the commissary, and the customary selling and bartering of food they can buy there or receive from visitors. The demise of the prison study might have silenced calls for a gold-standard trial that had the potential to end the controversy. But it didn't. When I talked to Alderman three months later, he had a new suggestion for an RCT, this time one in which people already consuming a low-sodium diet would be given either a salt tablet or a placebo and then monitored for heart attacks and strokes. Again, practical and ethical problems would certainly sink such a trial.

It is worth recognizing that public health measures are often taken in the absence of randomized controlled trials. Policy makers must rely instead on animal, epidemiology, clinical, and other evidence. Health officials have advised people to lose weight, stop smoking, avoid trans fat, and eat more fruits and vegetables, all without robust, controlled trials.

If asbestos researchers were to look at the battle over salt, they might quote the great New York Yankees catcher Yogi Berra, who purportedly said, "It's déjà vu all over again." The asbestos industry defended the safety of its product for decades after it was known to cause cancer (again, no randomized controlled trials). David Egilman, a clinical professor of family medicine at Brown University and then editor of the *International Journal of Occupational and Environmental Health*, described the asbestos industry's battle plan this way: "They can throw a lot of things at the wall and hope something sticks with the jury. . . . It forces people like me or other scientists to try to clean up each thing that was thrown at the wall, one at a time. And by the end of the day, that could be confusing to a jury or judge."[83] Sounds like salt to me.

Summarizing the Science

Most public health officials recognize that lowering sodium intake helps prevent cardiovascular disease. But some scientists have conducted large observational studies—that is, not controlled trials—that appear to indicate that consuming less than about 4,000 mg of sodium per day *increases* cardiovascular disease. That finding is welcomed by the salt and food industries and publicized in the media, but the research has been roundly criticized, including by an authoritative 2019 committee of the National Academy of Medicine.

The scientists who oppose lowering sodium insist that new, long-term, controlled trials must be done before consumers reduce their sodium intake and governments adopt policies to help them do so. (Some of the scientists who oppose lowering sodium have received small amounts of industry funding and collaborated with the food and salt industries; I address those situations in chapters 5 and 6.) But during the several decades in which researchers have called for such trials, the preponderance of persuasive evidence showing how lower sodium intakes would be healthful, not harmful, has apparently convinced funders that such expensive projects are unnecessary.

Whether or not you followed every twist and turn of the research I've described so far, I'll cut to the chase in chapter 4, where I summarize the evidence for consuming more sodium or less.

4   What All the Research Means

A modest reduction in population salt intake worldwide would result in a major improvement in public health—similar to the provision of clean water and drains in the late nineteenth century in Europe.

—Feng J. He, Graham A. MacGregor[1]

Confused by the competing claims? I hope not, but then again, I wouldn't be surprised if you were. Literally thousands of scientific articles have been published on salt, high blood pressure, and cardiovascular disease, so it *can* be confusing to dive deep into that sea of research, especially when the findings and the opinions of experts conflict so radically. And then the news media, websites, social media, and blogs, which sometimes have strong biases, convey some of that information to the public.

So how do expert committees reach their conclusions in the cases for and against sodium? Typically, by weighting a mass of diverse evidence by strength. Table 4.1 does just that by summarizing the strength of key research in support of or opposed to reducing sodium in the American diet.

In chapter 1 we saw that sodium intakes in human populations vary dramatically, from astonishingly small amounts by isolated, subsistence tribes, to excessive amounts in most industrialized countries, to enormous amounts in Turkey, parts of China, Japan, and certain other countries. But, bottom line, humans appear to be able to live quite well, virtually without hypertension or cardiovascular disease, with diets containing as little as a hundred milligrams of sodium per day—which is far less than the 1,500 to 2,300 mg of sodium recommended by the US Department of Health and Human Services, World Health Organization, and other public health authorities. Of course, it would be nearly impossible—and unnecessary—for

Table 4.1

Strength of evidence for and against reducing sodium intake, rated from 1 (low) to 5 (high)*

Key Evidence for *Reducing* Salt (strength)	Key Evidence for *Not Reducing* Salt (strength)
• Controlled trials show that consuming more sodium raises blood pressure (5) • In trials and observational studies, higher blood pressure increases the risk of cardiovascular disease (5) • Limited trials found that lowering sodium reduces the risk of cardiovascular disease (2)	• Some observational studies (based on NHANES, PURE, others) found that low sodium intakes were associated with higher mortality (1) • In limited trials, low-sodium diets together with restricted fluids and diuretics increased mortality in patients with heart failure (1)

*Based on the number and quality of studies.

healthy people living in a modern culture, with the temptation of salty prepared foods at every turn, to consume just a few hundred milligrams of sodium in a day.

Chapter 2 provided clear-cut evidence that blood pressure rises as sodium consumption increases, more so in African Americans and people with hypertension and less so in younger people with normal blood pressure. Overwhelming evidence also supports a second fact: the higher the blood pressure, the greater the risk of heart attacks and strokes.

Experts have long connected those two undisputed facts to conclude that the risk of cardiovascular disease increases as sodium intake increases and that the general population should consume less sodium. While that logic is not airtight, trials on salt and cardiovascular disease strengthen my confidence that the relationship is real.

The Trials of Hypertension Prevention (TOHP) and a large trial at a veterans home in Taiwan found that lower sodium intakes were accompanied by lower risks of cardiovascular disease. Further support for lowering sodium comes from the United Kingdom, Finland, and Japan, where government campaigns to lower sodium intakes were associated with fewer, not more, deaths due to cardiovascular disease—though other factors, such as lower smoking rates, might have contributed to the benefit. But as critics of lowering sodium argue, none of those studies demonstrated benefits from slashing daily consumption to 2,300 mg or less per day.

Contradicting most expert authorities, as we saw in chapter 3, are researchers who disagree that consuming less salt leads to less cardiovascular disease. Those researchers agree that consuming more than 5,000 mg of sodium per day increases the risk of heart attacks and strokes—but contend that intakes lower than 3,000 mg per day also increase the risk. With most Americans (and people in many other countries) consuming about 3,000 to 4,000 mg per day, they argue that lowering average sodium intakes to 2,300 mg or less per day could be deadly. The National Academy of Medicine (NAM) and others, however, found that the reports suggesting harm suffered from disqualifying limitations, including inaccurate measurements of sodium intakes and reverse causation, and had a "high risk of bias."[2] In 2016, Frieden, then the director of the Centers for Disease and Control, said those reports have created a "false aura of scientific controversy around dietary salt,"[3] and the NAM summarily dismissed them.

The argument boils down to interpreting a voluminous body of research, deciding where the balance of the evidence lies, and then judging how much evidence is enough to advise the public and call on companies to lower sodium levels. In the case of salt and cardiovascular disease, researchers have a rich lode of evidence to evaluate, including animal studies, comparisons of people in different countries and of people who migrated from one region to another, studies of aboriginal peoples, and controlled trials, most of which points toward cutting salt intakes.

Most of the world's leading health organizations and cardiovascular disease experts have concluded that a large number of increasingly refined studies have established that lowering sodium would yield huge health and economic benefits. Public health advocates warn of the risks of waiting for perfect proof before taking action based on the weight of evidence. In 1968 former surgeon general William H. Stewart said, in reference to controlling noise pollution: "Must we wait until we prove every link in the chain of causation? . . . In protecting health, absolute proof comes late. To wait for it is to invite disaster or to prolong suffering unnecessarily."[4] Similarly, in 1986, when the Princeton historian Theodore Rabb testified in Congress about the ozone hole, he reminded legislators: "Scientists are never 100 percent certain. . . . That notion of total certainty is something too elusive ever to be sought."[5]

Rabb also might have reminded legislators of a scientific aphorism popularized by Carl Sagan: "Extraordinary claims require extraordinary evidence." To effectively challenge the informed wisdom that reducing sodium levels would yield enormous health benefits, skeptics need much more than a small number of studies that are flawed and effectively rebutted by other research.

Almost all authoritative health organizations and academic experts agree that the evidence for lowering sodium—by individuals and throughout the food supply—greatly outweighs the evidence that lowering sodium would be harmful or without benefit. Every year that we—consumers, health officials, and the food industry—fail to reduce sodium consumption condemns many thousands of people to premature illnesses and deaths and unnecessary costs. The next chapter provides a portrait of one of the causes of that failure.

5   The Mouse That Roared: The Salt Institute

Salt is the flavor of life and this year we should all recognize its many benefits. . . . [Without salt] people will eat fewer vegetables, and by eating fewer vegetables, they will be less healthy.

—Lori Roman, Salt Institute president, quoted in *USA Today*[1]

If ever there was an entity worthy of the moniker "Big Salt"—an outspoken organization defending the reputation of salt and denying that typical consumption of salt causes death and disease—it was the Salt Institute. Don't be fooled by the scholarly sounding word "institute"—the outfit was really the salt industry's PR and lobbying arm. It was a nonprofit, but not a charity. The Internal Revenue Service categorizes it as a 501(c)(6) organization, one that aims to promote business interests.

Sounding as extreme as the most rabid conspiracy theorists, the Salt Institute took on the task of "promoting salt as a brand and educating the public on salt's positive health and environmental impacts."[2] It variously bragged: "No single ingredient does more positive things for food than salt."[3] In fact, salt is "the essence of life,"[4] "essential for life, health,"[5] and "the flavor of life."[6] And, it contended in large boldface print, **"LOW-salt diets may HARM you,"**[7] claiming as fact "that a low salt diet is significantly more harmful than a high salt diet."[8] I am glad to report that the organization did something in March 2019 that was wholly uncharacteristic of a trade association: it went out of business.

More than two decades ago seven prominent hypertension experts, including Paul K. Whelton at Tulane University School of Public Health and Tropical Medicine and Myron H. Weinberger at Indiana University School of Medicine, angrily charged that "basically, the Salt Institute, similar to the Tobacco Institute, is a group that attempts to manipulate scientific findings for its own commercial benefit, in this instance, to create doubt and confusion among Americans regarding the dangers of high sodium intake."[9]

Big Salt's members included Morton, Cargill, and other major salt manufacturers from around the world. (Ironically, some of the association's major members, such as Morton and Cargill, actually market reduced-sodium salts, but they represent a trivial fraction of the companies' overall sales.) But "big" it was not. The organization's budget was only around $2 million to $3 million a year, half the cost of one 30-second Super Bowl commercial, and it had only four or five staff members.[10] It was more like the "mouse that roared."

Still, when salt came under attack, you could count on the group to issue—and journalists to quote—a pithy, often sassy, statement proclaiming that salt is either innocuous or positively healthful. And the Salt Institute could magnify its impact by calling on members such as Cargill (the nation's largest privately held corporation with annual sales—from products such as sugar, refined oils, cotton, Diamond Crystal salt, and chocolate—of more than $100 billion) and friends throughout the food industry to defend salt.

Full disclosure: There was no love lost between the Salt Institute and my organization. The lobbying group once charged, for instance, "For years the Center for Science in the Public Interest has been using trumped up hysteria to try to get the federal government to control every recipe for almost every food manufactured in the United States."[11] And it accused me of being one of the leaders of the "anti-salt movement" (an accusation to which I proudly plead guilty).[12]

In 2010 I appeared on Comedy Central's *The Colbert Report* with Lori Roman, the head of the Salt Institute.[13] As Stephen Colbert prepared to introduce her, he explained how to distinguish between the Salt Institute and the Salk Institute, the research institute founded by Jonas Salk: the "Salk Institute cures polio; Salt Institute cures ham," he joked. But Roman didn't appreciate Colbert's humor, or his role as devil's advocate, when he gave me a chance to state some facts about salt and health. In response, she defended her organization's members' bread and butter by saying, "some of these facts have no basis in fact."

Roman was the president of the Salt Institute from 2009 until 2019. Prior to that, between 2006 and 2008, she was the executive director of the

American Legislative Exchange Council (ALEC), a group that campaigns for hard-right policies at the state level. Its members include conservative state legislators and corporate representatives. ALEC is an excellent training ground for someone who would be expected to challenge federal and local actions concerning salt. (Given that right-leaning position, it's not surprising to learn that in 2019 Roman became the president of the conservative American Civil Rights Union.)

Notwithstanding the organization's paramount goal of defending salt and salt manufacturers, the Salt Institute found room in its budget to support right-wing organizations.[14] It gave $2,500 to the Education Action Group, which advocates for government aid to private and religious schools,[15] and $15,000 to the Independent Women's Forum (IWF). That group's Board of Directors Emeritae, reflecting its political stance, includes Trump White House officials Kellyanne Conway and Larry Kudlow. In 2014, the IWF was railing against reducing sodium in school lunches[16] and the expansion of the federally funded school-lunch program, while it also advocated for informing consumers about the benefits of meat and dairy products.[17]

The Salt Institute made much bigger investments, however, in two officials it paid handsomely to focus like a laser on protecting salt's reputation and sales. Roman's salary and other compensation amounted to $449,000 in 2018.[18] That was one-seventh of the organization's total annual budget of about $3.3 million. Wilfred Nixon, the vice-president for science and environment, received $263,000.

The Salt Industry Defends Its Product

I was long puzzled by the Salt Institute's seeming preoccupation with defending salt in processed foods. After all, only 3 percent of the salt used in the United States finds its way into food.[19] Almost half is used on roads and more than one-third by the chemical industry. But, as one industry insider told me, it was to be expected that the industry would defend every single use of salt—every company and every industry defends *all* of its products. Three percent of salt sales is still almost four billion pounds, and food-grade salt may be much more profitable per pound than less-purified industrial salt. Still, Richard Hanneman, who preceded Lori Roman as the Salt Institute's president, told me that he spent most of his time on road salt and highway safety.[20]

But on food salt, Hanneman emphasizes that his organization concentrated on the science. He felt that neither side of the salt debate had conclusive evidence to support its position so that any "major change in diet was unjustified." He believes that sodium intakes are genetically determined and that no matter how hard the government tried it would not be able to reduce those intakes significantly. And dangers were lurking in lower-sodium diets—people would eat more food to obtain the sodium they needed, and that would lead to obesity.

The Salt Institute, the self-proclaimed "world's foremost authority on salt,"[21] found myriad ways to portray salt as being nutritionally just this side of spinach. It produced a variety of videos, pamphlets, and website content aimed at undermining public health recommendations to cut salt intake (and maintain industry sales and profits). It enticed the news media to quote its defense of salt at every opportunity. More than 30 years ago, for example, it told *Time* magazine: "It's easy to say cut back, but food just doesn't taste good without it. If we eliminate salt, we'll just see a lot more processed food being scraped into the garbage can."[22] Of course, no one advocates eliminating salt completely. A little bit is perfectly fine, and many manufacturers have reduced sodium substantially without sacrificing taste (see chapter 9).

In 2017, it sponsored a booklet called *Salt for Dummies*. Don't try to track it down, though. The publisher of the *Dummies* series, John Wiley & Sons, began in 2015 to market the brand to potential corporate clients so they could create "custom content [that] speaks directly to your customers."[23] So the booklet might have looked like a bona fide *Dummies* book, but it was really part of the lobby group's propaganda armamentarium.

The Salt Institute attacked the federal Centers for Disease Control and Prevention (CDC), one of the world's premier disease-fighting agencies, saying that "the CDC is wasting all your money" by discouraging people from eating salty foods instead of fighting infectious diseases. "Only a rabbit can eat a salad without salt."[24] Sometimes it was hard to take the group seriously, but it was deadly serious in opposing salt reductions.

The institute's rationale for doing nothing shifted as the science changed. In the 1980s, the group opposed lowering sodium in the general food supply, because only people who were salt-sensitive should worry about it.[25] As is now recognized, most people do not fall neatly into a "salt-sensitive" or "salt-insensitive" category, and, in any case, testing everyone periodically to see who was salt-sensitive would be astronomically expensive and totally impractical. Later the Salt Institute's argument shifted to the need for more research to prove that lowering sodium intakes would prevent, not promote, heart attacks and strokes.

More influential than the Salt Institute's sophomoric attacks on health advocates, the lobbying group, well, lobbied. (See also chapters 8 and 9.) For instance, a 16-page 2016 letter to the Secretaries of Agriculture and Health and Human Services charged that the sodium recommendations in the "Dietary Guidelines for Americans" for 2010 and 2015 to 2020 were "fatally flawed" and "systematically flawed" and should be withdrawn.[26] (Perhaps reflecting a keyboard with a stutter, "flawed" was used in that letter 14 times.) In 2018, the Salt Institute was already opposing any recommendation in the "Dietary Guidelines for Americans 2020–2025" to limit sodium when it said:

> Contrary to the government's current recommendations of a maximum of 2,300 mg/day of sodium, evidence indicates people on low sodium diets may place themselves at risk. Peer-reviewed research has shown that low-salt diets can lead to insulin resistance, congestive heart failure, cardiovascular events, iodine deficiency, loss of cognition, low birth weights, and higher rates of death.[27]

And should any local government dare to adopt sodium-reduction measures, the Salt Institute came down hard on it. In 2015, New York City became the first government to take regulatory action on salt. The city had the audacity to require menu warnings next to items at chain restaurants that contained more than a whole day's worth of sodium. The Salt Institute called that effort "misguided," "wrong," "could be harmful," "based on outdated, incorrect sodium guidelines," and "unnecessary."[28] The Salt Institute supported the restaurant industry's legal challenge to the law, but that gambit failed.[29] Fortunately, the city listened to experts at the American Heart Association and elsewhere and ignored the industry's pleas.

The Salt Institute sometimes bolstered its limited political muscle by hiring major Washington lobbying firms. For instance, it paid Patton Boggs a total of $220,000 in 2010 and 2011 and APCO at least $20,000 for lobbying to weaken or eliminate what the "Dietary Guidelines for Americans" said about salt (that effort failed).[30] A decade earlier, the trade group apparently had better luck—it applauded the US Department of Health and Human Services for eliminating a specific sodium-reduction goal from its "Healthy People 2000" report.[31]

In September 1996, the Salt Institute petitioned the FDA to repeal a regulation that allowed companies to state on their labels that low-sodium
foods, in the context of an overall low-sodium diet, could reduce the risk of
high blood pressure. "Our purpose in doing this is to remove what has been
an unfair discouragement for the general public to reduce dietary sodium
in hopes that it would reduce their hypertension or their risk of hypertension," said Hanneman.[32] Three months later the institute withdrew its
petition—before the FDA could reject it.[33]

In August 2006, Hanneman—along with two academic consultants,
Michael H. Alderman of the Albert Einstein College of Medicine and
Suzanne Oparil, a professor at the University of Alabama, Birmingham—
met with John O. Agwunobi, the assistant secretary for health at the Department of Health and Human Services. The meeting came shortly after the
FDA announced that it planned to hold a public workshop on the health
risks of a salty diet. Hanneman urged the government also to review the
health risks that might be caused by reducing salt intake.[34]

To obtain advice, gain spokespersons, and bolster its credibility, the Salt
Institute relied on its Health Council, a group composed of well-known
professors. Over the years members of the council included some of the
staunchest defenders of salty diets: McCarron, Oparil, Alderman, John Lar-
agh (New York–Presbyterian Hospital, Weill Cornell Medical College, New
York City), Alexander Logan (Mt. Sinai Hospital, Toronto), and Judith Stern
(University of California, Davis, nutritionist).

Academic scientists on industry committees typically claim to be independent and unbeholden to industry, but members of the Health Council
certainly sang from the "Defending Salt" hymnal. At least two of those
scientists have failed to disclose on multiple occasions their affiliation with
the Salt Institute (see chapter 6).

The Salt Institute paid council members honoraria of up to $3,000 a year,
though some did not receive any money, and encouraged them to get "out
of the closet" and speak out more boldly and publicly about their views on
sodium consumption.[35] Two former institute officials I spoke to could not
recall how much, if anything, they paid to the professors.

The lobbying group long maintained that a randomized controlled
trial (RCT) was needed to end the salt wars. We saw in chapter 3 how conducting such trials could provide useful information, but they are widely
seen as being unnecessary, probably prohibitively expensive, and, hence,

unlikely ever to be funded. But advocating for more research sounds so sincere and neutral that it can distract from the fact that just calling for the research could block federal education campaigns or regulatory measures indefinitely.

In 2018, researchers published an article in *Hypertension*, a top peer-reviewed journal published by the American Heart Association. The article, which I discussed in chapter 3, called for the RCT on prisoners.[36] At the end of the article, the authors declared "none" for conflicts of interest. But I discovered that the Salt Institute had given $25,000 to the professional organization of dietitians (the Academy of Nutrition and Dietetics, AND) for "development of a randomized controlled trial of cardiovascular outcomes."[37] Patricia Babjak, the CEO of the AND, told me:

> A portion of the funds were released to support the efforts of Dr. David McCarron [a co-author of the *Hypertension* article] and the study group that was organized with Duke University to develop the paper. . . . The balance of the funding has been earmarked for the Academy to assemble an advisory group to support the development of a protocol for a RCT to address the relationship between sodium intake and cardiovascular events.[38]

One of the authors of the *Hypertension* article, who requested anonymity in order to speak candidly, told me that he was not aware that anyone in the group had received any funding from the Salt Institute.

The Mouse's Last Squeak

On March 1, 2019, the Salt Institute quietly posted a little-noticed item on its website (see figure 5.1) to announce that it was disbanding! More than a century after its founding in 1914, and days before the publication of the National Academy of Medicine's report that dismissed some of the research showing risks of reducing sodium that the group relied upon, the Salt Institute said: "After careful consideration, the board members of the Salt Institute have decided to pursue the dissolution of the trade association, effective March 31, 2019."

Shortly after its announcement, I called the institute to ask why it was going out of business. All I got was an answering machine. (Members of the group's board of directors and Roman also declined via email to talk to me.) It seemed like quite a coincidence that the decision was made within days of the release of the NAM's report. But one knowledgeable person told me

March 1, 2019 By The Salt Institute

Salt Institute Statement

After careful consideration, the board members of the Salt Institute have decided to pursue the dissolution of the trade association, effective March 31, 2019.

The Salt Institute was first established in 1914 and has long advocated the numerous uses and benefits of salt, ranging from winter roadway safety and water quality to health and nutrition. Over the years, the Salt Institute has made a positive impact demonstrating the essential nature of salt in our daily lives through fact-based information, research studies and educational tools. The member companies are grateful for the expertise, dedication and support that the Salt Institute has provided since its inception.

The Salt Institute has laid the groundwork in helping the public understand the essential nature of our product and we know our member companies will continue to expand that knowledge base and focus their resources on delivering products, services and solutions to meet the needs of their customers.Thank you for your support over the last 105 years and best of luck to all our member companies.

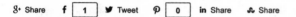

Figure 5.1
The Salt Institute's going-out-of-business notice.

that the decision to disband had actually been made the previous October. It was likelier that the salt industry, along with many major food manufacturers, understood that their ultimate customers—the general public—were increasingly concerned about their diets, and that it was time for the salt manufacturers and the food industry to stop fighting old battles. My informant also suspected that the member companies just wanted to cut their expenses, though the amount they paid the institute was relatively trivial.

And so what did staffers think were the organization's biggest accomplishments with regard to diet and health? Hanneman told me that they "defended the good name of salt." Morton Satin, the group's former vice president and science director, says the group succeeded in getting its message to the public and getting normally reticent scientists who are unconcerned about current sodium intakes to speak out more boldly. Roman, the president during its last decade, told me in her email: "We did our best to follow the science. Being ethical in every statement we made was of paramount importance to us. In the face of conflicting evidence, we called for more studies, which I feel was the logical and ethical thing to do."[39]

The disappearance of the Salt Institute eliminated the main industry defender of salt. Time will tell whether other industry groups, such as SNAC International, the snack-food industry's trade association, will fill in for it or if individual companies will take up the cudgels. But I doubt that any other trade association will defend salt with the zeal and persistence of the Salt Institute.

Salt Lobbyists Overseas

While the Salt Institute was laboring away in the United States, it had counterparts overseas. In France, Pierre Meneton, a cardiovascular disease researcher with the French National Institute of Health and Medical Research (Inserm), bearded the lion when he publicized the harmfulness of high-sodium diets. He blamed the salt producers' lobby and the food industry for misinforming health professionals and the media and stymying efforts to reduce sodium consumption.[40] Meneton estimated that high-salt diets were causing about 25,000 deaths per year in France.[41]

Around 2001, Meneton began to encounter some problems.[42] French media reported that Meneton was labeled a national security threat and was spied upon by the country's security services. The government allegedly bugged his office and cell phones and put his friends and relatives under surveillance, charges the government has denied but are supported by documents.[43] In her book titled *The French Vendetta*, the journalist Sophie Coignard concluded that the French food industry, which has much greater resources and influence than the salt industry, had persuaded the government to surveil Meneton.[44]

To Meneton, not publicizing his concerns about salt was unconscionable. "When I started to take an interest in this question [of high-salt diets]," he said, "the question was ignored by everyone, public authorities, journalists, professionals. This posed a major problem for me: What is the purpose of a scientist?"[45]

Meneton's troubles continued. In 2006, an official of the salt industry's lobbying organization, Comité des Salines de France (Salt Association of France), wrote to the director of Inserm, saying: "Recently we have alerted you to the immoderate and indiscriminate attacks launched on salt with no scientific basis by the monomaniac, Pierre Meneton. . . . We are obliged to draw your attention to an interview that this researcher has just granted, associating your institute with his anti-salt rantings."[46]

Meneton later said, "Another Inserm researcher, a nephrologist [kidney specialist] at the Necker Children's Hospital in Paris, publicly questioned my work. Everyone knows that he is paid by the salt industry as a scientific adviser."[47]

Clearly, Meneton had infuriated the salt industry by accusing it of deceiving the public about the health risks from salty foods. The industry also was angered that he gave an interview to *TOC*, a small-circulation French magazine, that was illustrated with an image of a salt packet emblazoned with the bold-lettered message "salt kills."[48] The industry then sued Meneton, the journalist who wrote the article, and *TOC's* publisher for defamation.[49] Ultimately, in 2008, a judge in the criminal court in Paris dismissed the case, saying that scientists who espouse a critical opinion cannot be sued under French defamation laws.[50]

Perhaps not surprisingly, when the industry organization presented its preliminary pro-salt position in court, its representative relied heavily on a few studies by Michael Alderman, the consultant to the Salt Institute in the United States.

Across the English Channel, the Salt Association has lobbied hard against the United Kingdom government's precedent-setting sodium-reduction campaign. Sounding like its American sibling, the British group said, "Recent research suggests that consuming too little salt may actually increase the risk of heart disease." It added:

> The public is increasingly asking "what should be our relationship with salt?" People are confused by the conflicting evidence. The war on salt has continued for decades, without firm evidence of any long-term health benefits from restricted salt diets. . . . We are urging the Government in the strongest possible terms to undertake new, population wide studies to determine the real effects of salt consumption on our health. Until then, the Government will be continuing to take risks with public health by its failure to acknowledge the essential role salt plays in maintaining a fit and healthy body.[51]

The British government ignored the salt lobby when it mounted its campaign to lower sodium intakes and created a character named "Sid the Slug" to help send the message. The Salt Association actually filed a formal complaint with an ad industry watchdog, the Advertising Standards Authority, about the Sid campaign, calling it "incorrect and potentially very damaging"—but the complaint was dismissed.[52] Lately, the Salt Association appears to be inactive (because of Sid or something else, I do not know).

I discuss in chapter 7 how the British government's salt-reduction campaign (including the hilarious efforts of Sid) helped lower sodium intakes and improve health in the UK and inspired as well the efforts to lower consumption in a growing number of countries. But first, in chapter 6, I explain how industry funding might cloud a research professor's objectivity.

6   Money and Science

The effects of industry funding seem to occur at an unconscious level, so much below the radar of conscious thought that the influence is not recognized.
—Marion Nestle, *Unsavory Truth*[1]

One of the standard ways that industry, be it makers of food, cigarettes, or pesticides, seeks to influence public opinion and public policies is to hire academic specialists to conduct research, provide advice, lobby government officials, give talks, and speak out in the media. The scientists who receive industry funding invariably take the side of industry: they downplay risks found in independently funded research or say that more evidence is needed before concluding that a product is harmful. Numerous academic studies have found that when companies sponsor research on artificially sweetened beverages, juice, milk, soft drinks, and the fake fat olestra, the outcomes are much likelier to favor the companies than when studies are independently funded.[2]

And so it is with salt. Companies such as Frito-Lay, the biggest maker of salty snacks, and the Salt Institute, the lobbying group funded by the salt industry (and the subject of chapter 5), have used scientists as paid or unpaid consultants. Indeed, Frito-Lay's former chief scientist, Dr. Bob I-San Lin, told me it was not difficult to "pay and persuade" scientists to help the company and to take a position that was consistent with the company's.[3] Funding might support research or pay scientists to be consultants. Sometimes the funding is disclosed in scientific papers or at conferences, but oftentimes not. Of course, receiving corporate funding does not guarantee that a person will take an industry-friendly position. And conversely, some academics have views supportive of particular products without receiving any funding from their makers. But make no mistake about the influence of funding. David Michaels, a professor at the George Washington University Milken Institute School of Public Health, is one of the most astute observers of the politics of regulation based on his experience as a top health official in the Clinton and Obama administrations. He states in his book, *The Triumph of Doubt*, "the funding source for any research—who's footing the bill—is a powerful motivator of anyone's reasoning."[4]

Most medical journals ask authors to disclose conflicts of interest to alert readers of possible biases. Disclosure is seen as a partial remedy for that perennial problem because it may lead readers to evaluate the articles with a more skeptical eye and enable them to reach their own judgments about the significance of the funding. But journals (and journalists) accept whatever information about conflicts of interest that scientists provide, and some may not provide full and honest disclosures. Consider the inconsistent statements about and by Michael H. Alderman, the hypertension researcher at Albert Einstein College of Medicine.

- August 1998: "Dr. Alderman said he doesn't accept industry money."[5]
- February 1999: "We do not have any connection with or receive funds from the food and salt industries or any related commercial interests."[6]
- August 1999: "I do not believe that the several thousand dollars I received five or more years ago [from the Salt Institute] would affect my integrity."[7]
- 2006: Alderman said he had never received funding from the Salt Institute.[8]
- 2011: The *New York Times* reported that he said "he once was an unpaid consultant for the Salt Institute but that he now did no consulting for it or for the food industry."[9]
- 2011: He acknowledged he "was a member of the Advisory Board of the Salt Institute from 1995 to 2008. During this time he attended an annual meeting most years, receiving a US$750 honorarium for the first meeting, and, he said, none thereafter."[10]
- 2019: His 42-page-long CV lists consultancies but not his work with the Salt Institute.[11]

In 2014, Feng J. He and Graham A. MacGregor, the British campaigners for less-salty foods, charged that Alderman, as co-author of an article in the

American Journal of Hypertension, "has once again failed to declare that he has worked over many years as a consultant to the Salt Institute. As [he was] editor-in-chief of the *American Journal of Hypertension,* this could be viewed as a very serious conflict of interest."[12] While the medical community does not have a uniform guideline for determining when authors no longer need to disclose past conflicts, Alderman's inconsistent statements hardly reflect full disclosure.

Alderman denies that his varied connections to the Salt Institute influenced his judgment. He told me, "It was the unexpected finding in my own research—never refuted, but frequently reproduced—that changed my mind from a believer [in cutting sodium] to a skeptic." I asked him if he regrets ever taking funding from the salt industry, and he told me, "Yeah, I think it's a mistake."[13]

Another long-time defender of salt is David A. McCarron, a former professor of medicine at Oregon Health and Science University and former unpaid associate researcher at the University of California, Davis (and recently a presumably unpaid but cheerful deliveryman for his wife's pet food company[14]). His assistance as a paid consultant to the salt industry is lauded in a tribute on his website by Dick Hanneman, the president of the Salt Institute:

> The Salt Institute has valued Dr. McCarron's consulting expertise for a quarter century and has appreciated the professionalism and responsiveness of his expert team. . . . Dr. McCarron has earned our respect and admiration for the quality of his counsel.[15]

Over the decades, McCarron wrote numerous articles putting "sodium into its correct context" and downplaying the role of salt in promoting cardiovascular disease.[16] He has contended that the salt–blood pressure "hypothesis has never been fully supported by either the researchers or the data in this area of investigation."[17] And he's claimed: "We have signals from many different sources telling us that maybe it is calcium and not sodium that is the problem."[18] At one time, McCarron was receiving $3,000 a year from the Salt Institute (possibly enough to reinforce his views on sodium, though only a pittance compared to the six-figure fees that some researchers get from drug companies[19]), and he served as a consultant at least through 2010.[20] (McCarron did not respond to my request for an interview.)

Around 2016, McCarron received funding from the Academy of Nutrition and Dietetics (AND, the professional organization of dietitians), which had obtained it from the Salt Institute.[21] The funding was for developing a protocol for a randomized controlled trial (RCT) on sodium and cardiovascular disease (I discuss these RCTs in chapters 3 and 5). McCarron co-authored an article proposing such a study—on prisoners—but failed to disclose the funding he previously received from the Salt Institute, Grocery Manufacturers Association (GMA, which since morphed into the Consumer Brands Association), and ConAgra Foods (maker of Chef Boyardee, Marie Callender's, and other salty processed foods).[22] (I spurred the journal to publish two corrections noting McCarron's relationships with GMA, ConAgra, and AND, but did not get it to disclose the Salt Institute.)[23] He also failed to disclose that funding when he spoke at a 2018 meeting that the National Academy of Medicine held on sodium.[24] One industry insider told me, "David McCarron has his whole career pegged on salt. And David McCarron is somebody that you [can] almost never convince there's anything wrong because . . . this is his life."

In a media interview, McCarron gave a laughable excuse for not acknowledging his industry connections in the article that proposed the prisoner study: "McCarron said that he left those positions off because, in his view, they were already widely known. 'It's common knowledge I have these relationships.'"[25]

Salim Yusuf of McMaster University Medical School in Hamilton, Ontario, has led the PURE research program that associated low sodium intakes with higher rates of deaths from cardiovascular disease than the higher intakes typical in industrialized countries. PURE studies have received a small amount of funding from Unilever (one of the more nutrition-conscious manufacturers) and the South African Sugar Association, but the great majority is from traditional medical research funders and the drug industry. Yusuf is also the executive director of the Population Health Research Institute (PHRI), which is affiliated with McMaster. Campbell Soup, ConAgra, PepsiCo, and other food-industry giants funded a PHRI nutrition conference in 2014, some of which focused on sodium.[26] But PHRI's main work relates to contracts with Bayer, Novartis, and other drug companies to conduct tens of millions of dollars' worth of research unrelated to salt.[27] (Yusuf declined my requests to discuss his group's research and funding.)

Some people assume that companies give professors money or perks (such as covering the costs of speaking at a conference in a nice place like Hawaii) to persuade them to change their views and defend industry. But that is a simplistic analysis. Often, in this chicken-or-egg situation, companies learn of professor whose views or research might be supportive of their products or practices. They then might cultivate those professors, perhaps inviting them to a conference or research facility or asking for advice on a letter they are sending to a government agency. If a professor expresses interest, company officials might deepen the relationship by asking the professor to be a consultant or offering to support a research project. Next thing you know, the professor is on television defending the industry or its products or arguing that a product has not been proven harmful—often without mentioning the corporate funding.

Some of the consulting fees, honoraria, and travel expenses that professors receive from industry are modest, but that does not mean they have no effect. Even small gifts—free lunches, stationery, drug samples—have been shown to influence doctors' attitudes and prescribing habits.[28] Is there any reason to assume that nutrition researchers would be any less influenced by consulting fees, free travel to conferences, or other gifts? Moreover, it is only human that when friendships develop, without money changing hands, it is hard to publicly criticize people.

Much as I am suspicious of the conflicts of interest that industry funding causes, it certainly is possible for professors to accept funding and still retain their integrity and objectivity. As food-industry critic and New York University professor emerita Marion Nestle has written, "Financial ties with food companies are not necessarily corrupting; it is quite possible to do industry-funded research and retain independence and integrity. But food-company funding often does exert undue influence, and it invariably *appears* to do so."[29] And to push this argument further, one might actually want companies to get advice from the most renowned experts. But many researchers do not want to risk being tainted by industry funding or even non-monetary relationships.

As an illustration of how complex the conflict of interest can be, it is fair to acknowledge, as defenders of industry funding sometimes contend, that non-industry funding could also lead to biases. Funding, or the desire for funding, from the National Institutes of Health, American Heart Association, or other non-industry agencies could distort a professor's views.

Knowing that such organizations have concluded that high-sodium diets are harmful, some professors might think they could enhance their chances of getting a grant by exaggerating the evidence that salty diets are harmful, understating gaps in the evidence, or avoiding doing research that might show that salty diets are not a problem.

While funding presents an obvious bias, intellectual bias might represent a more subtle influence. A researcher who conducted a study showing that something is, or is not, a problem may conduct further research with the hope of reinforcing that finding. That kind of bias can be a problem for any researcher, including ones who believe salty diets are risky or those who believe them to be safe.

In the previous two chapters I offered an inside look at how lobbyists operate and examined how biases in industry funding can affect researchers. Let's now look at the efforts by dozens of countries around the world to reduce sodium intake.

7 Less-Salty Diets around the Globe

Globally, 1.65 million deaths from cardiovascular causes . . . were attributed to sodium intake above 2,000 mg per day. . . . These deaths accounted for nearly 1 of every 10 deaths from cardiovascular causes.

—Global Burden of Diseases Nutrition and Chronic Diseases Expert Group, *New England Journal of Medicine*[1]

Hypertension is a global problem. The condition causes more deaths than any other single factor. According to the World Health Organization (WHO), the number of people with uncontrolled hypertension jumped from 594 million in 1975 to 1.13 billion in 2015. Two-thirds of them lived in low- and middle-income countries, and less than one out of five had their hypertension under control.[2] The WHO and others have also estimated that raised blood pressure causes about 10 million deaths per year, or about 17 percent of all deaths.[3] Although many factors such as obesity and aging populations contribute to that toll, salty home-cooked meals or processed and prepared foods are certainly a major factor.

The massive Global Burden of Disease study, which involves more than 3,600 researchers around the world and is based at the University of Washington in Seattle, has looked at the relationship between diet and cardiovascular disease in 195 countries.[4] It concluded that high sodium intake was the greatest cause of diet-related deaths—about 1 million to 5 million per year—with diets low in dietary fiber and fruit not far behind. Those three dietary problems were responsible for half of all diet-related deaths. Another report pegged the number at 1.1 million to 2.2 million deaths per year, including almost 90,000 in the United States.[5] In response to such evidence, a number of governments are working aggressively to lower sodium intakes, and some multinational and local companies have started to market less-salty foods.

A young nonprofit organization called Resolve to Save Lives is spurring progress in low- and middle-income countries, starting with China, Ethiopia, Thailand, Vietnam, and the Philippines. It is funded by major foundations and headed by Tom Frieden, the former director of the Centers for Disease Control and Prevention. One of its three goals is to prevent millions of deaths by lowering sodium levels in the food supply.[6]

More and more governments around the world are recognizing the health problem and the cost problem. Governments and individuals spend billions of dollars a year treating hypertension and its consequences. Lowering sodium levels in the overall food supply could save a good chunk of those expenses. And a growing number of major manufacturers both acknowledge the public health benefits of lowering sodium and anticipate that if they do not voluntarily reduce sodium now, they will be forced to do so in the future.

Fortunately, the controversy over whether consuming less sodium would be good or bad that has slowed progress in the United States has not infected the rest of the world. Elsewhere, it is generally accepted that people should gradually, but greatly, reduce their sodium intake.

Finland was a salt-reduction pioneer, for instance, because of the extremely high sodium consumption of its residents (one-fourth greater than the amount Americans consume). Beginning in 1979, Finland's government sponsored a huge public education campaign, which was supported with legislation and other measures.[7] It pressured companies to market healthier products by lowering both sodium and saturated fat. Finland also allowed a heart-healthy symbol to be used on packaged foods with less than specified levels of sodium and required a warning notice on foods with excessive levels. It achieved a major reduction in sodium of at least 1,600 mg per person per day, or about one-third.[8] Rates of heart attacks and strokes declined by about two-thirds, despite increases in obesity and alcohol consumption. Unfortunately, since 2002 the Finnish effort has flagged, as have further reductions in sodium consumption.

Campaigns in northern Japan, where diets were among the world's saltiest, yielded decreases almost as big.[9] Lower sodium intake coupled with medications, community-based education, and other actions combined to lower the stroke rate by more than 85 percent.[10]

Currently, dozens of countries, ranging from Turkey to Argentina to Thailand, are working to reduce sodium in the food supply.[11] Countries have used education, regulations, and taxes to cut sodium. Hungary, for instance, slapped a small tax on salty snacks and condiments. Fiji imposed a 32 percent tariff on monosodium glutamate. Turkey, where sodium intakes averaged 7,200 mg per day, used education and voluntary limits to reduce consumption by 16 percent over four years.[12] Table 7.1 lists some of the growing number of international efforts to limit sodium.[13]

Battles over sodium have been waged in the United Kingdom for more than a quarter century. In 1994, after much debate, a government advisory committee on food policy recommended a one-third reduction in salt intake, from 3,600 mg per day to 2,400 mg per day. How did the food industry behave? Fiona Godlee, editor of the *BMJ*, described it in unusually sharp language for an august medical journal:

> The food industry has lobbied fiercely against the threat to its profits. . . . Rather than reformulate their products, manufacturers have lobbied governments, refused to cooperate with expert working parties, encouraged misinformation campaigns, and tried to discredit the evidence.[14]

Worse, Britain's chief medical officer cast doubt on the evidence linking high sodium intakes to high blood pressure and stressed that the committee's recommendation was not going to be accepted as government policy.

But the battle over salt was just starting. The United Kingdom has been fortunate to have a persistent, knowledgeable, passionate—and effective—physician wage a multifaceted campaign to lower sodium consumption. Literally for decades, Graham A. MacGregor, a physician trained as a kidney specialist, together with his steadfast colleague Feng J. He, a physician and epidemiologist, have chastised industry for harming consumers and chastised the government for allowing industry to do so. MacGregor might well be called the Rachel Carson of salt reduction. As a professor of cardiovascular medicine at the Wolfson Institute of Preventive Medicine at Queen Mary University of London, he conducts original research and is a prolific author of scientific papers. In addition to that, he is a strategist, lobbyist, and publicist dedicated to preventing cardiovascular disease in the United Kingdom and around the world. In 2019 he was honored for his long and impactful career by being appointed a Commander of the Most Excellent Order of the British Empire—not quite knighthood, but close.[15]

Table 7.1

International actions to limit sodium

Argentina	A 2013 law set modest sodium reductions for 18 categories of meats, bread products, cheeses, and soups to be achieved by 2015. For example, the law limits average sodium in hamburger meat to 850 mg and in instant soups to 352 mg per 100 grams (3.5 oz.). If achieved, such cuts would cut sodium consumption by about 350 mg per day and prevent an estimated 19,000 deaths over 10 years. Some provinces banned saltshakers from tables at restaurants, but that has not been well enforced.
Australia	Twenty sodium-reduction targets were set for nine food categories: breads, breakfast cereals, simmer sauces, soups, processed meats, savory pies, potato chips, extruded snacks, savory crackers, and cheese. Participating companies (more than 35) determine individually which products to reformulate and the extent of reduction. By 2013 the average sodium level in breads was reduced by 9%, breakfast cereals by 25%, and cured meats by 8%.
Austria	Many bakeries committed to reduce the salt content of bread products by 15% by 2015.
Bahrain	Reducing sodium in bread, most of which is produced by a government-owned bakery.
Belgium	A 1985 rule limited the sodium content in bread to 480 mg per 100 grams. In 2009 the government set voluntary goals for 13 food categories.
Brazil	In 2011, the food industry agreed to reduce sodium across 16 food categories by 2.5% to 19.5%. Full implementation is set for 2020.
Bulgaria	In 2012, mandatory limits were set for bread (480 mg of sodium per 100 grams), cheese, meat and poultry products, and lutenica (a vegetable relish product).
Canada	A Sodium Reduction Strategy was finalized in 2012, with modest results through 2018. A plan for front-of-package warning notices was proposed but not finalized.
Chile	Requires "High in Salt" warning labels on foods with more than 400 mg per 100g (or 113 mg per oz.) for solid foods and 100 mg per 100 ml (or 240 mg per 8 fl. oz.) for soups, beverages, and other liquid foods.
Ecuador	Requires prominent label notices to indicate that foods are high, medium, or low in sodium (and sugar and fat).
Finland	Since 1992, a "high in salt" notice (not very prominent) has been required on foods with more than a specified amount of sodium.
Greece	Greece limited the salt content in bread (1.7% salt by dry weight) and tomato products like juice, concentrate, and paste.
Hungary	A tax is levied on a small number of salty foods and condiments with sodium contents above specified levels. In the first four years, that tax (plus taxes on soft drinks, energy drinks, candies, and other foods) raised $219 million for public health spending.

Table 7.1 (continued)

Israel	Requires warning notices on solid foods with more than 500 mg of sodium per 100g (and 400 mg for liquid foods); those limits will drop by 100 mg in 2021. Warnings are also required on foods high in saturated fat and sugar; a voluntary healthy symbol is allowed on qualifying foods.
Kuwait	Goal was to reduce salt in bread by 10% (actual reduction was at least 20%), with other reductions in cheese, corn flakes, pastries, potato chips, French fries, sandwiches.
Mexico	Requires Chilean-like warning labels on foods high in sodium and other nutrients.
Netherlands	The maximum salt content for bread is 1.8%, with voluntary limits for other categories. Significant sodium declines were seen in some food categories.
Paraguay	A 2013 resolution mandated a 25% sodium reduction in bread, the main source of salt for Paraguayans.
Peru	Requires Chilean-like warning labels on foods high in sodium and other nutrients.
South Africa	In 2013 limits were set on sodium in bread, breakfast cereals, butter and spreads, savory snacks, potato chips, cured and uncured processed meats, dry soups, and gravies. Implementation deadlines were set for June 30, 2016, and June 30, 2019. Sodium was to be reduced from 2010 levels in bread by 28%, cereals by 37%, and cured meats by 46%. When the 2016 targets were implemented, two-thirds of products already met their targets and many more products had salt levels close to the target. Effort not evaluated.
Turkey	Limits on sodium in bread (which provides one-third of Turks' sodium) and some processed foods like tomato paste; banned sale of chips in school canteens in 2011. Sodium intake dropped 20% from 7,200 mg/day in 2008 to 5,800 mg in 2012.
United Kingdom	Voluntary salt-reduction targets were finalized in 2006 and updated several times. The 85 targets applied to processed meats, bread, cheese, convenience foods, snacks, and other foods. Sodium consumption declined by more than 10%.
United States	In 2016 the FDA proposed voluntary sodium targets (with 2- and 10-year time frames) for more than 150 food categories, but they were not yet finalized as of spring 2020. New York City and Philadelphia require warning icons on menus for high-sodium (2,300 mg or more) meals at chain restaurants.
Uruguay	Requires Chilean-like warning labels on foods high in sodium and other nutrients. In 2015 it banned saltshakers, mayonnaise, and ketchup at restaurants in Montevideo and saltshakers from schools nationwide. Montevideo restaurants must offer at least 10% of menu items without added salt.

MacGregor was incensed that the UK government buckled under pressure from the food industry, which had threatened to withdraw funding it gave to the ruling Conservative Party. So in 1996 MacGregor created a nonprofit advocacy group supported by leading sodium experts called Consensus Action on Salt and Health (later changed to Action on Salt).[16] The group successfully pressured the British government to develop a multifaceted sodium-reduction campaign. According to MacGregor, "This required some fairly strong-arm tactics to persuade government officials to take action which they eventually did."[17] He and his colleagues supported the government campaign with efforts to "name and shame" companies that did not lower their sodium levels.[18] Later, because salty diets were a problem globally, MacGregor broadened his scope by creating World Action on Salt and Health and enlisted professors from around the world.

Largely because of pressure from the activist professors, several members of Parliament and the Labour government took aim at salt. In 2003 the United Kingdom became the first major country to mount a systematic, but still voluntary, campaign to reduce sodium. In 2006 the government's Food Standards Agency, which was relatively new and determined to make a difference, specified sodium levels for about 80 categories of processed and restaurant foods that it asked industry to achieve in the next four years.[19] The government expected companies to have the average sales-weighted sodium content at or below those levels. And companies were asked to limit the sodium content of any new products to those levels. The UK followed up with three sets of tighter targets in 2009, 2011, and 2014, and proposed a fifth set in 2020 with a 2023 deadline.[20] Their latest goal is to reduce Britons' average sodium intake to 2,800 mg per day.

Then instead of leaving those recommendations moldering on bookshelves, where most voluntary recommendations end up, the government mounted a creative advertising campaign, featuring the memorable "Sid the Slug," to urge consumers to choose lower-sodium foods (see figure 7.1). Salt, of course, is famously used to kill slugs. To play on that, one TV commercial showed Sid in a parking garage, where he freaked out at a woman loading grocery bags into her car. His father—"dead now," the slug said—had once offered him some good advice: "Stay away from fast cars, loose women, and SALT."[21]

But more important than the ad campaign, the UK government publicly and privately pressured companies to lower sodium levels. As I discussed in

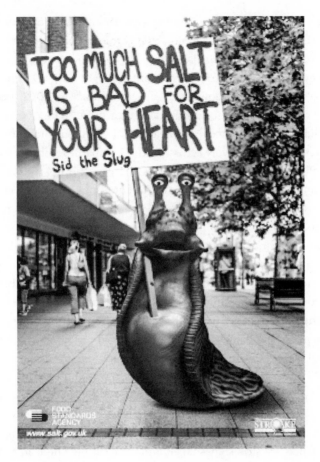

Figure 7.1
Sid the Slug was a key spokescharacter in the UK's salt-awareness campaign.

chapter 2, after five years lower-sodium diets were preventing 6,000 premature deaths per year. Several years later, further declines were calculated to be preventing as many as 9,000 deaths per year.[22]

Unfortunately, after a 2010 election that put the Conservative Party in charge, a reorganization moved responsibility for the salt campaign from one department to another, and interest flagged. Instead of pressuring industry to use less salt, the government and industry created a weak Public Health Responsibility Deal, and the campaign lost momentum.[23] The government contended that the looser arrangement would be more effective and less costly. But the pace of declines in sodium consumption stopped declining, with researchers estimating that thousands more people each year between 2011 and 2025 would suffer cardiovascular disease.[24]

The effectiveness of the British campaign to reduce sodium is indicated by a survey of major fast food restaurants (Burger King, Domino's, KFC, McDonald's, Pizza Hut, Subway) in six countries.[25] In 2012, researchers examined company nutrition information for more than 2,000 fast foods in Australia, Canada, France, New Zealand, the United Kingdom, and the United States. Sodium levels across all the companies' offerings averaged 25 percent higher in the United States than in the UK and 36 percent higher than in France, where the government also was pushing companies to cut the salt. For instance, in late 2019, Chicken McNuggets in McDonald's home country had 150 percent more sodium than in the UK. Burger King Onion Rings had over six times as much sodium in the United States. And Subway's Italian B.M.T. sandwich had 17 percent more sodium in the United States than in the UK.[26] Yet some fast foods had more sodium in the UK while others, such as the Big Mac, had equal amounts.

More than 70 countries have followed Britain by setting targets—usually voluntary, a few mandatory—for sodium levels in certain foods (table 7.1).[27] But several countries are taking a different approach. They are requiring foods with more than a specified level of sodium (and calories, sugar, and saturated fat) to bear prominent warning labels on the fronts of packages (see figure 7.2).[28] Chile was the first country to require warning labels as part of a broader program to encourage healthier diets beginning in childhood. Its labels are stop sign–shaped and state simply "high in sodium" or other nutrient. If a food is high in more than one of those nutrients, the label must show two, three, or four warning notices. Also, Chile has banned unhealthy foods from school cafeterias, limits cartoons on packaging, taxes sugar drinks, and restricts junk-food advertising on television.

Peru, Mexico, and Uruguay adopted labels like Chile's. Israel has required similar warning icons to steer consumers away from foods high in sugar, salt, or saturated fat (though not calories), and also created a voluntary "healthy food" icon to attract people to healthier foods. Brazil is considering warning labels,[29] as is Colombia.[30] In 2018, Health Canada proposed four options for a warning notice, but that measure has been at least temporarily shelved.

Front-of-package warning notices can be much more effective than the Nutrition Facts labels used in the United States—which (for starters) are not

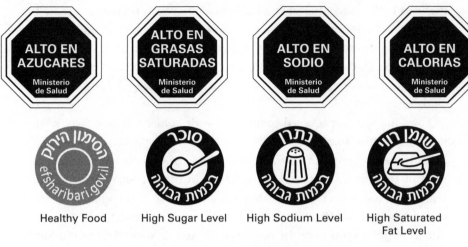

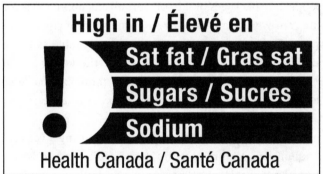

Figure 7.2
Front-of-package warning labels. Top: Chile's labels for foods high in sugar, calories, saturated fat, and sodium; middle: Israel's "healthy food" symbol and warning labels for foods high in sugar, sodium, and saturated fat; bottom: one of several formats that Canada has considered.

placed on package fronts with recognizable icons but rather appear in small print on the side or back, and usually list more than a dozen nutrients. But numbers alone do not highlight problem nutrients in terms people can easily grasp, such as "high in sodium." The Chilean health minister Carmen Castillo said the new law has had "a tremendous impact on public health."[31] Before the legislation took force, she said, businesses rushed to reformulate one-fourth of processed foods. A study published in 2020 found that sales of beverages high in sugar or other problem nutrients declined by 24 percent after the labeling and advertising law was passed, but the net change in calories from all beverages purchased was only 7.4 per day (that study did not include beverages sold at restaurants).[32] In another recent report from Chile, University of Chile researchers found that sales of sugary breakfast cereals dropped by 11 percent and sugary juices by almost 24 percent.[33]

Lowering salt in packaged foods, by fiat or bolder labeling, may work in countries like Britain and Finland where most people rely on packaged foods and eating out. But several billion people around the world still cook most of their meals from scratch at home. In India, about 85 percent of salt comes from salt used in cooking and at the table.[34] In contrast, Americans get only about 10 percent of salt that way. Health officials in cook-at-home countries need to devise novel ways to reduce sodium consumption. Because people buy packages of salt, one promising approach is for stores to offer products in which one-third or so of the sodium chloride is replaced by potassium chloride, a salt not quite as salty as table salt (see the section titled "Potassium Salt and Other Tricks of the Lower-Sodium Trade" in chapter 9). A drawback is that "lite salt" is more expensive and would have to be subsidized by the government in order to encourage people to choose it.

While other countries from Turkey to Chile are using a variety of means to lower sodium levels, until recently it has been talk and argument, not action, in the United States. We can only wonder how warning labels on foods, strict limits on sodium, or even voluntary limits, if adopted years ago, might have prevented thousands of strokes and heart attacks. I discuss in the next chapter how tough it has been to improve American salt policies.

8 Policy Paralysis in the United States

It is clear . . . that we as a society and we as health professionals must address the sodium issue, and we must do it now.
—Arthur Hull Hayes, MD, FDA commissioner, 1982[1]

Much of the key scientific research on salt has been conducted in the United States and sponsored by the National Institutes of Health (NIH). But while some countries are taking the findings of that research seriously and lowering sodium in their food supplies, the United States has moved at a snail's pace. Consumers can help themselves by reading labels and visiting websites in their quest to consume less sodium, but our salt-filled food environment—a *toxic* food environment—makes it almost impossible to eat packaged or restaurant foods and still limit sodium.

We each should certainly eat more unprocessed foods, use Nutrition Facts labels, and put our saltshakers in the cupboard. But we consumers shouldn't have to bear the entire responsibility for coping with a high-sodium food environment. As the Institute of Medicine (IOM, now the National Academy of Medicine) has emphasized, "it is unlikely that the average consumer will be able to successfully reduce sodium intake without changes to other components of the food environment."[2] The only way to achieve healthy sodium intakes on a national scale is through public health actions.

Official committees going as far back as the historic 1969 White House Conference on Food, Nutrition, and Health have urged industry and government to take steps to reduce the sodium content of foods—starting with baby foods—to help prevent hypertension. (See box 8.1 for a timeline of significant policy activities.) The conference's final report stated:

Box 8.1
Timeline of policy activities related to salt

1969   White House Conference on Food, Nutrition, and Health calls for sodium labeling and reduced use of salt by food processors.

1977   Senate Select Committee on Nutrition and Human Needs recommends that people consume about 2,000 milligrams (mg) of sodium per day.

1978   CSPI petitions the US Food and Drug Administration (FDA) to require sodium labeling on all packaged foods (and a warning notice on the highest-sodium foods), revoke the "generally recognized as safe" (GRAS) status of salt, and limit amounts in processed foods.

1979   FDA's Select Committee on GRAS Substances (SCOGS) concludes that salt cannot be considered GRAS.

1980   The US Department of Agriculture (USDA) and Department of Health and Human Services (HHS) publish the first "Dietary Guidelines for Americans," which urged consumers to "avoid too much sodium." Updates published every five years provided similar, but increasingly specific, advice.

         HHS said that companies should reduce sodium in processed foods by 20 percent and that average sodium consumption should be 1,200 to 2,400 mg per day by 1990.

1981   FDA announces a 5-point plan to educate consumers and encourage companies to lower sodium levels.

         CSPI petitions FDA for warning label on packages of salt.

         5,000 health professionals urge FDA to limit sodium in processed foods.

1982   FDA rejects CSPI's 1978 petitions to label sodium content and reduce sodium levels.

1983   CSPI sues FDA for not limiting sodium in foods.

1984   Court permits FDA to defer action on CSPI's 1978 petitions.

         FDA requires that beginning in 1986 sodium content be listed on all foods that bear nutrition labeling (about half of all foods).

1990   Congress passes the Nutrition Labeling and Education Act, which requires labeling of sodium (and other nutrients) on almost all packaged foods.

2005   CSPI asks the court to require FDA to take final action on CSPI's 1978 petitions to revoke salt's GRAS status and limit sodium levels, but the court denies that request.

         CSPI re-petitions FDA to revoke the GRAS status of salt and limit sodium in processed foods to safe levels.

Box 8.1 (continued)

2007   FDA holds public hearing to obtain public comments on CSPI's petition.

2009   New York City, in partnership with many other health departments and nonprofit organizations, announces the National Salt Reduction Initiative to press companies to lower sodium levels.

2010   The Institute of Medicine recommends that the FDA revise the GRAS status of salt and set gradually declining mandatory limits on sodium in packaged and restaurant foods.

2011   FDA holds public meeting on how to reduce sodium consumption.

2012   USDA requires stepwise sodium reductions in school meals to take effect in 2014, 2017, and 2022.

2015   CSPI sues FDA for not acting on CSPI's 2005 petition to restrict sodium levels.

New York City requires warnings on high-salt foods at chain restaurants.

2016   FDA denies CSPI's 2005 petition, but settles CSPI's 2015 lawsuit by proposing voluntary 2- and 10-year sodium targets for processed and restaurant foods.

2018   Philadelphia requires warnings on high-salt foods at chain restaurants.

USDA delays until 2024 further reductions in sodium levels in school meals.

Commissioner Gottlieb says FDA will finalize its 2-year sodium targets in 2019.

2019   New York and five other states, CSPI, and Healthy School Food Maryland sue USDA to reinstate its 2012 requirement for lower sodium levels in school meals. In 2020 the judge ruled against USDA.

Evidence has been accumulating that high intakes of dietary salt from infancy onward may be an important factor in initiating and aggravating hypertension. . . . More informative labeling of food as to salt content is needed. . . . Food processors should be encouraged to minimize the amount of salt.[3]

The conference did not recommend a specific sodium intake, and it had no power to force action. But in the same year, the NIH advised that "stringent sodium restricted diets (less than 2,000 mg a day) bring about some reduction in blood pressure in about one-third of those with hypertension."[4]

Partly because of the 1969 report and public criticism, the baby food industry started to clean up its products. In 1975, Frank Nicholas, the savvy chief executive of Beech-Nut, a smaller competitor of Gerber, saw a great sales opportunity. He purged the salt from all the company's baby foods.[5] That action generated huge, favorable publicity for the company and forced Gerber and Heinz to stop adding salt to at least some of their baby foods.[6]

In 1968, the Senate created the Select Committee on Nutrition and Human Needs, which was chaired by Senator George McGovern (D-SD), who worked collaboratively with Senator Robert Dole (R-KS). The committee initially focused on poverty and hunger and spurred major expansions of the food stamp and school nutrition programs, but it then expanded its focus to include nutrition for the general public. After numerous hearings featuring testimony from leading nutrition experts, in 1977 the committee issued a groundbreaking report, "Dietary Goals for the United States." The report focused on diet's contribution to heart disease, cancer, and other chronic diseases. It expressed concern, among many other matters, that "millions of children and youth are moving toward hypertension." The report concluded:

> The evidence indicates that a systematic effort to reduce dietary sodium chloride intake and increase dietary potassium intake would result in the amelioration of much suffering among those who are prone [to hypertension] and would increase both duration and quality of life for many millions of people.[7]

The committee then bit the bullet and made one of the world's first specific recommendations for sodium intake: people should consume about 2,000 mg a day.

The Senate report ignited a firestorm of controversy about what Americans should be eating. Fortuitously, the publication of the report coincided with the beginning of President Jimmy Carter's administration, which sought to reduce the toll of diet-related disease. But "Dietary Goals" was still a report from just one Senate committee and did not have the force of law. To move the ball forward, in 1980 the US Department of Agriculture (USDA) and Department of Health and Human Services (HHS) made the centerpiece of their diet-improvement efforts the publication of a slim pamphlet called "Dietary Guidelines for Americans." The report helped shift public attention from deficiencies of vitamins and minerals to excesses of foods that promote chronic diseases. It gave official endorsement to a diet with fewer calories and less sugar, saturated fat, and salt. It connected high-sodium diets to high blood pressure and said that Americans "take in much more sodium than they need."

Every subsequent edition of the "Dietary Guidelines for Americans," which by law is updated every five years, has recommended limiting sodium intake, with the 1995 edition supporting a limit of 2,400 mg of sodium per day. In 2005, the report dropped the recommendation slightly to 2,300 mg for most healthy people under about 50 years old. But for individuals with hypertension, African Americans, and middle-aged and older adults—that's more than half the population—it lowered the limit to 1,500 mg per day. In 2015, the "Dietary Guidelines" narrowed that advice to people with pre-hypertension and hypertension, which also is well over half the population.

My organization, the Center for Science in the Public Interest (CSPI), fired its opening salvo in the salt wars in 1977. It started with the hiring of a recently minted nutritionist with a master's degree from Cornell University, Bonnie Liebman, and a crash project of reviewing the evidence on the health effects of high-sodium diets. Some of the research was equivocal or did not find a problem, but much of it indicated that high-sodium diets were harmful. Some of the nation's leading hypertension experts were deeply concerned about Americans' sodium intakes. For instance, Edward D. Freis, a senior investigator at the Washington, DC, Veterans Administration Hospital, wrote, "The evidence is very good, if not conclusive, that reduction of salt in the diet to below [800 mg] a day would result in the prevention of essential hypertension and its disappearance as a major health problem."[8] Jeremiah Stamler, the Northwestern University School of Medicine hypertension expert, said that habitual salt intake sets the stage for hypertension. "It therefore," he wrote, "makes good sense to encourage the American people to eat less salt and encourage the food industry to help by reducing the salt that is so ever present in commercial products."[9]

With sentiment like that from medical leaders, in 1978 the CSPI formally petitioned the FDA to implement a suite of actions that would begin solving the sodium problem. We asked the FDA to:

- Require sodium content to be listed on all food packages. Also, foods with 200 to 799 mg of sodium per serving would have to state "Highly Salted" on the fronts of packages, along with an image of a saltshaker. The labels of even saltier foods would have to add, "In some people, a high salt (or sodium) diet may contribute to high blood pressure."[10]

- Strip salt of its legal status as a "generally recognized as safe" substance and reclassify it as a more rigorously evaluated and regulated "food additive."

- Limit the sodium content of processed foods by either (a) setting a uniform limit on the milligrams of sodium per 100 grams (or per 100 calories or per serving) in all foods or (b) setting different limits for different categories of foods.[11]

In 1981, the CSPI filed another petition that called on the FDA to require a notice (an admittedly rather wordy one!) on canisters of salt:

The Surgeon General has determined that, for many people, a diet high in sodium or salt may produce high blood pressure. High blood pressure increases the risk of heart attack and stroke. The public is advised to limit salt consumption by cooking with only small amounts and refraining from adding salt to food at the table.[12]

Small packets of salt could state: "The Surgeon General has advised the public to eat less salt."

Those petitions marked the first time that someone called on the FDA to fulfill its public health mandate and adopt specific policies to solve the sodium problem. Little did we know at the time that those petitions were only the first step of a journey that would last more than four decades—and that journey still continues. As an indication of what the FDA's receptivity to our petitions might be, shortly before we filed our petitions, the agency's acting director of nutrition, John Vanderveen, told me that the large amounts of salt in processed foods might be beneficial, because they protect very active people from sodium depletion.[13] Coincidentally, at about the same time, Sanford A. Miller, the director of the FDA's Center for Food Safety and Applied Nutrition—and Vanderveen's boss—told me that high levels of salt in packaged foods were a major nutrition problem and should be limited.[14]

The GRAS (Generally Recognized as Safe) Review

Let's now take a little detour back to 1969. That was not only the year of the White House conference on diet and health, but also the year that the FDA banned cyclamate, an artificial sweetener suspected of causing cancer. Cyclamate was not an official food additive, but rather an ingredient considered by the FDA to be "generally recognized as safe," or GRAS. GRAS substances were supposed to be familiar ingredients that everyone "knew" were perfectly safe, like vinegar, vitamin C (ascorbic acid) . . . and salt and sugar. Because of the public uproar over a synthetic and probably dangerous chemical like cyclamate being considered safe, President Richard Nixon ordered the FDA to review the safety of all GRAS substances.[15] To conduct the review, the FDA asked the Federation of American Societies for Experimental Biology, a consortium of scientific societies with mostly academic members, to establish a Select Committee on GRAS Substances, or SCOGS.

The committee took a decade to review the safety of over 370 substances and concluded that almost all were safe. But in 1979, the year after CSPI's initial petitions to the FDA, SCOGS shook the food world by concluding:

> It is the prevalent judgment in the scientific community that the consumption of sodium chloride in the aggregate should be lowered. . . . The Select Committee agrees and favors the development of guidelines for restricting the amount of salt in processed foods.[16]

It went on to say in its linguistically convoluted way that the evidence was not sufficient to determine that the adverse effects reported from current usage of salt were not deleterious. In other words, current uses of sodium could not be considered "generally recognized as safe"—exactly what CSPI's petition contended.

The FDA usually responded "reasonably quickly" to SCOGS reports (most of which required no real response), but because of "significant controversy" over the salt decision the FDA needed to prepare strategy documents, according to Miller.[17] The FDA needed to consider "a great number of legal, technical, and administrative issues." Changing the regulatory status of such a ubiquitously used ingredient, and possibly other sodium-containing ingredients, certainly would be complicated, but FDA probably also feared that the food industry would try to block action, including by suing the agency.

And, indeed, industry fervently wanted to stop the FDA from limiting salt in foods, including in potato chips. One example involved Frito-Lay— the nation's biggest snack-food maker, which even back then had sales of more than $1 billion a year.[18] Dr. Robert I-San Lin was the chief scientist at Frito-Lay between 1975 and 1982. Now in his mid-eighties and living in California, he still has a memory that would put an elephant to shame. He told me that his supervisor wanted him to testify at a public meeting convened by the SCOGS committee and deflect or deny health concerns about salt. But he refused because he believed that Americans were consuming too much salt. His supervisor told him "testify or pack up and leave," but he managed not to do either. Instead, another Frito-Lay employee, along with two academic consultants to the snack-food industry, spoke at the meeting. One of those consultants, John Laragh, a professor at Cornell University Medical Center, testified: "We don't know what the ideal intake of sodium chloride is. But we do know that . . . compromising the intake can be dangerous."[19] In other words, don't mess with the salt in foods. Lin says now, "We could defeat the FDA and stop them from taking action on SCOGS's advice. . . . I could whack them down easily,"[20] though at the time he told his supervisors that he was "very reluctant to put up a fight with the Committee on salt . . . [because] none of the following arguments [against using less salt] are invincible."[21]

Other Regulatory Inaction

In 1981, the Reagan administration appointed Dr. Arthur Hull Hayes to head the FDA. Because Hayes headed the hypertension clinic at the Hershey Medical Center in Hershey, Pennsylvania, I was hopeful that the agency would act boldly to tackle the sodium problem. But in the context of an administration that was philosophically opposed to regulation, Hayes and FDA adopted a largely voluntary plan that encouraged companies to drop salt from cooking instructions, label sodium on packages, reduce sodium levels in processed foods, and produce more low-sodium foods.[22] The key word there is "voluntary." Then-congressman Al Gore (D-TN), who had held a hearing in 1981 on a bill to require labeling of sodium, predicted that the voluntary approach was "almost certainly doomed to failure."[23] And he was right, partly because it is impossible to get several hundred million consumers to read labels carefully before they buy a bottle of salad dressing, bag of chips, or can of soup, and companies did not experience much pressure to lower sodium levels. Stronger medicine was needed to help cure the sodium problem.

At Gore's hearing, Representative Robert Walker (R-PA) objected to a labeling bill, telling me when I was testifying, "I'm a little concerned about a process that has a Big Brother approach." I responded, "I don't

like Big Brother any more than you do. But I find when I want to eat processed foods that the salt content is dictated by another Big Brother—or Big
Aunt—Betty Crocker."[24]

Even Commissioner Hayes said at Gore's hearing, "I have made it abun-
dantly clear [to food industry executives] that if sufficient positive action
is not forthcoming, I would feel compelled to pursue a mandatory solution."[25] (Jumping ahead for a moment, in 1986 the FDA found that only
about half of foods had sodium labeling;[26] I'm not aware of any report that
measured changes in the number of new lower-sodium foods or the sodium
content of existing products.)

Representative Gore's bill attracted broad support from fellow Demo-
crats and such groups as the American Heart Association (AHA), American
Association of Retired Persons (AARP), and American Medical Association
(AMA). But to get a vote on the House floor, the bill first had to be approved
by the Health and the Environment Subcommittee of the Energy and Com-
merce Committee. Chairman Henry Waxman and Gore thought they had
the votes, but then the food industry turned the screws.[27] A congressional
aide reported that the AMA's resolve dissolved when "the food industry
reminded the doctors that the AMA didn't like being regulated any more
than it did." And industry lobbyists expressed their displeasure directly to
members of Congress. In particular, Campbell Soup and Procter & Gamble
reportedly persuaded two key Democratic congressmen (James Florio and
Thomas Luken), who represented the districts in which those companies
were headquartered, to drop their support. Waxman acknowledged the
obvious: "We are having difficulty getting the votes to pass this legislation
because of industry pressure."[28] The bill was withdrawn in 1982.

In 1982, Hayes spoke at a conference sponsored by the AMA. "It is clear,"
he said, "that we as a society and we as health professionals must address
the sodium issue, and we must do it now."[29] In a formal statement, the
FDA acknowledged that it "agrees with [the SCOGS GRAS review] that 'a
reduction of sodium chloride consumption by the population will reduce
the frequency of hypertension.'"[30] It also acknowledged that setting limits
on sodium "would accomplish the desired goals" of reducing hypertension.
But the agency rejected setting limits "because the Commissioner believes
that a voluntary program will produce the desired results with less regulatory burden." The FDA issued an ultimatum: "If no significant progress
occurs toward these goals in a reasonable time, the agency will consider

additional regulatory actions." But the FDA did little over the next three decades.

The FDA, under the leadership of a hypertension expert, had an opportunity to save thousands of lives, but in 1982 it denied both CSPI's labeling and "limits" petitions.[31] The FDA said it would defer any action on the GRAS status of salt until it saw whether labeling and voluntary actions would reduce sodium to safe levels. As a consolation prize, however, in 1984 it at least required any foods with nutrition information on their labels or foods that were fortified with extra nutrients—about 30 percent of the dollar value of foods regulated by the FDA—to include sodium along with calories and other information.[32]

In the face of the FDA's denial of its petitions, in 1983 CSPI, represented by attorneys at the Georgetown University Law School, sued the agency. We contended that the FDA failed to fulfill its legislative mandate by not requiring sodium labeling and not setting limits on sodium in processed foods. The next year, however, the FDA persuaded the court to set aside the lawsuit so the agency could see whether sodium labeling did, indeed, lead consumers to choose lower-sodium products and companies to lower sodium levels.

The food industry wasn't going to just sit around when salt was in the crosshairs of the public health community and the FDA was expressing concern about salty diets. In the 1980s, Frito-Lay, a division of PepsiCo, tried a new strategy: shift blame from too much sodium to too little calcium. In a memo labeled "Frito-Lay's confidential information," Frito-Lay's Bob Lin reported that David A. McCarron (a key figure in chapters 3 and 6), then a professor at the University of Oregon Health Sciences Center, had asked for funding for work aimed at showing that calcium, not sodium, was the key dietary culprit in causing hypertension. Lin wrote, "An effective promotion of 'Calcium Antihypertension Theory' may release the pressure on sodium for the time being."[33]

Lin recommended giving McCarron a grant of $10,000 to $20,000 ($26,500 to $53,000 in 2020 dollars) and cooperating with the Salt Institute, thinking that the resulting research could provide "powerful ammunition" for the company. But Lin presciently warned, "I don't believe proper calcium intake can prevent/ameliorate most types of hypertension, so even if the 'Calcium Theory' campaign is successful, the [sodium] issue will come back in the long run." Lin also criticized McCarron's own research: "From

[a] scientific point of view," he said, "there is much to be desired. . . . There are potholes."[34] And, in fact, during a phone call Lin told me: "I doubted that McCarron was a real expert on salt and hypertension, and knew that he downplayed the link between them."[35] Lin did not recall whether McCarron actually conducted a study, but McCarron certainly publicized the notion that calcium, not just sodium, was a major cause of hypertension.[36] (McCarron did not respond to my requests for an interview.)

Speaking more broadly, Lin believes that industry has fought so hard against effective government actions to reduce sodium consumption because of a basic philosophical principle. PepsiCo (and presumably other industry giants) "fight against any government intrusion into business freedom."[37] That would apply to salt reduction, food labeling, pollution controls, and many other matters. But internally, Lin was trying hard to reduce salt in Frito-Lay products. He tested techniques including using finer salt crystals and using electrostatically charged salt particles that would spread more evenly on chips and increase the salty sensation.

To say that progress was slow in the 1970s and 1980s would grossly overstate the pace of change. One likely reason was that the FDA was afflicted by a severe case of conflicts of interest. The revolving door between the food and drug industries and the FDA spun faster than a carousel on amphetamines: a commissioner left for the drug industry, a deputy commissioner became the vice-president of the food industry's major trade association, the head of the foods division came from a food manufacturer and left to become an industry consultant, another head of the foods division joined the soft-drink industry's trade association, the head of nutrition left for a major candy company, and one chief lawyer went to the vegetable-oil industry while another came from and went back to a law firm representing food and drug companies. Such officials molded the mind-set and decisions of the agency.

After the court put CSPI's sodium lawsuit in abeyance, and the voluntary labeling program was in place and without apparent effect, CSPI sought other ways to educate people about sodium. We began a decade-long effort to win passage of a law that would require more informative food labeling with fewer deceptive health and nutrition claims. Thanks especially to Representative Waxman and Senator Howard Metzenbaum (D-OH), that effort culminated in the 1990 Nutrition Labeling and Education Act, the law that requires nutrition labels on almost all packaged foods. The list of labeled nutrients includes sodium. The restaurant industry, however, "vociferously opposed" the legislation unless restaurants were excluded, which they were (unless they made deceptive health and nutrition claims).[38]

Nutrition Facts labels have been invaluable to millions of consumers who are watching their intakes of sodium, calories, cholesterol, or other nutrients, but they have not led to the kinds of improvements we had hoped to see, either in the nutritional quality of foods or in shoppers' choices. A decade after it became law to label processed foods with Nutrition Facts, Americans were still consuming the same amount of sodium. So in 2005 CSPI focused once again on sodium. We published a report, "Salt: The Forgotten Killer,"[39] and sued the FDA for never taking final action on our 1978 petitions to revoke salt's GRAS status and limit sodium levels in foods.[40] Back in 1984 when the court denied CSPI's initial lawsuit, District Court Judge June L. Green ruled that the FDA "must make a decision on the GRAS status of salt" after its voluntary programs "have been in effect for a reasonable period of time and FDA has had an opportunity to assess their impact."[41] Twenty years certainly gave companies and the FDA that "reasonable period of time," yet over those years, sodium consumption hardly changed. Unfortunately, the court ruled that our petition had gathered 27 years' worth of dust and we would have to file a new petition with the FDA, which we did later in 2005.[42] The new petition highlighted the voluminous medical research that had accumulated in the intervening years. This time the world seemed more ready to listen. (Except, of course, the irrepressible Salt Institute, which told the FDA: "There is no justification to change the GRAS status of salt. . . . Prudence dictates that we tread very carefully in any consideration of a change in the regulatory status of salt to ensure that we do not do the population more harm than good.")[43]

Though the scientific evidence of salt's harmfulness had become even more decisive, federal officials continued to avoid taking bold actions to protect the public's health. Amazingly, in 1990, long after the "Dietary Guidelines for Americans" and other authoritative publications stated that too much salt increases blood pressure, the FDA's Vanderveen (who had become the full-fledged director of nutrition) said, "There is no conclusive evidence that salt consumption causes hypertension. It's only a hypothesis."[44] And when the officials took any action, it was minimal and had no effect on consumption. Mounting effective regulations and hard-hitting educational campaigns was beyond the pale for FDA officials. The basic reasons were obvious: industry opposition and costs.

FDA officials were not the only ones who failed to tackle sodium. The USDA regulates the labeling and safety of meat and poultry products ranging from pork chops to frozen pepperoni pizzas, which contribute about one-fifth of the sodium we consume. To encourage action in that arena, I met with several top officials in 2005 to express my concerns about sodium.[45] But when I said that salty USDA-regulated foods, and implicitly the USDA, were responsible for thousands of premature deaths every year, it was like waving a red cape in front of a bull. Dale Moore, the Secretary of Agriculture's chief of staff, was outraged and stormed out of the meeting. Richard Raymond, the Under Secretary for Food Safety, responded dismissively, "people will eat what they're going to eat" and should just read labels. So much for action by the USDA.

But, as Alexander Pope wrote almost three hundred years ago, "hope springs eternal in the human breast." I continued to harbor hope that the United States government would protect the public. The next chapter explains the latest developments.

9 Progress at Last!

Given the overwhelming scientific evidence, pursuing voluntary reductions of sodium in the food supply is warranted and overdue.

—Thomas R. Frieden, MPH, MD, Director of the Centers for Disease Control and Prevention, 2016[1]

Little was happening on the salt front in somnolent Washington during the first decade of the twenty-first century, despite prodding from two of the largest health organizations. The American Medical Association (AMA) pointed out what health experts all knew:

Even motivated individuals find it difficult to moderately reduce sodium intake because most sodium consumption derives from salt added during food processing and by restaurants. Therefore, any meaningful strategy to reduce population sodium intake must rely on food manufacturers and preparers to reduce the amount added during preparation.[2]

The AMA called for at least a 50 percent reduction in sodium in processed foods and restaurant meals over the next decade in order to slash stroke and heart attack rates. A few years later, another major organization of health professionals, the American Public Health Association (APHA), called for a major decrease in sodium by 2021. Both recommendations were ignored in Washington.[3]

New York City and Allies Challenge Companies

Several local health officials, distressed by the high rates of cardiovascular disease in their communities, decided that it was time to take on salt and not wait for the federal government to act. In 2009, New York City's

Department of Health and Mental Hygiene, the most action-oriented health department in the country, spearheaded a new effort to cut sodium intakes. To pressure companies to use less salt, the health department created the National Salt Reduction Initiative (NSRI), which ultimately was supported by over one hundred nonprofit health organizations and local and state health authorities.[4] The goal was to reduce sodium in packaged and restaurant foods by 25 percent over five years.[5] The NSRI, analogous to the British plan, developed a set of voluntary sodium targets for 61 categories of packaged foods and 25 categories of restaurant foods. NSRI announced modest two-year and tougher four-year recommended reductions ranging from 15 to 40 percent, depending on the category. Those were not maximum amounts for any given product, but the sales-weighted averri for a company's products in each category. The goals were based on foods some companies were already marketing, so New York officials knew that the goals were achievable. Officials then met with company and trade association officials to encourage them to meet the targets.

The food industry did not exactly rally en masse in support of the NSRI. The Grocery Manufacturers Association (GMA), the packaged-food industry's powerful lobbying arm, said it supported a voluntary, gradual approach to reducing sodium consumption to 2,300 mg per day, but carped that the "food industry continues to have a number of outstanding issues" with the initiative.[6] In its 23-page letter, GMA complained about virtually every aspect of the program. It said, for starters, that New York should focus on the whole diet and lifestyle instead of just one ingredient. Its members "strongly" felt that New York should not even be mounting a "national" initiative, but should let the federal government do so—never mind that the federal government had done nothing for decades, and that dozens of other cities and states across the country and numerous national health organizations supported the NSRI.

Next, GMA criticized the specific goals for many food categories, such as charging that the 40 percent reduction goal for breakfast cereals was "too aggressive" and that a 25 percent reduction in cold cuts would impair the industry's widespread practice of incorporating water into processed meats. Of course, if companies disagreed with the targets that affected some of their products, they could ask for changes or simply ignore the purely voluntary NSRI. (In January 2020, GMA changed its name to the Consumer Brands Association, representing a broader range of companies than makers of grocery goods, and stopped lobbying on food safety and nutrition.)

In the end, more than two dozen manufacturers and chain restaurants, both local and national, agreed to meet the NSRI targets for at least some of their foods. Kraft, Heinz, Mars, Starbucks, and Subway were some of the largest participants. Mondelēz International, a spinoff of Kraft Foods and maker of Oreo cookies and Triscuit crackers, reduced sodium in Nabisco's Teddy Grahams Honey flavor crackers by one-third, from 150 mg to 100 mg per serving. Subway reduced the sodium in two of its most popular sandwiches, the Subway Club and Italian B.M.T., by about 30 percent.

The city saw progress in many food categories. In 2009, when the targets were established, no categories met the 2012 or 2014 targets. By 2014, 16 of 61 categories (26 percent) met the 2012 targets and 2 of those (3 percent) met the 2014 targets. The period between 2009 and 2014 found a "modest" 7 percent decrease in sodium in all packaged foods, but that was far short of the 25 percent goal.[7] The pressure exerted by the NSRI dovetailed nicely with the pressure that other countries were putting on industry.

The key takeaway from the NSRI was that focused government attention could spur sodium reductions. But then a development occurred that moved the action from New York City to Washington, DC.

A Salutary Recommendation from the IOM

Long before the New York City–led program, CSPI had encouraged Congress to fund a report not on whether Americans were consuming too much sodium, but on how to lower sodium levels. Representative Rosa DeLauro (D-CT) and Senator Tom Harkin (D-IA), two of the most stalwart health advocates then in Congress, got Congress to fund the Centers for Disease Control and Prevention (CDC) to prepare a report on how sodium intakes could be lowered.

The CDC and other agencies within the US Department of Health and Human Services (HHS) called on the Institute of Medicine (IOM, now the National Academy of Medicine, or NAM) of the National Academy of Sciences in 2008 to undertake that study. In 2010, the NAM issued its landmark report, "Strategies to Reduce Sodium Intake in the United States," that immediately energized the policy debates.[8] The report pointed out the "staggering" health costs—$73.4 billion in 2009—related to hypertension.

Jane E. Henney, a professor of medicine at the University of Cincinnati and former commissioner of the US Food and Drug Administration (FDA) who chaired the IOM committee, lamented, "For 40 years we have known about the relationship between sodium and the development of hypertension and other life-threatening diseases, but we have had virtually no success in cutting back the salt in our diets."[9] "The vast majority of the US population is consuming sodium at levels that are simply too high to be safe."[10]

The top recommendation in the IOM report was that "the Food and Drug Administration should expeditiously initiate a process to set *mandatory* national standards for the sodium content of foods" [emphasis added]. The IOM also recommended that those limits should apply to both packaged and chain-restaurant foods and be decreased gradually every several years.

In defending the need for mandatory limits, the report said that voluntary initiatives "are challenged by the inability to ensure that there will be compliance and they do not guarantee a level playing field for food producers. Additionally, it is likely that volunteers will drop out as reductions become more challenging over time." The IOM emphasized that "adopting an exclusively voluntary approach in the United States may have limited success and questionable potential for long-term sustainability based on past US experience."[11]

That echoed what Richard Kahn, the chief scientific and medical officer of the American Diabetes Association, told the FDA several years earlier: "Voluntary action has clearly not worked to reduce the sodium content in processed foods. . . . So to continue along with another twist of some voluntary standards or voluntary mandate, so to speak, it's not going to work at all."[12]

Predictably, anti-regulatory forces attacked the IOM's recommendations. Conservative talk show host Rush Limbaugh, sounding like a latter-day Paul Revere, decried (falsely), "they're going to take away our salt shakers."[13] The Salt Institute, of course, weighed in. Morton Satin, the group's vice president and science director, charged that the IOM report ignored research that questioned the health benefits of widespread salt reduction. "This whole thing doesn't seem to have been well thought out," he said of the 400-plus-page report. Satin argued that the government should promote a balanced diet rather than a lowered salt intake—a boring message that has never had any effect in either balancing diets or lowering salt.[14] The next year, the Salt Institute was back at it with more rhetorical flair when the FDA and US Department of Agriculture (USDA), spurred in part by the IOM report, invited comments from the public on reducing sodium intakes: "Yet, at a time when the overwhelming evidence is against population-wide salt reduction, the same FDA is preparing to turn consumers into 300,000,000 guinea pigs with an untested, ideology-based, risk-prone dietary intervention."[15]

Typical of industry's comments was one from the National Frozen Pizza Institute. "NFPI supports the goal of achieving gradual but significant voluntary reductions in the sodium content of the US food supply under the leadership of the federal government. . . . It should take into account the potential impact of sodium reduction on food safety, functionality, cost, consumer acceptance, nutrition, and overall public health."[16] The pizza makers say, in effect, that sure, they want to lower sodium levels. But then they give every excuse as to why it shouldn't and couldn't be done.

Would consumers support mandatory limits on sodium, as the IOM recommended, or would they oppose "nanny state" health measures? The CDC sponsored a survey of almost 10,000 consumers to answer that question. It found that a remarkable 82 percent of consumers supported policies to limit sodium at fast-food restaurants.[17] Close behind, 56 percent of people surveyed supported policies to limit sodium in packaged foods, with another 24 percent neutral.

The FDA Awakens

The day before the IOM report was released, the *Washington Post* stated that the FDA was developing voluntary guidelines for companies to reduce sodium that "would eventually lead to the first legal limits on the amount of salt allowed in food products."[18] The IOM's recommendations and the *Post* story hit the food industry like a bombshell and certainly got the FDA's attention, too. But instead of going down the IOM's recommended *mandatory* route, FDA commissioner Margaret Hamburg immediately said that her agency would set *voluntary* targets. "We believe we can achieve some substantial voluntary reductions," she said. (What was going on here? Let's not forget, as I noted in chapter 8, that 30 years earlier FDA commissioner Arthur Hull Hayes said: "If sufficient positive action is not forthcoming, I would feel compelled to pursue a mandatory solution.")[19]

So, the FDA pulled together a team of scientists, economists, lawyers, and policy experts to shape a voluntary sodium-reduction plan. Their challenge: the FDA had to figure out sensible targets for every segment of the food supply, which consists of well over 100,000 packaged products.[20] The FDA said, though, that less than 10,000 packaged foods accounted for more than 80 percent of sales.[21] Add to that mix many thousands of dishes offered by tens of thousands of restaurants.

The FDA's staff proceeded with the task, but it was slow going, partly a consequence of its complexity, partly because of the inherent slowness of bureaucracies (more about that later in this chapter). Meanwhile, forces outside the agency sought to accelerate its work or stop it.

From inside the government, CDC director Tom Frieden weighed in with a series of memos and emails. According to someone familiar with their contents, the missives were extremely forceful, reflecting Frieden's increasing frustration with the slowness.

Michael M. Landa—the director of the FDA's Center for Food Safety and Applied Nutrition who had overseen the FDA's sodium-reduction proposal—retired in January 2015. But by March he was expressing his dismay about the FDA's slow pace. Landa wrote to the Secretary of the Department of Health and Human Services, Sylvia Mathews Burwell, and urged swift action: "There should be no further delay in issuing draft voluntary sodium reduction targets, whether to help set a 'level playing field' to facilitate industry reduction efforts or to lay the groundwork for mandatory limits, should the targets fail."[22] Seven months later Landa rebuked his former agency directly, telling it:

> The Federal government's failure to take any substantive action in response to the [2005] Citizen Petition [from CSPI] is incomprehensible, and it would be irresponsible to wait any longer. . . . What is the Federal government waiting for? Sodium reduction talk from the Federal government is cheap and has long been getting cheaper.[23]

At the same time, the threat of sodium guidelines did not go without notice in Congress. One of the key opponents of the FDA's guidance was Representative Andy Harris (R-MD), an anesthesiologist turned legislator. Though he did not receive significant campaign contributions from the food industry, Harris was typical of the anti-regulatory, pro-corporate Tea Party legislators who poured into Congress in 2011.[24] At a congressional hearing in 2015, Harris hauled out the much-criticized PURE study I discussed in chapter 3. He told FDA commissioner Hamburg:

> That study actually indicates that if you are a healthy person you actually have an increased cardiovascular risk of salt restriction. . . . That's not clear. I mean, I think you know that the party line is that salt is bad and decreasing salt is good, but it appears that's not really true.[25]

That was representative of how flawed research can be used to muddy the waters, confuse consumers, and impede policy changes.

Like Frieden and Landa, I, too, felt the public had waited long enough for the FDA to act. After all, the Obama administration's last year was fast approaching, and there was no way to predict what the next administration would do. So on October 8, 2015, CSPI, represented by the Public Citizen Litigation Group, sued the FDA in federal court.[26] We charged that the FDA unlawfully had not responded to CSPI's 2005 petition calling for mandatory sodium reductions. That lawsuit led to a negotiated agreement between the government's lawyers and our lawyers that set a deadline of June 1, 2016, for the FDA finally to respond to our petition.

Target Time at FDA

And exactly on schedule, on June 1, the FDA proposed voluntary targets. Progress at last! The FDA provided goals for more than 150 categories of foods—both packaged and restaurant. They ranged from flavored potato chips to semisoft blue-veined cheese to frozen pizza with meat, poultry, or seafood.[27] In setting targets, the FDA made sure that the lower sodium levels were practical for each food category and would not compromise the safety of any food. While the targets would still have to be finalized after a period of public comment, the proposal was a giant step forward.

The official name of the FDA's proposal is "Voluntary Sodium Reduction Goals: Target Mean and Upper Bound Concentrations for Sodium in Commercially Processed, Packaged, and Prepared Foods: Guidance for Industry—*Draft Guidance*." I'll refer it to as the FDA's guidance, plan, or targets.

The FDA proposed easy targets for industry to meet two years after they were finalized. Many foods were already meeting those targets, and the FDA did not anticipate any food safety or taste problems. If the entire food industry adhered to the two-year targets (an unlikely occurrence), the FDA estimated that Americans' average sodium consumption would drop from 3,400 mg to 3,000 mg, a moderate 12 percent reduction.

The FDA also proposed much more ambitious targets to be met in 10 years. Full adherence to those targets would reduce average consumption to 2,300 mg, about one-third less than people now consume and in line with the "Dietary Guidelines for Americans" recommendation. Reaching those goals would prevent tens of thousands of premature deaths each year. The FDA said, "A consensus exists that reducing sodium intake to 2,300 mg/day is a viable, achievable, and effective strategy to reduce the incidence of [cardiovascular disease]."[28]

To buttress its case in anticipation of opposition, the HHS and FDA had undertaken an economic analysis of potential savings that would result from lower sodium intakes. (To obtain the document I had to file a request under the Freedom of Information Act and then wait more than a year.) The numbers are staggering. Cutting about 1,300 mg (about one-third) of sodium out of the average diet and getting close to 2,300 mg, according to the report, would save $142 billion over 20 years in reduced or delayed medical costs.[29] The healthier and longer lives that Americans would enjoy would be worth an additional—and astonishing—$3.6 trillion over 20 years. Even if the FDA overestimated the benefits by several-fold—because lowering sodium would not happen overnight, and the assumptions might have overstated sodium's effect on blood pressure—I'm sure that the medical savings alone would dwarf the estimated cost to companies of reformulating some of their products.

FDA's blueprint was a variation of the ones developed in the United Kingdom and by New York City. It includes two kinds of targets, with one specifying sales-weighted average levels of sodium for each food category. ("Sales-weighted" means that the sodium content of an individual product is weighted by the volume of it sales—popular products are given more weight than poor-selling ones.) Those targets establish a benchmark for a whole category (for example, breakfast cereals made by various companies), but not for individual products (Kellogg Corn Flakes). Note that some companies could do nothing, but instead rely on their competitors to lower sodium sufficiently for the category to meet the target. The second kind, to help ensure that no individual product had huge amounts of sodium, sets maximum (voluntary) sodium levels for all products in a category.

Maximum levels are important because they encourage companies to refor-mulate their saltiest products—and enable health officials, journalists, con-sumer groups, and consumers to identify foods containing grossly excessive amounts of sodium.

To understand how the two kinds of targets would operate, consider white bread.[30] The FDA found that in 2010 the average bread (weighted by sales) had 523 mg per 100 g (or 148 mg per 1-ounce slice). At least one brand had 700 mg per 100 g. The two-year targets seek to lower that aver-age to 440 mg, with no bread containing more than 570 mg. FDA's 10-year target aims to bring the industry-wide average down to 300 mg per 100 g, with no bread having more than 460 mg.

Similarly, the average sodium level for all canned, ready-to-eat (not con-densed) soups, weighted by the volumes of each soup sold, would (assum-ing that all the major companies met the guidelines) drop from 265 mg per 100 g (equivalent to 636 mg per cup) to 230 mg in two years and 200 mg in 10 years. Also, no ready-to-eat soup would have more than 310 mg per 100 g after two years and no more than 260 mg after 10 years. For compari-son, Campbell's Chunky Beef with Country Vegetables soup now contains 360 mg per 100 g. If Campbell followed the FDA's guidance, the soup would have no more than 260 mg per 100 g in 10 years.

The CDC's Frieden was one of many who cheered FDA's announcement. He wrote in the *Journal of the American Medical Association* "that a decrease in sodium intake by as little as 400 milligrams a day could prevent 32,000 heart attacks and 20,000 strokes annually."[31] The American Heart Associa-tion (AHA)'s CEO Nancy Brown applauded the FDA's move and urged the agency to finalize the targets soon (see box 9.1 for a look at the valiant salt reductions efforts of the AHA).[32] "These new targets will spark a vital, healthy change in our food supply, a change consumers say they want," Brown said, adding that lowering sodium levels could eliminate 1.5 million cases of uncontrolled hypertension and save billions of dollars in health-care costs over the next decade.[33] CSPI, too, applauded, saying, the proposal "provides clear goals by which companies can be held accountable. And, it helps level the playing field for those companies that are already trying to use less salt in their foods."[34]

As welcome as the FDA's action was, comparing a few of the FDA's targets to those of Britain indicates how far behind the United States has fallen. For instance, the FDA's short-term, sales-weighted target for breakfast cereals is

---

Box 9.1
Salt hero—American Heart Association

The American Heart Association (AHA) has been the only major health charity or professional organization that has stayed on the sodium battlefield through the decades. Its credible spokespersons—under the leadership of CEO Nancy Brown and backed by the association's stellar reputation—have testified at government hearings, pressed for strong government recommendations, and lobbied Congress to require healthier school meals. Its physician allies have regularly, publicly, and loudly rebutted flawed scientific reports. Its Heart-Check program, by licensing companies to use the familiar heart-shaped logo on labels of heart-healthy foods, encourages companies to improve their products and enables consumers to choose healthier foods. On the educational front, the AHA has done everything from publishing low-sodium cookbooks, to sponsoring clever online videos on reducing salt, to publicizing "The Salty Six" processed-food categories: bread and rolls, cold cuts and cured meats, pizza, poultry, soup, and sandwiches. In recent years, the group has consistently supported the sodium limit of 1,500 mg per day for most adults as stated in the 2010 "Dietary Guidelines for Americans."

---

550 mg per 100 grams,[35] whereas the average sodium content for cereals in Britain is already 176 mg.[36] Similarly, American breads have about 500 mg per 100 g, and the FDA's proposed goal is 430 mg. British breads already average 380 mg per 100 g, with a 2023 goal of 340 mg.

Industry, Trade, and Food Giants Respond to Targets

Industry did not exactly embrace the program like a long-lost friend come home. Even though industry got its prize of an entirely voluntary proposal, some companies still feared that it could lead to mandatory regulations and subject companies to lawsuits if they did not meet the targets. I believe those concerns are akin to Chicken Little's worries, but they led some industry officials to consider the voluntary targets to be little better than mandatory limits.

The Salt Institute blasted its predictably hyperbolic salvo at the FDA: "The issuance today of new 'voluntary' sodium reduction mandates by the FDA is tantamount to malpractice and inexcusable in the face of years of scientific evidence showing that population-wide sodium reduction strategies are unnecessary and could be harmful."[37] (Several months earlier, the industry group predicted that the FDA was going to issue guidelines because of "long-term pressure from the Center for Science in the Public Interest," not because of the massive amount of scientific evidence it disagrees with.)[38] Of course, the FDA did not issue any "mandate" and its guidance was only a proposal. Its final guidance would be entirely voluntary and could be ignored by any or all companies (an obvious defect in the eyes of those who hope that sodium consumption would be reduced rapidly and substantially).

The snack-food industry's trade association, SNAC International, also criticized the FDA for proposing a new policy before a "real scientific consensus is reached."[39] It said that the modest two-year goals for snack foods were far too ambitious (100–300 mg too low), and wanted the agency to eliminate the upper-bound targets entirely.[40] It contended that the National Academy of Medicine should conduct a new review before the FDA did anything. In fact, in 2019 that organization published just such a report—a scientific consensus—that recommended that healthy adults consume less than 2,300 mg of sodium per day, exactly what it recommended more than a decade earlier. SNAC did not dispute (or applaud) the NAM's conclusions, but said that it supported stepwise reductions provided that they were small and voluntary.[41]

The GMA was more measured, but also raised concerns about endangering people who might consume too little sodium. The group said, "Like others inside and outside of government, we believe additional work is needed to determine the acceptable range of sodium intake for optimal health. This evaluation should include research that indicates health risks for people who consume too much sodium as well as health risks from consuming too little sodium."[42] With almost all Americans consuming far more sodium than is recommended, being concerned about under-consumption is like being concerned that a roller coaster will crash into your home.

The GMA's official responses to the FDA were 15-page and 74-page epistles reminiscent of its statement about New York City's NSRI. The association complained that two years did not give companies enough time to revise their recipes and that many proposed reductions were too steep.[43]

Other trade associations and individual companies also put in their two cents.[44] General Mills, Red Lobster, and the National Restaurant Association all asked the FDA to extend the two-year targets for another one to three years. As for the longer-term targets, the American Bakers Association said, "We believe that ten years, for certain products, is not a feasible timeframe for complying with the proposed targets." It asked that that target date be extended. The American Butter Institute and American Cheese Society asked the FDA to drop their entire food categories from its program.

Refreshingly, several leading manufacturers welcomed the FDA's plan. Mars, which makes some salty Uncle Ben's rice products in addition to its non-salty candy bars, said, "Mars applauds FDA for releasing its draft voluntary guidelines on sodium and we look forward to providing additional comments on the recommendations. At Mars, we have been working on reducing sodium in our products since . . . 2010."[45] Two weeks earlier, Nestlé, PepsiCo, and Unilever had joined Mars in urging that the FDA propose sodium targets.[46] Interestingly, those industry giants, except for PepsiCo, quit the GMA and created the Sustainable Food Policy Alliance to support more progressive food and environmental policies. In 2019, that alliance also applauded the NAM's updated recommendation for lowering sodium to an average of 2,300 mg per day, saying, "Food companies can and should do more to reduce sodium in food products. Reducing sodium levels can be a powerful public health action to lower blood pressure, a leading risk for heart disease."[47]

Flaws in the Ointment

I was delighted that the FDA had finally taken a big step forward on the sodium issue, even if its proposed guidance was voluntary. But one prominent flaw would limit the plan's impact: the 8-year gap between the 2-year and the 10-year goals. That is different from the voluntary plans developed by the NSRI and the United Kingdom, which phased in gradually lower targets every two or three years. Similarly, Chile had two-year nutrient targets for its food-labeling standards and then tightened them after two years and again after one more year.

Mary R. L'Abbé, the former director of the Bureau of Nutritional Sciences at Health Canada and now a professor at the University of Toronto, says that the lack of interim targets means that sodium reduction would likely quietly slide off the agendas of both industry and government after the first flurry of activity. She worries that "10 years is really almost a way of burying something sometimes. There's a lot of in-house corporate expertise that you lose if you just pick up and start and stop."[48] Government and industry experts likely would move on to pressing new issues. And journalists, legislators, and the public would probably forget about the whole thing.

The National Hispanic Medical Association said in 2016, "If anything, the FDA should set a more aggressive timetable; after all, this is only *voluntary* guidance." As it pointed out, "Establishing the 10-year targets in 2017 would mean 17 years between the long-term sodium-reduction goals and the 2010 baseline."[49] Now, as I write in 2020, it is clear that industry would have had more than 20 years to reach the 10-year targets, assuming that those targets are finalized.

Separate from the long-drawn-out timetable, the National Medical Association (the organization of African American physicians) pointed out a serious weakness in how the targets applied to restaurants.[50] It said, "many restaurant meals are enormous, with some providing one or more days' worth of sodium, even though their sodium content per 100 grams may not be excessive." It urged the FDA to set maximum sodium levels *per serving*, not just *per 100 grams*, for three key food categories: Sandwiches, Mixed Ingredient Dishes, and Other Combination Foods.

New White House, New Scrutiny

Unfortunately, because the Obama administration took so long to propose the sodium targets, it did not have enough time to obtain comments from industry and consumers and finalize the sodium targets before the president left office in January 2017. Once Donald Trump was elected president, I assumed that it would be a long, long time before the targets were finalized. President Trump was far more enthusiastic about repealing laws, regulations, and voluntary guidances than adopting new ones—no matter how many lives they might save. But, remarkably, the new commissioner of the FDA, Dr. Scott Gottlieb, was not a shrink-the-government crusader like many other high-level appointees. He was seriously interested in fulfilling his responsibilities as a health official.

In March 2018, Gottlieb expressed his concerns about diets high in sodium. He said that "researchers have estimated that reducing sodium intake by one-half teaspoon [about 1,200 mg] a day could prevent nearly 100,000 premature deaths a year and up to 120,000 new cases of coronary heart disease, 66,000 strokes, and 99,000 heart attacks." He added, "There remains no single more effective public health action related to nutrition than the reduction of sodium in the diet." Gottlieb said that the FDA planned to finalize the two-year targets in 2019.[51]

But the salt wars took an unexpected turn when Gottlieb resigned from his position in March 2019 and was not replaced until December. Also in 2019, the snack-food industry, including PepsiCo (Frito-Lay), ConAgra (Slim Jims, Orville Redenbacher's), Campbell (Pepperidge Farm cookies), and others, was hatching a plan to delay the finalization of the targets. The American Bakers Association, American Frozen Food Institute, International Dairy Foods Association, North American Meat Institute, and National Restaurant Association were also part of that effort, according to *Politico*, the news outlet focusing on politics.[52]

One knowledgeable person (who would discuss the issue only on an anonymous basis) said that much of the food industry "was terrified" that the Trump administration would finalize the sodium targets. So the trade associations, doing business as the Sodium Coalition, lobbied the FDA and the White House to keep the targets in abeyance until Trump administration economists conducted a new estimate of the costs and benefits of the FDA's program. That could easily delay the final program for another year and give industry more time to kill it completely (such as by getting Congress to include a fatal sentence in an appropriations bill). As of spring 2020, the FDA's four-year-old, life-saving plan was still not finalized.

But wait. Why is the White House involved—isn't the FDA an independent agency? By law it is, but in reality its parent agency, the Department of Health and Human Services, and the White House scrutinize every major action the agency wants to undertake.

Meanwhile, that same insider told me that SNAC apparently was telling the White House and other parts of the government about its own assessment of the costs—but not the benefits—of complying with the sodium guidelines. That person understood that the costs were "grossly exaggerated." The industry group told *Politico* that it was merely trying to be helpful: "We believe an OMB review will be a helpful part of the policymaking process." Laura MacCleery, CSPI's policy director, was more candid, telling *Politico*, "It's unfortunate that there's a last-ditch attempt to throw sand in the gears."[53] (SNAC did not respond to my emailed questions.)

Big Questions: Why the Voluntary Path and Long Gestation?

Considering the utter failure of voluntary action in the past, *why did the FDA once again go the voluntary route?* And—considering that CSPI petitioned the FDA in 1978 and 2005 to lower sodium levels in the food supply, that the agency's SCOGS advisory committee concluded in 1979 that salt was not "generally recognized as safe," and that the Institute of Medicine in 2010 recommended that the FDA set mandatory limits on sodium—*why did the FDA take so many years to propose targets?* The answers are complicated—and good examples of why it takes a lot longer to adopt new federal policies in real life than in a one-hour TV drama.

I was initially sorely disappointed that the FDA was not setting mandatory maximum sodium levels. Such limits for all foods in a category, even if they would affect only a minority of products, have at least three advantages over a voluntary approach. First, they would have teeth and ensure that all companies actually trimmed sodium in their saltiest products. Second, the FDA could easily enforce them. And third, they would provide a level playing field—companies that made the effort to lower sodium would not have to compete with companies that spared themselves the effort and expense. Kraft Food's Senior Vice President of Research and Nutrition, Todd Abraham, said that Kraft lost sales when it reduced sodium but other companies did not.[54]

On the other hand, FDA officials recognized that just setting maximum limits on sodium would not spur companies to reduce levels in the great majority of foods already below those limits. In fact, companies that used less sodium might even feel they had permission to add more salt up to the maximum. The FDA wanted to accomplish more. Complementing maxima with targets for entire food categories would give companies a benchmark for cutting the sodium in large fractions of their portfolios.

I have since been persuaded that the voluntary approach was inevitable. Mike Taylor, who was the FDA's Deputy Commissioner for Foods at the time and a strong public health advocate, defended the voluntary approach. FDA officials felt they lacked "the data to justify specific limits for each of the many categories of food products." However, Taylor felt that even a voluntary program would represent major progress.[55] He added, "Importantly, of course, FDA did do a lot of technical homework to produce the voluntary targets, and my hope was that there would be learning and additional data collection that could in the future support mandatory limits."[56] He might have added that most other nations' salt-reduction initiatives are voluntary.

Landa, another dedicated health proponent, regarded even the voluntary guidance as "a fairly heavy lift" both scientifically and legally and believed that an actual regulation to limit sodium "would not have gotten off the ground" because of implacable industry opposition—but it would have been tough even without that opposition.[57] For one thing, libertarians would have waved the "nanny state" flag.

Companies fearing that strict legal limits on sodium content would necessitate expensive reformulations of salty foods, impair their products' taste, and reduce sales might well have gotten their friends in Congress to shut down the whole sodium-reduction initiative. In contrast, setting voluntary targets would shrink all the pitfalls and still impose pressure on industry to cut the salt.

But even the FDA's voluntary scheme was temporarily handcuffed by Congress. Representative Harris sponsored a measure that prevented the FDA from working on its 10-year guidelines until the NAM had issued a report on the safety of cutting sodium to 2,300 mg per day. The appropriations legislation for 2017, 2018, and 2019 included a measure that

> prohibits the FDA from using funds provided . . . to develop, issue, promote, or advance any regulations applicable to food manufacturers for population-wide sodium reduction actions or to develop, issue, promote or advance final guidance . . . for long term [10-year] population-wide sodium reduction actions until the dietary reference intake report with respect to sodium is completed.[58]

The administration's slowness in proposing its guidance is another story. After all, the FDA scheme for targets was similar to what the United Kingdom and New York City had done, so the agency was not breaking any new conceptual ground. But what seemed all too slow from the outside was par for the course, or even rapid, for people whose watches worked on government timetables.

To help understand the administration's concerns and emphasize the urgency of reducing sodium, in 2012 the AHA, APHA, and CSPI met with White House staffers. Across the table were several officials, including Sam Kass, a restaurant chef who had been the Obamas' personal chef before he became the White House Senior Policy Advisor for Healthy Food Initiatives and a chef at 1600 Pennsylvania Avenue. In other words, he was the nutrition chief at the White House, the first such person to have that role. The officials explained that competing priorities inevitably slowed down the release of sodium guidelines. But at that time, the FDA's proposal for voluntary guidelines was nowhere near completion or headed to the White House.[59]

I don't know if we impressed them with the importance and practicality of lowering sodium across the entire food supply. But I do remember well one awkward moment when a member of our delegation stated with utmost confidence that manufacturers and restaurants could easily lower salt levels by simply omitting salt from all their recipes. That person—as I soon discovered—had no idea who Kass was or that Kass had more than a little experience cooking delicious meals in some very prestigious kitchens. I bet Kass got a good laugh out of that faux pas.

In February 2014, those same health groups, plus the AMA, met again with White House officials to press for action on salt. At that time, the FDA still had not sent a proposal to the White House. One official asked what we thought about setting targets for only key—not all—sources of sodium and also said that the administration was not likely to move ahead on salt before it acted on heart-disease-promoting trans fat (which the FDA banned a year later). Another official criticized the health groups for exaggerating the risks of high-sodium diets and warned that even a voluntary reduction program could trigger the ire of companies that suspected that voluntary recommendations could lead to mandatory requirements.

In doing research for this book, I asked former officials familiar with the "sausage-making process" inside the government why it took so long to propose the guidelines. Several talked to me on the condition of anonymity. At the FDA, Michael Landa and others emphasized the sheer enormity of the task. Staffers had to evaluate the range of sodium levels in products that spanned more than 150 categories, identify sensible and defensible average and maximum levels for each category, make sure that sodium's preservative and other functions were not lost, and determine that the whole initiative jibed with the law. Another reason was bandwidth: the FDA's staff had other major priorities competing for their time—implementing a complicated new food safety law, banning partially hydrogenated vegetable oil (the source of artificial trans fat), and making controversial revisions to the Nutrition Facts label. The sodium guidelines sometimes got pushed aside.[60] From the White House's perspective, Kass said, "it took [the FDA] years to get us a proposal."[61]

Adding to the scientists' challenge was the bureaucratic problem. The government's process for issuing *anything* is complicated and slow. The FDA's foods division first must develop a plan and get buy-in from the commissioner's office. (The draft document was almost cleared to go upstairs in July 2013.)[62] The agency then needs to circulate it to and get agreement from sister agencies, such as the CDC, USDA, and the National Heart, Lung, and Blood Institute (part of the National Institutes of Health). Next, its parent agency, the Department of Health and Human Services (HHS), has to approve the plan. HHS staffers told me they as well had too much work and too little time, but the department always supported, not nitpicked, the FDA's draft plan.

After going up and down the departmental ladder at HHS, a draft proposal has to pass muster at the White House, which typically asks for changes or an economic analysis that would show that the whole endeavor was worth the trouble. Competing priorities there may have played a role, too. First Lady Michelle Obama, the most ardent advocate for better nutrition ever to occupy the White House, was pressing especially hard for requiring calorie labeling at chain restaurants, updating the Nutrition Facts labels, and promoting children's health through healthier school meals and the Let's Move program, though she also championed sodium reductions. And the White House considered implementing the Affordable Care Act (Obamacare) its absolute top priority, with any other health issues being a distraction or obstruction, according to one former administration official. That person wished progress could have been faster, but did not question the strategic focus on Obamacare. Kass, however, disagreed with the "competing priorities" problem. He said, "I just think it's inaccurate. . . . We can walk and chew gum at the same time."[63] From the FDA's perspective, though, Commissioner Hamburg "felt like there were a million pushbacks and 'slow walks' of reviews."[64] (Several former White House officials who might have rounded out the picture did not respond to my interview requests.)

Kass told me that everyone in the White House was on board with the sodium plan. But, he added, "It just takes time to do a piece of policy that is that complicated. . . . At every turn it was a priority." The GMA, ConAgra, and others were lobbying the White House to drop or water down the sodium-reduction plan, but that did not appear to have been a major impediment. For Kass, a bigger concern was the FDA's estimate of the possible costs of the plan to industry. He was shocked by the magnitude of the costs—billions of dollars. "It was astronomical," he said, a "f***ing disaster." Kass feared that disclosure of those costs—even though the benefits might be hundreds of times greater—would trigger a firestorm of opposition from Republicans in Congress and the food industry. That "could potentially kill this project," Kass said, adding that the FDA "did a great job on a very, very complicated piece of policy." Then he suggested how the cost estimate and political risk could have been kept significantly smaller:

> They treated [the guidance] as if this would be a law and that every company would have to change their products, which dramatically inflated the perceived costs of the effort and, in our opinion, left the policy really susceptible to attack, and made it quite vulnerable, both as a policy and also how Republicans could potentially use it to put forward laws that in the future could ban the FDA from taking this kind of action.[65]

I fervently wanted to obtain the FDA's estimate of the potential costs to industry, but even a Freedom of Information Act request couldn't pry the document out of the agency.

Kass was right that the voluntary nature of the sodium-reduction program means that some companies would do nothing or make smaller reductions than the guidelines call for—greatly shrinking industry's actual costs. Consequently, the White House had the FDA rework its economic estimates, adding further delay.

Though all those explanations make sense, another official who is knowledgeable about the Obama administration's regulatory practices thinks they downplay industry's role. That official spoke of two factors he felt had a major impact on the sodium effort. First, industry was more opposed to sodium limits, even if voluntary, than to food safety, school meals, and other matters because those limits could ultimately lead to requirements that would force companies to reformulate large percentages of their products. Second, and more generally, this person told me, the administration was excessively risk-averse and could have made more and faster progress on many issues.

The process to propose sodium reductions was frustratingly slow, but there was no villain or cabal that sought to undermine the FDA's effort to lower sodium consumption. Rather, it was a case of how the Washington policy-making apparatus works when it comes to anything that is complicated, controversial, and consequential. As Kass said, "It took longer than everybody wanted, but we got it done. And I think that's what's most important."[66] True, but the matter was not really "done." It took the administration so long to propose the guidelines that there was no time to finalize them, and the matter has languished for four years.

School Cafeteria Fights

One of the important battlefields in the salt wars is schools. Health advocates have long focused on the nutritional quality of school meals, because some 30 million children eat low-cost or free lunches per day, and 15 million children eat breakfast at school.[67] For decades, the meals needed improvement and updating to be consistent with the "Dietary Guidelines" as required by law. All too often they were brimming with excess calories, sodium, and saturated fat and deficient in vegetables and whole grains. Recall from chapter 2 the research indicating that higher-sodium diets in infancy and childhood lead to higher blood pressure as children grow older. Reformers hope that eating healthier meals in school would accustom children (along with their families) to eating healthier meals outside of schools, too.

Health advocates in government (especially First Lady Michelle Obama, Secretary of Agriculture Tom Vilsack, Senator Tom Harkin, and Representative Rosa DeLauro) and out (including Margo Wootan, my long-time colleague at CSPI, and the coalition of local and national nutrition organizations, National Alliance for Nutrition and Activity, that she created) waged long battles to improve school meals. Their efforts led to the passage in 2010 of the Healthy Hunger-Free Kids Act, which mandated more-nutritious school meals.[68]

In 2012, the USDA, which oversees school meals, adopted an ambitious schedule for improving them. New regulations required schools to serve more fruits, vegetables, and whole grains and to use less salt. The USDA told schools that they would have to reduce sodium levels in three stages over the next decade, with Target 1, 2, and 3 deadlines of July 1, 2014, 2017, and 2022—hardly a rushed schedule. Target 2 aimed to reduce sodium 24 percent below the 2014 level, and Target 3 aimed to cut sodium by an ambitious 48 percent below the 2014 level.[69]

Almost all schools met the relatively easy 2014 Target 1 goals, but then the school-food industry swung into action and lobbied Congress hard to block further improvements.[70]

Schwan's Company supplies about 70 percent of the pizzas—notoriously salty foods—served in K–12 schools. The company's social responsibility report states that Schwan's Food Service "works . . . to continuously improve on our great-tasting, wholesome foods for students."[71] Sadly, Schwan's was one of the companies that fought the hardest against lowering sodium levels. Considering its products, its opposition was not a great surprise.

But opposition to the cutbacks came not just from industry. The School Nutrition Association (SNA), which represents some 58,000 people who direct school-food programs and prepare those meals, took a surprising position. In keeping with its wholesome-sounding name, the group claims that its members "have been providing America's students with healthy, balanced school meals that help them succeed in the classroom and beyond."[72] In fact, until recently the SNA campaigned for healthier meals, but then it joined the opponents.

So why, you might ask, would a "nutrition association" oppose improved nutrition? The group said that many students would have scraped their less-salty meals into the garbage bins and eaten fewer cafeteria meals, reducing revenues.[73] I think, though, that it is more likely that this is an occasion to "follow the money." Around 2012, the SNA got $6.7 million, or two-thirds of its total revenue,[74] from companies that sell foods to schools: Campbell, Del Monte, Domino's Pizza, General Mills, Kellogg, Kraft Heinz, Land O' Lakes, PepsiCo, Perdue, Schwan's, Tyson, Uncle Ben's, and dozens of others.[75] (That's now down to about half its revenues.)[76] In 2012 and 2013 those commercial interests flexed their muscles and got the SNA to change its tune.[77] (One other money issue: the SNA pays its CEO, Patricia Montague, about $400,000 per year in salary and benefits.)[78]

The SNA fired its lobbyist of more than three decades, Marshall Matz of OFW Law and a long-standing and widely respected nutrition and anti-hunger advocate. In his stead, the SNA hired a major Washington lobbying firm, Barnes & Thornburg, which represents the pesticide industry, McDonald's, and Kellogg. The SNA even filed an ethics complaint, which was ultimately dismissed, with the DC Bar that could have led to the disbarment of Matz and a law partner.[79] The stunning reversal of the SNA's stance on nutrition led to a mini-revolt, with 19 former presidents of the group urging Congress to stay the course and not interfere with the USDA's plan.[80] Stanley C. Garnett, who had run the USDA's child nutrition division, said that the SNA "sold their souls to the devil."[81]

The industry forces succeeded in delaying the 2017 and 2022 sodium reductions until the matter was studied further. Congress used the appropriations process to temporarily prohibit "funds from being used to implement regulations requiring a specified reduction in sodium in federally reimbursed meals, foods, and snacks sold in schools."[82] But the SNA continued to lobby for a permanent delay to allow "school nutrition professionals to continue serving healthy, nutritious meals that students will eat."[83] They contended that meeting the tougher sodium standards would not only be expensive, but would be impossible without some kind of technological breakthrough.

Major industry players supported SNA. In a letter to USDA, 14 trade associations—from the American Association of Meat Processors to the Wheat Foods Council to SNAC International—avowed, as somberly and sincerely as a funeral director, how "it is vitally important for scientific consensus to be the basis for our US policies." They then called on USDA secretary Sonny Perdue not to require any further reductions in sodium until the NAM updated its sodium recommendations.[84] The 2019 NAM report was exactly what they said they wanted—but it recommended almost exactly the same sodium intakes as before—except *lower* ones for children 4 to 13 years old. I have not seen any indication that industry, now that it got the report it had demanded, will support to new sodium limits in school meals.

The USDA did not wait for the new NAM report, but granted the industry's wish in 2018 when it delayed the 2017 Target 2 requirements until 2024. It also eliminated the original 2022 Target 3 deadlines. The agriculture department, newly a subscriber to Orwellian phrasing, professed that it "remains committed to strong nutrition standards for school meals"[85] and that its lengthy delays actually "empowered local schools with additional options to serve healthy and appealing meals."[86] The USDA earlier said it wanted to revise its nutrition standards so as to "make school meals great again," playing off President Trump's favorite slogan. That, officials said, would prevent greater food waste by children who balked at eating more whole grains and vegetables and less-salty foods.[87] The SNA applauded the USDA for its revised rule.[88] But CSPI's Wootan said, "The Trump rollbacks are recklessly putting kids' health in jeopardy."[89]

The argument for rolling back the health-oriented rule was totally undercut by 2019 research—conducted by USDA itself.[90] The department's Food and Nutrition Service found that the initial 2014 changes led to much healthier school meals *without* increasing plate waste. But the study had no effect on the USDA's policies.

The USDA's actions appeared to be illegal and have been challenged in court. The law requires the nutritional quality of school meals to be based on the "Dietary Guidelines for Americans." It also requires the USDA to provide cogent responses to comments that people submitted in response to the proposed rule changes (96 percent of the 85,000 comments favored sticking to the original sodium restrictions). To force the USDA to reinstate the original sodium limits, in April 2019 New York State, along with California, Illinois, Minnesota, New Mexico, Vermont, and the District of Columbia, sued the USDA in federal court for not giving a rationale for ignoring the law and the outpouring of public support.[91] New York attorney general Letitia James, said, "The Trump Administration has undermined key health benefits for our children—standards for salt and whole grains in school meals—with deliberate disregard for science, expert opinion, and the law."[92]

On the same day two consumer groups, Healthy School Food Maryland and CSPI, filed a similar lawsuit.[93] One year later, in April 2020, a federal judge struck down USDA's rule, declaring that the USDA failed to allow the public notice to comment on possibly gutting the standards.[94] That decision mooted the states' lawsuit still in court.[95]

Notwithstanding the USDA's degradation of school meals, in 2020 Secretary Perdue had the chutzpah to say, "Food ought not be political. Goodness. If we can do anything in a bipartisan way it should be about feeding kids."[96]

The Trump administration's delays are one reason why many kids are still eating high-sodium Campbell soups marketed to schools.[97] On a per-cup basis, Campbell's Classic Minestrone provides 670 mg of sodium, Reserve Red Lentil Vegetable provides 890 mg, and Chunky Beef with Country Vegetables a whopping 1,520 mg. In supermarkets, Campbell's kid-oriented soups—such as Marvel Avengers soups or Disney Princess Jasmine Soup—contain no more than 480 mg per cup. (The recommended daily limit for children 4 to 8 is 1,500 mg; for children 9 to 13 it is 1,800 mg.)

Fortunately, many school districts are reducing sodium regardless of what industry's friends in Washington do. A few are meeting the Target 2 levels, but the Target 3 goals are more aspirational than realistic for now.

Tamara Yarmon is the nutrition director of Omaha Public Schools, which has more than 50,000 students. To achieve Target 2, she says that several changes have been key: cooking more foods from scratch, such as gravies, dressings, chili, and sloppy joes; buying lower-sodium breads, chicken nuggets, and other foods from local or national suppliers; offering more fresh vegetables; and having a low-sodium seasonings bar.[98]

Stephen O'Brien, Director of Strategic Partnerships and Policy for New York City's Department of Education, says that meeting the Target 2 levels is challenging because chefs and manufacturers must adjust ingredients in numerous dishes while still delivering meals that are tasty and accepted by students. But, he says, schools need to make the effort, and New York's school meals largely meet Target 2 numbers. If New York City's schools, with more than a million ethnically diverse students who have equally diverse taste preferences, can serve tasty, moderate-sodium meals, then presumably other school districts could.

The Dallas school district's executive director of food service, Michael Rosenberger, says that Dallas's meals also are close to meeting Target 2 levels. He uses as much fresh and locally grown foods as possible. But many of the foods he buys from processors or obtains through the USDA's commodities program, such as breaded chicken tenders or pizza, he says, are too high in salt.

Cities Pass Laws

Federal and state governments certainly have public support for setting nutrition requirements for schools. But getting restaurants to offer nutritious dishes is a much greater challenge. Part of the problem is that many people throw their health concerns to the wind when they eat out. That might have been okay when eating at restaurants was a special event, but now Americans get one-third of their calories at restaurants, cafeterias, and other places outside the home. The calorie labeling now required on menus and menu boards at chains with 20 or more outlets nationwide should encourage diners to think before they order. That might encourage some establishments to shrink their often humongous, high-calorie servings, simultaneously shrinking the amount of sodium, saturated fat, and sugar they contain. While sodium is not listed on menus, chain restaurants are required to provide, upon request, brochures that list all the same nutrients that are on food labels.

Many large American cities have high percentages of African Americans, and African American adults have among the highest rates of hypertension in the world—40 percent.[99] That is one of the reasons why a few cities are trying to reduce sodium consumption. First New York City in 2015 and then Philadelphia in 2018 demonstrated one way that local or state governments

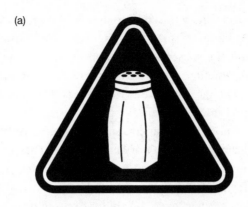

(a)

(b) **⚠ SODIUM WARNING**

Figure 9.1
Saltshaker warning icons: Sodium warnings required next to high-sodium items on menus at chain restaurants in (a) New York City and (b) Philadelphia.

could educate consumers and chain restaurants, decrease sodium intakes, and fight hypertension. Both cities require a saltshaker icon to be depicted on menus and menu boards next to any food or meal that has more than a whole day's worth of sodium—2,300 mg (see figure 9.1). Philadelphia's version also requires the words "SODIUM WARNING," printed in red or black, to the right of the icon.[100] "Heart disease and stroke are robbing too many Philadelphians of their lives and their ability to work and support their families," said Mayor Jim Kenney. "A sodium warning label gives people information they need to help keep themselves healthy."[101]

A whole day's worth of sodium is, if anything, an enormously generous threshold for triggering a warning notice. But even so, the litigious National Restaurant Association sued New York to kill the Board of Health's mandate, charging that it was "arbitrary and capricious" and "filled with irrational exclusions and nonsensical loopholes."[102] To the association's dismay, the justice presiding over the case, Eileen Rakower, upheld the saltshaker warning, saying: "Information is power." The association's lawyer, Angelo Amador, was quick to announce not only the NRA's plan to appeal but also its intention to "seek interim emergency relief" given the emergency as he saw it: "Today's decision by the court to uphold this arbitrary, onerous, and costly mandate is a blow to small business owners."[103] Now, four years after the court loss and the subsequent lost appeal,[104] I haven't heard a single word about small restaurants experiencing any harm. And that makes total sense, because only large restaurants, with at least 15 stores nationwide, are covered by the two cities' ordinances.

At least one major chain, Panera, supported New York City's warning notice. Ronald Schaich, the CEO of Panera, said, "There are a number of items on [our] menu, not a lot, that have high salt levels or that are indulgences and . . . that is OK as long as you are clear, you're making that choice, you're aware of it and you have the ability to make it on your own."[105] If only more industry officials felt that way! In response to the menu notices, Panera lowered the sodium in three items at its locations nationwide—the soup bread bowl (by 290 mg), the Bacon Turkey Bravo Sandwich (by 740 mg), and the Italian Combo Sandwich (by 630 mg).[106] But several other items, including a large Baja Mac & Cheese (2,330 mg) and Chicken Noodle Soup Bread Bowl (2,150 mg), remain sodium shockers.

A gentler approach to inform consumers and, ideally, change their behavior is a public education campaign. Policy makers often propose such campaigns because they rarely offend companies (and corporate campaign contributors). But in the face of massive advertising and tempting unhealthy foods, health education campaigns are generally expensive and ineffective. One scientific review concluded that an education campaign that included intensive counseling might have a small effect on people with hypertension, but was "unsuited" for population-wide efforts.[107]

Philadelphia's health department decided to take a different approach to education. In 2013 it started a campaign aimed not at consumers but at Chinese restaurants, which serve six million meals a year. The campaign focused on salt because Philadelphia is saddled with a higher rate of hypertension than other big cities. Its goal was to get the restaurants—where foods are generally absurdly salty—to cut the salt and monosodium glutamate (MSG), the flavor enhancer.[108] Philadelphia has over 400 independently owned Chinese restaurants, and half of them participated in the program. Temple University researchers found that after three years, 206 take-out restaurants reduced sodium by an average of 36 percent in Shrimp and Broccoli, 28 percent in Chicken Lo Mein, and 19 percent in General Tso's Chicken.[109] Overall, the participating restaurants reduced sodium by almost one-third. Restaurateurs, take notice: Grace Ma, director of the Center for Asian Health at Temple University's Lewis Katz School of Medicine, said that a taste test showed that customers could not even detect the lower sodium content.

Industry Begins to Awaken

For decades, most food manufacturers and restaurants never paid attention to the amount of salt and other sodium-containing additives they used. But especially after the United Kingdom's Food Standards Agency in the mid-2000s began pressuring companies to use less salt, many multinational companies began to realize that they needed to put that issue on their agendas. And if they were going to use less salt in the UK, some felt they should do it elsewhere. Adding to the pressure in the United States were New York City's 2009 National Salt Reduction Initiative and, especially, the call by the IOM in 2010 for mandatory limits on sodium.

ConAgra, General Mills, Kellogg, Kraft, Nestlé, and other major manufacturers began lowering sodium levels in some of their products, as did some large chain restaurants, including Arby's, Boston Market, Denny's, and McDonald's. (No data are available for independent restaurants, but I doubt that many have lowered sodium levels.) Table 9.1 shows some of the promised or actual reductions. Notwithstanding the reductions, though, many of these companies' products are still loaded with sodium.

Some of the sodium reductions have been dramatic. For instance, digging through my old files, I found that since 1978 the sodium content of Wishbone Italian Salad Dressing was reduced from 362 to 170 mg per tablespoon. Nabisco cut the sodium in Wheat Thins from 370 to 180 mg per ounce and in Cheese Nips crackers from 480 (in 1972) to 150 mg. General Mills cut the sodium in Cheerios from 330 (in 1984) to 140 mg and in Wheaties from 370 (1984) to 185 mg per ounce. Sodium in Campbell's Tomato Soup was reduced from 760 to 480 mg per cup. Since the early 1980s, Frito-Lay reduced sodium from 260 to 170 mg (35 percent) per ounce in its Lay's Classic Potato Chips. And three Hungry Jack Complete 4-inch pancakes used to have 1,150 mg, but now have only 480 mg (thanks, in part, to several potassium- and calcium-containing ingredients used in place of sodium-containing counterparts, a substitution I discuss later in this chapter). Admittedly, those are cherry-picked examples—many

Table 9.1

Company commitments to lowering sodium*

Food Manufacturers		
Company	Year	Commitments or Achievements
Barilla	2013	The company reduced salt by 11% across its portfolio.
Campbell	2010	By 2011, 71 Pepperidge Farm breads will have 25% less sodium than regular breads, rolls, bagels.
	2016	Sodium in more than 792 products has been reduced by 5–33%. Sodium in SpaghettiOs canned pastas was cut by up to 35%.
ConAgra	2013	Before 2006, sodium was cut by 20–30% in Kid Cuisine foods, 19% in the Chef Boyardee line, and up to 40% in Marie Callender's foods. Sodium was reduced in 80% of its products by 20% since 2010.
	2016	By 2016, sodium in Orville Redenbacher's Microwave Popcorn–Butter was reduced by 33%, Chef Boyardee Beef Ravioli by 34%, and Hunt's Original Diced Tomatoes by 49%.
General Mills	2016	By 2020, General Mills met its goal of 20% reductions in all of its key product categories, including breakfast cereals, frozen pizza, and baking mixes.
Heinz	2016	Between 2010 and 2014, Heinz decreased sodium 10–40% in key retail products, including a 15% reduction in ketchup.
Kellogg	2017	By 2016, sodium in breakfast cereals was reduced by an average of 33%; 84% of cereals had 150 mg or less per serving.
Kraft	2012	Sodium was reduced by an average of 10% across its portfolio by 2013.
	2014	Reductions included Kraft Original BBQ Sauce (40%), Lunchables (average of 25%), Teddy Grahams Honey Graham Snacks (25%), Oscar Mayer Beef Bologna (25%), Kraft Singles American Slices (18%).
Mars	2015	Reduced sodium by 25% globally.
Nestlé	2014	Sodium was lowered in Stouffer's Mac & Cheese by almost 15%, 12–31% in California Pizza Kitchen pizzas, in Lean Cuisine from an average of 1,000 mg (10 products in 1981) to less than 600 mg per package.
	2015	Reduce sodium by 10% across DiGiorno, Tombstone, California Pizza Kitchen, Jack's, Hot Pockets, and Lean Pockets by 2016.

Table 9.1 (continued)

Food Manufacturers

Company	Year	Commitments or Achievements
	2018	Reduce sodium by an average of at least 10% over 2017–2020 in foods that are not aligned with the WHO recommended limit of 2,000 mg per day. That is in addition to the more than 20% reductions since 2005.
Nissin	2016	Nissin reduced sodium 25% by reducing salt and eliminating MSG in Cup Noodles' most popular flavor, chicken, from 1,430 to 1,070 mg.
PepsiCo	2013	Reduced sodium in flavored potato chips by an average of about 25%.
	2016	The 2025 goal is that at least 75% of its global-foods volume will not exceed 1.3 milligrams of sodium per calorie (in 2018 58% of foods met that level). Between 2006 and 2020 the average sodium per serving in key global food brands will have been reduced by 25%.
Sara Lee	2010	Reducing sodium by an average of 20% over five years in Ball Park franks, Jimmy Dean frozen breakfast meals, Hillshire Farms lunchmeat, Sara Lee breads.
Unilever	2013	In 2013 it gradually cut sodium in some soups and other products by up to 40%.
	2018	In 2018 sodium levels in 66% of its foods (by volume) were consistent with WHO recommended intakes of 2,000 mg per day.
Walmart	2011–2016	From 2011 to 2015 Walmart cut sodium in its private-label foods by 18% (shy of its 25% goal). A new goal set in 2016 was to reduce sodium by another 20%.

Restaurants

Company	Year	Commitments or Achievements
Boston Market	2010	Sodium in poultry gravy cut by 50%; reduced sodium in "fresh, all-natural chicken" and stuffing by 20% and mashed potatoes by 26%. Customers did not notice any difference.
	2012	Will reduce sodium by 15% menu-wide by the end of 2014.
Burger King	2008	Limited sodium in kids meals to 600 mg.
	2010	Reduced sodium in ketchup (25%), ham (40%), Chicken Tenders (30%).

Table 9.1 (continued)

Restaurants

Company	Year	Commitments or Achievements
Darden (Olive Garden, LongHorn Steakhouse, other restaurants)	2016	A 2011 commitment to reduce sodium company-wide by 10% over 10 years blossomed into a 19% reduction by 2016.
McDonald's	2012	Reduced sodium in Grilled Chicken patty by 45%, Crispy Chicken patty by 50%, across product line by 11%. Its 2012 goal was to reduce sodium by an average of 15% across nationally available foods by 2015.
Sodexo (food service management)	2011	Reduce average sodium content in top 100 recipes by 25% over the next two years and by 50% over the next five years. Company has nutrition standards intended to lower sodium.
Subway	2013	Eight Fresh Fit 6-inch sandwiches that had more than 1,000 mg of sodium were reduced by an average of 32%.
Taco Bell	2017	An overall 15% sodium reduction since 2008, including 32% less in chicken, 6% less in ground beef, 12% less in steak, and 50% in sauces. Taco Bell is aiming for a 25% reduction across its menu by 2025.

*Information gathered from company reports and news articles without third-party verification.

products had the same sodium levels over the decades, and a few even had more sodium—but it is nice to see some major reductions.

Walmart, the supermarket behemoth, might have made a bigger dent in the salt problem than any other company—or than all other companies. In 2011, as part of a broader nutrition program, Walmart said it would reduce sodium in its house brand by 25 percent by 2015[110] and press national brands to do the same. It did not quite reach that goal, but the 18 percent reduction in four years was still impressive.[111] Sam Kass, who negotiated with Walmart for months to get strong commitments, told me in 2019, "in terms of what's actually so far taken out, more sodium, there's no question that the Walmart agreement did more for that than the FDA has at this point."[112]

Looking more broadly at the food supply, several studies have measured changes in sodium levels. In one, researchers did not find any change in sodium consumption, be it from foods prepared at home or outside the home, between 1999 and 2012.[113] More recently, the USDA and CDC started a Sentinel Foods Surveillance Program, which examined a large and diverse group of processed and restaurant foods.[114] They reviewed labels and conducted laboratory tests to identify changes over roughly a four-year period. Based on the labels, sodium changed in one-third of the products, with about twice as many decreases as increases. The researchers said that some of the decreases were likely due to the use of potassium salts, such as in refrigerated biscuit dough. I have more to say about potassium later in this chapter.

The biggest study, and the one with the most optimistic results, looked at the sodium content of packaged (but not restaurant) foods between 2000 and 2014. Based on the purchases by 172,000 households at grocery stores, the sodium "density"—the amount of sodium per 100 grams (3.5 ounces) of food—declined by 12 percent over those 15 years.[115] That decline has not yet been reflected in the National Health and Nutrition Examination Survey (NHANES). Despite their welcome finding, the researchers cautioned: "The slow rate of decline in sodium from store-bought foods suggests that more concerted sodium reduction efforts are necessary." With sodium declining at the glacial pace of less than 1 percent per year, it would take several decades to reach the goal of 2,300 mg per person per day.

Progress has been even slower—or nonexistent—in restaurants. Researchers at Boston University and Tufts University found that fast-food meals have become less healthful over the years. Over a 30-year period, between 1986 and 2016, the sodium content of entrées and desserts at 10 major fast-food chains increased by almost one-third and of side dishes by an astonishing 82 percent.[116] (Portion sizes and calorie counts generally increased, too.) Another study reported that the average sodium content of menu items at large chain restaurants did not change at all between 2012 and 2016.[117] The one glimmer of hope was that items newly introduced in 2016—except for entrées at fast-food restaurants—were slightly lower in sodium than items that had been eliminated after 2012. A huge limitation of those two studies is that sodium levels were not sales weighted. That is, it would make a big difference if a new, lower-sodium (or higher-sodium) item were a huge sales success at a large chain or a poor-selling item at a smaller chain.

Clearly, the restaurant industry and foodservice operators more generally need a good kick in the pants. One group that is trying to make a difference is the Culinary Institute of America (CIA), one of the nation's leading culinary schools. It has co-sponsored annual Menus of Change conferences with the Harvard T.H. Chan School of Public Health.[118] Their goal is to encourage individual chefs, large restaurant companies, hotels, airlines, and other institutions to provide healthier meals and options that are plant based. The CIA and Harvard speakers give great health and culinary advice to companies whose meals reach millions of mouths.

The CIA recognizes that adding a little bit of salt can intensify the flavors of many meals, but decries "that the foodservice and food manufacturing sectors have long been too reliant on salt to do the heavy lifting to create high flavor impact and customer satisfaction." Its informative (and beautifully designed) Menus of Change annual reports note that a single sandwich or entrée might contain more than a whole day's worth of sodium. But occasionally even the CIA drops the ball. The same website that says "it's possible to create flavorful dishes without adding a lot of salt or using high-sodium ingredients" also has recipes for several foods, such as Vietnamese Summer Rolls and Moroccan Chicken Pita Sandwiches, that are loaded with salt.[119]

Supermarkets could play a more significant role in helping their customers improve their diets. For one thing, most supermarkets carry house brand packaged foods. Those foods usually mimic the national brands as closely as possible in terms of taste and nutrition, but the stores could tell their house-brand suppliers to nudge sodium levels downward. They also should sell lower-sodium products at the same price as the standard ones. I discovered that a large Midwestern supermarket chain was selling lower-sodium condensed Tomato and Cream of Mushroom soups for $1.19 per can compared to $0.79 for the regular soups—a 50 percent premium.[120]

Corporate Salt-Cutting Techniques

Cutting salt is not brain surgery. The simplest way to lower sodium levels is to simply use less salt. In one experiment, researchers lowered the salt content of bread by 5 percent each week for a 25 percent total reduction without any decrease in participant acceptance.[121] In another taste test, the salt content of chili was lowered by 40 percent without a reduction in acceptance.[122] Cutting substantial percentages of sodium in processed meats and certain soups had no effect on acceptability either.[123] It is simply a myth that cutting salt would inevitably cut taste.

Outside the academic testing lab, some manufacturers and restaurants have realized they were using unnecessarily large amounts of salt and that reducing salt modestly had no effect on taste or acceptance. Consumers often don't notice modest reductions of 10 to 25 percent even if they result in a slightly less-salty taste.

Makers of crackers have found a nice trick for lowering sodium while maintaining acceptance. They simply salt just one side of the crackers. Obviously, that tactic won't work in soups or stews.

An easy way for restaurants to reduce sodium (and help our waistlines), without affecting taste one whit, would be to reduce their humongous serving sizes. At a restaurant like Denny's or IHOP, a single meal could involve chewing through two pounds of food. Executives at one large chain, though, told me that some long-time customers rebel when served meals that are just 5 or 10 percent smaller.

Another low-tech way to reduce sodium is to use salt crystals with a modified shape or size. One such salt is Cargill's Diamond Crystal Kosher Salt. It is made by a method called the Alberger process, which results in pyramid-shaped hollow crystals. Salt processed that way provides the usual salty taste, but it lacks some of the "useless" salt in the middle of the crystals that may never touch the tongue when used on potato chips, French fries, nuts, pretzels, and other foods where much of the salt sits on the surface. A given volume of Diamond Crystal Kosher Salt has half as much sodium as regular table salt and 40 percent less than Morton's Kosher Salt.

Martin Breslin directs the culinary services at Harvard University, which serves 25,000 meals a day. He swears by Diamond Crystal Kosher Salt as a great way to cut sodium. He was able to cut the sodium in many of his 7,000 recipes simply by switching from regular salt or regular kosher salt to Diamond Crystal's salt and using the same number of teaspoons or tablespoons. Despite the lower sodium levels and less-salty taste, Breslin did not receive any complaints from students and other diners. He estimates that that one simple step cut sodium levels almost across the board by about 30 percent.[124] (Changing the ingredient was easier than rewriting the recipes with half as much regular salt.) He also worked with local bakers and suppliers of deli meats, Indian dishes, and sauces to reduce sodium levels in their products.[125] In some cases, those companies switched to the lower-sodium recipes not only for Harvard, but for all their customers.

Another special kind of salt consists of microscopic crystals that are up to one one-hundredth the size of regular crystals. They deliver an intense burst of saltiness to taste buds. Manufacturers claim that their "micro" salt (such as SodaLo) can cut sodium by 25 to 50 percent in bread, cheese, sausage, potato chips, and other foods.[126] One thing I've found, though, is that while makers of salt substitutes ballyhoo their products, food manufacturers sometimes discover that they simply don't work as promised.

Compass Group, which serves nine million meals a day at university, corporate, and other cafeterias throughout much of the world, has been at the forefront of providing healthier meals that also protect the environment. Deanne Brandstetter, the company's vice-president of nutrition and wellness, described her company's starting point: "Our first strategy for reducing sodium in our menu offerings should be reducing some of our portion size[s]. Research shows the more calories you consume, the more sodium you consume. Many of our portions offer too many calories as well as too much sodium."[127]

Morrison Healthcare, a division of Compass Group, operates the foodservices in more than 650 hospitals and healthcare systems. It has worked with suppliers to obtain sodium reductions ranging from 10 percent in dressings to 49 percent in roast turkey. It has used thinner sandwich buns, cutting the calories and sodium in half. Morrison also has a "Great Living" menu for patients that cuts sodium almost in half—from 4,500 to 2,300 mg per day.[128] Reducing sodium requires careful work by chefs, but there's no reason that every cafeteria and restaurant could not make similar reductions.

Norbert Bomm, Corporate Executive Chef for R&D at Morrison Healthcare, has his own palette of approaches for reducing sodium.[129] He says the biggest impact came from using no-salt-added canned tomatoes and flavoring them with McCormick's salt-free seasonings, which he called "absolutely mind-blowing." He uses pureed black beans and white beans in soups. More generally, he uses local, seasonal, fresh fruits and vegetables wherever possible and prepares more foods in-house instead of relying on outside suppliers.

Food marketers typically like to reduce sodium quietly instead of bragging about it on the fronts of labels or restaurant menus, because they think consumers believe that "less salt" means "less taste." As former Unilever scientist Doug Balentine (now Senior Science Advisor for Global Nutrition Policy at the FDA) told the *Wall Street Journal*, "Once you start saying you've taken salt down, it's basically equal to, 'it's not going to taste good.'"[130] Hence, companies prefer to make "stealth" reductions in salt. I'm hopeful that the public's attitude will change to "that's terrific" as people recognize the harmfulness of high-sodium foods and the tastiness of lower-sodium foods.

In most cases, *how* companies adjust their recipes to lower sodium are usually deep, dark secrets. But Heinz's British division lifted the veil of secrecy regarding some of its recipe changes. Tristan Robinson, then the company's nutritionist, said that Heinz worked hard to meet the UK government's expectations for lower-sodium products.[131] For example, the company markets Pasta Shapes in Tomato Sauce for young children. Because those children's taste buds had been shaped by no-salt-added toddler foods, Heinz simply eliminated about 60 percent of the salt. No other changes were necessary, and kids apparently were no less happy with the less-salty product.

In other cases, Heinz had to reformulate in ways that compensated for the reduced salt. To offset the elimination of MSG and one-fourth of the salt in its traditional Cream of Chicken Soup, the corporate chefs needed to add 40 percent more chicken. They were able to chop the sodium content of its Cream of Tomato Soup in half and use less oil and sugar by adding at least 12 percent more tomatoes. And to cut almost half the sodium from its Big Soup Chicken & Vegetables, the chefs used less salt, dropped the MSG, and added 28 percent more chicken and 5 percent more vegetables. Such changes might increase costs and the prices consumers pay a bit, but few consumers would complain about getting more chicken and vegetables and less salt and MSG.

In the mid-2000s the food conglomerate ConAgra Foods made serious efforts to lower sodium levels. Pat Verduin, who led Product Quality & Development for the company, told me recently, "For a product line like Marie Callender's, we were able to reduce salt levels with little impact on the flavor. In other product lines, we had to make more significant formula adjustments to reduce salt and match the flavor expectations of our consumers."[132] The company also made major reductions in Kid Cuisine, Chef Boyardee, and other lines. Besides just using less salt, ConAgra adjusted spice levels, added potassium salt, and employed natural sodium enhancers.

Revolution Foods, the school-cafeteria operator, has huge experience in satisfying some of the most vocal critics—kids. Unlike food manufacturers and restaurants, companies that provide school meals are required to meet the USDA's nutrition standards. Cliff Lyles, Revolution's executive chef, starts modifying recipes simply by reducing the salt content until a taste panel of kids says that a food tastes bland. To further cut the sodium he will add ingredients that provide a "sense of salt without having salt." Those may include vegetable concentrates, onions, carrots and other root vegetables, herbs, spices, and sharp cheeses—ingredients that give meals a "heartier, richer, full-flavor profile that helps eliminate the need for salt." Lemon and lime juices (and citric acid) work well for spicy, lower-salt dishes such as Cilantro Lime Rice, Orange Chicken, and Chile Verde. Revolution has not yet used potassium salt to cut the salt.[133] (In my conversations with chefs, few were even aware they could use potassium salt to reduce sodium.)

Researchers have long maintained that children who get accustomed to a modest reduction of saltiness are more willing to accept another reduction. But Lyles says that taste buds have strong expectations when it comes to such familiar foods as hot dogs, hamburgers, and chicken noodle soup. Those are the toughest foods in which to reduce salt. As Campbell has done, foodservice chefs overcome the problem by creating whole new lower-sodium recipes.

Even a prison system is using some of the same culinary devices. Deserae, the lead cook and an inmate at the Coffee Creek Correctional Facility in Wilsonville, Oregon, says that using flavorful fresh vegetables is one of her major ways of reducing sodium and creating appealing meals.[134] Oregon prisons have also switched to beef and chicken soup bases that are 89 percent lower in sodium.[135] The Oregon Department of Corrections says that such measures led to a 17 percent reduction in sodium consumption.

Those of us looking to rely less on processed foods can use many of the same salt-reducing tricks in our homes that companies, and an occasional prison, use. I'll expand on that in chapter 11.

Taste and Taste Perception: Lessons from Campbell Soup

In some cases, reducing sodium may require some sophisticated culinary substitutions, and major companies need to move cautiously. Campbell Soup Company's former director of research and development, Lisa

Thorsten, notes that salt affects all five dimensions of taste—salty, sweet, bitter, sour, and umami (savory or meaty tasting). Removing too much salt can result in unpleasant-tasting or bland foods unless other ingredients can be adjusted to compensate, whether by boosting the perception of saltiness or enhancing other taste perceptions that depend on an interaction with salt. Company chefs then need to experiment, such as by adding herbs and spices, natural or artificial flavorings, or roasted instead of boiled ingredients—all of which may increase costs. At home, it's easy for a disappointed cook to suffer through, or toss, a lousy-tasting meal. The stakes are far higher for companies churning out millions of packages of food a year.

In the 1980s and 1990s, Campbell was one of the only companies that invested in research to lower sodium levels. Thorsten told me that lowering sodium is "in the DNA" of Campbell's R&D and marketing departments.[136] Sodium was probably so much on Campbell's mind because so many of its soups were so high in salt and used as "don't eat" examples by nutritionists. A typical cup of soup contains about five times as much sodium as an ounce of potato chips. One obvious reason for that difference relates to portion size: it takes a lot more salt to season an eight-ounce serving of soup than a one-ounce serving of chips.

Over the years, Campbell lowered sodium in products ranging from "red-label" condensed soups to V8 juice to SpaghettiOs. When Bonnie Liebman, Greg Moyer, and I wrote *Salt: The Brand Name Guide to Sodium Content* in 1983, Campbell soups typically contained around 1,000 mg of sodium per cup.[137] In 2008, with much fanfare, Campbell announced it was reducing the sodium in 36 Select Harvest soups and a dozen "kid favorites" from an average of 700 to 800 mg per cup to 480 mg. Douglas R. Conant, Campbell's President and Chief Executive Officer, said,

> This is another significant step in our leadership in sodium reduction. Our lower sodium products continue to outperform expectations . . . but we will not rest here. Our journey to lower sodium across Campbell's portfolio will continue with the goal of making soup the ultimate healthy simple meal.[138]

But then the roof caved in. Thorsten said, "Almost the moment the Select Harvest products hit store shelves, the phone started ringing." The consumers were "crazy angry and disappointed," describing the new taste as "bland" and "like dishwater." Sales sunk, and so did the company's commitment. The cause of the debacle, according to Thorsten, was that in its rush to lower sodium levels Campbell failed to do taste testing with existing consumers of the soups.

Unfortunately, Campbell didn't just "rest here," but reversed course. In 2011, the company boosted the sodium in Select Harvest soups back up to about 650 mg per cup.[139] The CEO-elect (and now the former CEO) Denise Morrison, who had made the original call to cut sodium to 480 mg, explained that Campbell wanted to give consumers more choice by increasing the sodium content. In reality, that gave consumers *less* choice because people can add salt to their foods, but they cannot take it out. Instead of continuing to focus on "sodium innovation," Campbell said it would shift to taste-oriented innovation." A few years later it threw in the towel on the Select Harvest line, though some lower-sodium flavors were reincarnated as Homestyle or Healthy Request soups.[140]

It is possible that taste was not the only problem with Campbell's soups, but also consumers' *perception* of taste. In one investigation, which supported Balentine's observation, declaring "Now Reduced Salt" on the front label led a taste panel of consumers to believe that the soups would not taste as good as soups without the label.[141] If Campbell had alerted consumers to the change so that they would expect a different flavor from the one they had before, Thorsten said, perhaps consumers would have been more accepting of the change in order to obtain the benefits of the lower sodium content.

Fortunately, the Campbell story did not end with Select Harvest. In 2018 the company's vice president for research and development, nutritionist Joshua Anthony, emphasized that Campbell recognized the importance of lowering sodium, but also that "taste is still king." The company could not force people to consume healthier products that did not taste good. Still, he reported that between 2009 and 2017 the percentage of Campbell's products with 480 mg or less of sodium per serving jumped from 45 percent to 71 percent.[142] He explained that reducing sodium was hardest in the traditional red-label condensed soups, because consumers have such strong taste expectations based on years or decades of experience. Chicken Noodle soup, in particular, which has few ingredients and is watery, is an especially tough case. It was easier to develop new products, including ready-to-eat soups (such as Lightly Salted Santa Fe Vegetable Soup), so the company could gradually create new, less-salty norms.

To help Campbell and other food manufacturers use less salt and avoid sales debacles, and to help home cooks too, it would be great to have safe and tasty salt substitutes that performed some or all of the technical functions of salt, such as preservation and texture. Sprinkling such substitutes into our food, analogous to using non-caloric sweeteners like aspartame and stevia, could be a big help in lowering sodium consumption. To understand why ideal salt substitutes have never been found, let's visit our taste buds.

The largely plant-based diet our ancestors consumed tens of thousands of years ago was extremely low in sodium. But sodium is absolutely essential for life. So evolution probably favored the development of a pleasant sensation when animals ingested salty foods, as well as a hormonal means of retaining the necessary amount of sodium in the body. Babies begin to develop a taste for salt at around three months.[143] We may be hard-wired from a very young age to crave salt, but that doesn't mean that we are condemned to eat dangerously salty diets. In fact, people can easily adjust to foods containing moderately less sodium over two or three months.[144] After that, conventionally salted foods often taste too salty.

Surprisingly, given our vast scientific knowledge about the workings of the human body, just how our tongues perceive salt is complicated and still poorly understood. Taste buds scattered around our tongue and on our palate contain taste cells that detect substances that convey the five basic tastes. The primary way we detect salt involves a sodium receptor located on the surface of taste cells. That receptor is known as ENaC, which stands for epithelial sodium channel (Na is the symbol for sodium). When those taste cells are stimulated by sodium ions in foods and beverages, nerve cells at the base of the cells are activated and carry a signal to larger nerves and then to the brain, which registers the salty taste.

But the sense of taste is more complicated than just stimulation of ENaC. In animal studies, researchers blocked the ENaC taste cells, but the animals still detected salt.[145] That indicated that animals have other means of tasting sodium chloride, as well as potassium chloride and other salts. Some researchers hypothesize that low levels of sodium (and potassium) activate other taste cells and trigger a pleasant taste sensation—but high concentrations of sodium (and moderate and high levels of potassium) are perceived as tasting *unpleasant* or even repulsive. Some research suggests that that mechanism involves taste cells that also detect sour and bitter foods. But Gary Beauchamp, Emeritus Director and President of the Monell Chemical Senses Center, warns that human taste buds may be very different from those in animals—for instance, cats do not even have any functional taste receptors for sweetness—and that a lot more research needs to be done to truly understand how we detect a salty taste.

Because the ENaC channel is highly specific to tiny sodium ions, researchers doubt that they will find any other safe atom, ion, or molecule that would taste just like salt. Lithium, which has been used at low levels for more than half a century to treat bipolar disorders, was a possibility because it is even smaller than sodium. It tastes perfectly salty—but is toxic at levels only slightly higher than the therapeutic doses.[146] Potassium ions are a little larger than sodium ions, have a somewhat salty taste, and may be the closest we get to a versatile, inexpensive salt substitute.

Potassium Salt and Other Tricks of the Lower-Sodium Trade

If you remember the periodic table from Chemistry 101, you might recall that potassium falls right under sodium. The similarities between the two atoms indicate why potassium and sodium share some of the same qualities. As I have suggested earlier, potassium chloride, or potassium salt, as it is increasingly called, is the best partial substitute for sodium chloride.

Potassium-rich substances have a long, if accidental, history of use as a seasoning. Some hunter-gatherer tribes around the world have used the ashes from burnt plants as a condiment.[147] The ashes contain several hundred times more potassium than they do sodium, and the urine of members of the tribes that use "culinary ashes" contains far more potassium than sodium. Our Paleolithic ancestors probably consumed around 10,000 mg of potassium per day, several times as much as Americans consume, indicating that it is safe to eat.

A physician with the World Health Organization (WHO) studied two tribes that lived in the Amazon basin of Brazil. The Mundurucú were the more acculturated of the two and their blood pressure rose with age, similar to most people in modern cultures. That may have been, in part, because they used salt as a condiment, whereas the other tribe, the Carajá, whose blood pressure did not rise with age, used potassium-rich plant ashes.[148]

Far from the Brazilian rainforests, some food manufacturers use potassium chloride (also called potassium salt) to replace one-fourth to one-half of regular salt, depending on the food. Not only does that cut the sodium, but it adds potassium, an essential nutrient that counteracts the effects of excess sodium in the body. Manufacturers buy the potassium salt and mix it in whatever proportion they want with regular salt and other ingredients.

NuTek Food Science, a small company based in Omaha, Nebraska, is the only marketer of potassium salt I know of that is a real crusader for reducing sodium consumption. It markets potassium salt, its sole product, mostly to manufacturers (Salt for Life is its consumer version). NuTek told the FDA in 2016 that its potassium salt helped companies lower sodium by an average of 34 percent in 19 different foods, from American cheese to hot dogs to white bread.[149] All those foods were either being marketed or ready to launch. Significantly, 17 of those 19 foods met the FDA's 2-year sodium targets, and 12 of the 19 even met the FDA's 10-year targets. Clearly, potassium salt could play an important role in reducing sodium consumption.

One prominent example of the nutritional benefits of using potassium salt is obvious in the marketplace. Tomato soup, Campbell's second most popular soup—with sales of 85 million cans each year[150]—is one of the company's lowest-sodium condensed soups, with 480 mg per cup. Other condensed soups average around 800 mg. Tomato soup's ingredients include both potassium salt and regular salt.

If potassium salt is such a great substitute for some of the table salt in foods, one might ask why it is not more widely used. The ingredient has two noteworthy limitations: The first is taste—it is somewhat less salty than regular salt, and it has a strong, unpleasant metallic taste when too much is used. But companies are discovering that they can use an amount that contributes to a salty taste and doesn't impair a food's flavor. Second, potassium chloride costs at least five times as much as table salt. That sounds like a lot, but on a per-serving or per-package basis, the extra cost is trivial. NuTek says that it would cost less than one extra penny to season a large, 13-ounce bag of potato chips that costs around three or four dollars. There's another reason that limits the use of potassium salt, though, and that is inertia: it is both a nuisance and an expense for companies to test different amounts of potassium salt in various products and perhaps adjust the amounts of other ingredients.

But Brian Boor, NuTek's chief strategy officer, offers a different explanation for many companies' disinterest in using potassium salt. Boor, who travels the world talking to large manufacturers and chain restaurants, believes that the greatest impediment to wider use of potassium chloride is the "clean label" movement.[151] Under pressure from consumers wanting foods made without additives, companies have been replacing ingredients that have chemical-sounding names and shortening their ingredient lists. Adding something that smacks of being a "chemical"—which potassium chloride is, of course—is the last thing most companies want to do. Also, some people might associate potassium chloride with chlorine bleach, or even with chlorine gas, which was used as a chemical weapon in World War I. Campbell Soup's Joshua Anthony has echoed Boor's concern, saying that the public's chemophobia was one of the things that made it difficult to replace some of the sodium chloride, which, of course, is also a chemical. (Chemophobia can't be too powerful a deterrent, though, because Campbell is using potassium chloride in a variety of soups, presumably without affecting sales, and a growing number of companies are doing the same.)

To reduce the clean-label problem, in 2016 NuTek petitioned the FDA (and foreign governments) to allow potassium chloride to be listed on food labels as "potassium salt." Mars, Nestlé, Unilever, Campbell, Walmart, GMA, the city of Philadelphia, the Academy of Nutrition and Dietetics, CSPI, and many others supported that petition.[152] Not surprisingly, the since-shuttered Salt Institute came out squarely against it, charging that allowing potassium chloride to be labeled as potassium salt would lead to "consumer confusion" and was illegal.[153] That opposition was a bit ironic, because the major salt manufacturers, all members of the Salt Institute, also market potassium salt.

In 2019 the FDA responded to NuTek's petition by proposing a synonym for potassium chloride—not "potassium salt" but "potassium chloride salt." That was bureaucracy in action.[154] Never mind that no one has heard of the term—it does not address the "clean label" problem. The food industry, CSPI, and others argued that allowing "potassium chloride salt" would not encourage companies to use potassium chloride. As of spring 2020, the FDA had not decided what to call it.

To see the potential impact of salt substitutes on nutritional values, I reviewed the sodium and potassium levels in three categories of food in which some brands contained, and others did not contain, potassium chloride.[155] This is what I found:

- Ready-to-serve soups: 154 soups containing potassium chloride averaged 18 percent less sodium and 92 percent more potassium than 229 soups without it.

- Condensed soups: 129 varieties made with potassium chloride had 34 percent less sodium and 240 percent more potassium than 190 varieties without it.

- Microwave popcorns: the 63 products with potassium chloride averaged 23 percent less sodium and 139 percent more potassium than 94 varieties without it.

Some of the manufacturers undoubtedly made other changes in their recipes when they added potassium chloride and subtracted regular salt, such as adding more vegetables, sugar, or flavorings. But the use of potassium chloride probably deserves much of the credit for the lower sodium levels and certainly for the higher potassium levels. In some food categories, companies might be replacing not salt, but ingredients like sodium bicarbonate or monosodium glutamate with their potassium counterparts.

Increasing potassium consumption is an unadulterated benefit for healthy adults. The FDA considers potassium chloride "generally recognized as safe" and permits it to be used without limit in any food.[156] At least in people with hypertension, higher potassium intakes reduce blood pressure, as I discussed in chapter 2.[157] Numerous studies also found an association between increased potassium and fewer strokes,[158] although the NAM's 2019 recommendations on sodium and potassium intakes did not consider them to be of high enough quality to say definitively that their findings were correct.[159]

While potassium is beneficial or innocuous to the great majority of people, too much of that nutrient—from salt substitutes or from bananas, beans, potatoes, and other foods naturally rich in potassium—can endanger certain people. Most prominently, that includes people with advanced chronic kidney disease (CKD), who are not able to excrete excess potassium. That leads to increased potassium in blood, or hyperkalemia, which can cause an irregular heartbeat or a heart attack. Patients with CKD represent under 0.5 percent of adults.[160] In addition, people taking certain antihypertensive drugs, including potassium-sparing diuretics, ACE inhibitors, and ARBs, need to guard against excess potassium. Those people need to talk with their physician or other healthcare provider about their diets.

A recent computer-modeling study of the health impact if the entire Chinese population used potassium-enriched salt at home provided reassuring news.[161] An international team of cardiovascular disease experts estimated that replacing 20–30 percent of salt with potassium salt would yield huge benefits: 460,000 fewer deaths each year, or one in nine deaths from cardiovascular disease. Even among CKD patients, three lives would be saved due to lower blood pressure for every life lost due to higher potassium intake and hyperkalemia.

In any case, sticking to a safe diet in the United States just became easier for CKD patients now that potassium is listed on Nutrition Facts labels. (The new labels also may encourage some companies to use potassium salt because they could tout the higher potassium content.)

If potassium salt became widely used as a salt substitute, health officials definitely would have to monitor for any harm to consumers.[162] If problems were discovered, the FDA might have to set limits on the substance's use or require a warning notice. But even if potassium salt replaced as much as one-fourth of the regular salt added to processed and restaurant foods, an unrealistic assumption at least in the short run, that would boost average potassium intake only from 2,800 mg to 3,500 mg per day. That is just a bit over the 3,400 mg that the NAM committee said in 2019 is an Adequate Intake for healthy men and somewhat over the 2,600-mg Adequate Intake set for women. The potassium statement on Nutrition Facts labels is currently based on a Daily Value of 4,700 mg per day, the NAM's previous recommended daily intake. Healthy people do not have to worry about consuming too much potassium.

Besides potassium salt, several substances that do not contain potassium also may serve as salt enhancers and allow companies to use less salt.[163] They include such flavor enhancers as MSG (the infamous but poorly substantiated cause of headaches or skin flushing that some people complain about after eating at a Chinese restaurant), hydrolyzed vegetable protein, yeast extracts, the nucleotides 5-IMP and 5-GMP, and the amino acid arginine. Those ingredients do not necessarily taste salty but can bring out some of the tastes that salt brings out, including umami. All those substances are much more expensive than regular salt and potassium salt.

A very different approach for reducing salt would be to find substances that make salt taste saltier. A company in California, Senomyx, is trying to do just that. Senomyx, now part of a larger Swiss firm, develops substances that increase the sensitivity of taste buds or that provide a strong flavor punch of their own. It already markets ingredients that make sweetness-detecting taste buds more sensitive to sugar, thereby allowing manufacturers to use less of it. It also found two substances that it says can reduce or eliminate MSG.[164] But so far, despite years of trying, Senomyx has not found substances that sensitize the taste buds that trigger the "salty" sensation in our brains and would enable companies to use less salt.[165] A safe and effective product could be the holy grail of sodium reduction, but don't expect such ingredients to be discovered for many years, if ever.

Instead of counting on an unlikely technological or culinary breakthrough—or a sudden, increased consumer responsiveness to "cut the salt" campaigns—to bring about population-wide reductions in sodium consumption, in the next chapter I will offer some recommendations for national policies that could reduce sodium right now.

10   Action Plan for Better Health

The best way to proceed is to start with a voluntary salt reduction policy with the threat of regulation/legislation.

—Feng J. He and colleagues, *Journal of Human Hypertension*, 2014[1]

The scientific evidence is crystal clear that lowering sodium consumption greatly improves health. That is something that almost all experts agree on—indeed, have agreed on for many years. And there is widespread recognition that lowering sodium would save tens of thousands of lives, along with many billions of healthcare dollars, per year.

Health officials traditionally placed their sodium-lowering bets on conducting weak, brief education campaigns to encourage consumers to choose less-salty foods. Such efforts convey an impression of promoting health, but at the same time do not offend industry. But that approach proved a dismal failure in reducing average sodium intakes, even after Nutrition Facts labels provided information on all packaged (though not restaurant) foods. More effective measures were needed, namely sodium reductions by food manufacturers and restaurants to make "the healthy way the easy way" for consumers.

The World Health Organization (WHO) and the governments of the United Kingdom, Chile, Canada, Turkey, South Africa, and elsewhere are increasingly placing their bets on pressing the food industry to cut the salt. Some companies have responded positively by using less salt and more vegetables, fragrant spices, or potassium-containing salt substitutes, as I explained in chapter 9. Progress can be accelerated by setting mandatory, not voluntary, limits on sodium in major sources of sodium or requiring warning notices on high-sodium foods.

Progress has been slow in the United States, but the US Food and Drug Administration (FDA) has laid the groundwork for significant progress by proposing voluntary sodium targets for companies to reach within 2 years and 10 years. If and when those targets are finalized, the FDA should not expect that all companies would quickly lower sodium levels. Based on his experience in the United Kingdom, professor and advocate Graham A. MacGregor emphasizes the importance of having health officials maintain strong pressure on industry to reformulate their foods, including the use of the bully pulpit.[2] And simultaneously, he says, the agencies also should be open to valid industry arguments that certain goals are impractical or might introduce food-safety risks.

Because the FDA commissioner is too busy to focus full-time on this one issue, the *FDA should appoint a "Salt Czar" who would use the agency's bully pulpit* to exhort companies to decrease sodium levels in their products. That person, along with other FDA staff, would have to have many meetings with companies and trade associations over a long period of time to emphasize the huge health benefits that would be obtained by reducing sodium and to persuade them to cooperate. The Salt Czar should publicly applaud companies both big and small that reached or did better than the targets— and do some public naming and shaming to let the laggards, and the public, know how serious the agency was about sodium reduction. With the support of staff members the Salt Czar could provide technical assistance to companies (especially smaller ones) having a hard time lowering sodium, and could revise targets that were unrealistically ambitious.

The FDA should have a robust program for periodically *monitoring sodium levels* in the overall food supply and in the categories of foods subject to its targets. It would have to determine the sales-weighted average sodium content in each of the 150+ food categories. It also would need to identify how many (and which) individual foods exceeded the "upper-bound" (maximum) sodium targets for each category. Journalists and health groups should do the same to keep companies' feet to the fire.

Meanwhile, the Centers for Disease Control and Prevention will be conducting its ongoing National Health and Nutrition Examination Surveys (NHANES), which would provide the data to determine whether the sodium targets actually led to lower consumption. Though analyzing those surveys takes a year or more, they are essential to evaluating the effort and suggesting possible improvements.

But what if companies don't even achieve the eminently achievable two-year targets? In that case, the FDA, or Congress, could impose incentives that would encourage compliance. The Institute of Medicine (IOM), now the National Academy of Medicine, suggested in 2010 that special "informational label" notices could be used to encourage companies to lower sodium.[3] One approach would be to *require products that exceeded the upper-bound targets to bear a label notice* stating, "FDA Notice: The sodium content of this food exceeds the FDA's recommended limit."

The FDA—and, for meat and poultry products, the US Department of Agriculture—could adopt a broader labeling program that would *require bold front-of-package warning notices on foods high in sodium*, as well as on foods high in calories, added sugars, and saturated fat. Such labels are being used and appear to be effective in Chile, with several other countries requiring similar labels.

Labeling could be extended to restaurants by *requiring saltshaker icons on menus* of chain restaurants for items that contain more than a certain amount of sodium, as New York City and Philadelphia require. Instead of waiting for federal action, local and state agencies could require such notices.

The 2010 IOM committee recommended mandatory national standards for the sodium content of foods. If industry was clearly not meeting the FDA's sodium targets, the FDA could *make the upper-bound targets mandatory instead of voluntary*. Such a requirement, which would affect only the saltiest foods, could be for all food categories or only certain major sources of sodium, such as bread, pizza, processed meats, sandwiches, and soups. Industry would fiercely oppose that measure and warning labels.

A major defect in the FDA's plan is that the timeframe is far too protracted and does not include enough periodic step-downs in sodium. The plan would leave 8 years between the deadlines for the 2-year and 10-year targets. Without the pressure of targets that became progressively more stringent every one to four years (as in the United Kingdom, South Africa, Chile, and National Salt Reduction Initiative), sodium reduction almost certainly would drop off the FDA's and industry's agendas.[4] The IOM suggested tightening the targets every three years. Hence, the FDA should *issue an intermediate set of targets* set halfway between the 2- and 10-year levels; such 6-year targets would keep the pressure on companies to reformulate their products (or drop some of their saltiest products), while still providing time for the FDA to evaluate the progress in reducing sodium intakes and make necessary adjustments for the next deadline.

Potassium chloride could replace about one-fourth of salt in many foods, but some companies fear that consumers perceive that ingredient as a "chemical" to avoid. To facilitate the use of that ingredient, the FDA should *allow potassium chloride to be listed as "potassium salt"* on food labels, as numerous companies and health organizations have encouraged it to do.

The USDA should help lower children's sodium intake and accustom their taste buds to enjoying less-salty foods by *setting a 2022 deadline for the Target 2 limits on sodium (which had been delayed from 2017 to 2024) and reinstating its cancelled Target 3 limits for 2025.*

Federal, state, and local agencies should *use their purchasing power to encourage companies to market lower-sodium foods.* For example, giant purchasers, such as the Department of Defense and Department of Veterans Affairs, should choose only those products that met the FDA's targets.

One reason that progress on salt came earlier in the United Kingdom than almost anywhere else is that a prominent academic, MacGregor, has devoted a substantial portion of his time to criticizing companies marketing excessively salty foods, waging successful media campaigns to inform consumers, debunking misleading studies, and spurring improved government policies. We need *one or more American medical experts to make the same kind of commitment to public campaigning.*

Finally, consumer education. Local, state, and federal health agencies should sponsor *hard-hitting media campaigns emphasizing the risks of salty diets and encouraging people to read labels and choose lower-sodium foods. Primary care physicians should advise patients,* especially those suffering hypertension and heart disease, how to lower sodium consumption (or refer patients to registered dietitians). And, of course, *consumers should be encouraged to adopt an overall healthier diet immediately* based primarily on fruits, vegetables, nuts, beans, whole grains, seafood, low-fat and fat-free dairy foods, and unsalted meat and poultry. I'll now put on my chef's toque and give you a few tips on how to do so, without sacrificing taste.

11 Protecting Your Own Health

Reducing sodium in our diets is a health strategy proven to prevent heart attacks and strokes. By paying attention to the sodium in our diet, we can take one more step towards controlling our own health.

—*Harvard Health Blog*[1]

Going on a healthier, lower-salt diet is, in theory, one of the easiest lifestyle improvements you could make. But the food environment conspires against you. Most packaged foods are loaded with salt, and restaurant meals contain even more. Even your taste buds conspire against you—they clamor for that salty taste. Still, if you want to make the effort to lower your risk of disease, you can slash the sodium content of your diet. The information in this chapter will help you get started.

But first, what *is* your sodium intake? And for that matter, what's your blood pressure? Should you worry? If your blood pressure is under 120/80 mm Hg, you don't have to worry much about blood pressure *now*. And if it is *well under* 120/80, such as 100/60, you may never have to worry— though if you are still in your 40s, 50s, or 60s your blood pressure might rise as you age. After all, more than 80 percent of Americans 75 and older, and as many as 90 percent of Americans ultimately, develop high blood pressure.[2] Moreover, salty diets may contribute to problems other than ones related to high blood pressure, such as kidney stones and osteoporosis. Thus, almost regardless of what your blood pressure is now and how old you are, it would be worth consuming less sodium. But the higher your blood pressure is, especially if you are on the younger side, the more important it is to cut back (*and* lose weight if you're heavy *and* exercise more *and* eat more fruits and vegetables *and* possibly take blood pressure–lowering drugs).

Tips for Reducing Sodium in Your Diet

A good way to start reducing your sodium intake is to estimate how much sodium you consume. You could use the form in this section—see table 11.1 ("My Sodium Intake")—to help you keep track of all the foods you eat for a whole day or, better, a whole week. Make half a dozen photocopies so you can see a pattern in your salty food choices, and determine your average intake, over time.

Tracking my own sodium intake was enlightening because it highlighted the hefty contribution of bread: I like to toast half a bagel in the morning, often eat a sandwich or two for lunch, and maybe have another slice at dinner—so bread provided a lot more than 6 percent—the national average—of my sodium. The supermarket brand of whole-wheat sandwich bread that I was eating had 135 mg of sodium in a 1-ounce slice. Altogether, bread was contributing over 700 mg of sodium to my daily diet—until I switched brands.

On packaged foods, the Nutrition Facts labels will tell you how many milligrams of sodium each serving contains. Just be sure to adjust the number if your own serving size differs (I often use a kitchen scale to measure how much I'm eating). And be aware of what sodium-related terms on packages mean. For instance, "reduced sodium" foods are not "low" in sodium but have at least 25 percent less than their conventional counterparts. Though companies don't brag about it on labels, foods that contain 460 mg or more of sodium per serving are considered "high" in sodium.[3] Box 11.1 includes FDA definitions of sodium-related terms on food labels.[4]

It is easy to check labels at the grocery store and look for lower-sodium brands. The differences between brands are often startling. That provides clear evidence that many companies could reduce sodium levels dramatically—and that consumers could reduce their sodium intake dramatically—without rendering their foods unpalatable. And consuming the less-salty foods could gradually lower consumers' preference for salty foods. For example:

• **Bread and rolls** are the biggest sources of sodium in the average diet, not because they are so high in sodium per slice, but that people eat so much of them. On a per-ounce basis Schmidt Old Tyme 100% Whole Wheat Bread has 75 percent more sodium than Pepperidge Farm 100% Whole

Table 11.1

My sodium intake form   *Date*:

Food	Sodium (mg) per Labeled Serving	My Serving Size	Amount of Sodium I Ate
Breakfast			
Lunch			
Dinner			
Snacks			
TOTALS			

Box 11.1
FDA definitions of sodium-related terms on food labels

- **Sodium-free**—less than 5 mg of sodium per serving and contains no salt
- **Very low sodium**—35 mg or less per serving
- **Low sodium**—140 mg or less per serving (5% of sodium's Daily Value)
- **Reduced (or Less) sodium**—at least 25% less than the regular product
- **Light in sodium; Lightly salted**—at least 50% less than the regular product
- **No salt added; Unsalted**—no salt is added during processing—but these products may not be salt/sodium-free unless stated
- **High in sodium**—460 mg or more (20% of sodium's Daily Value)

Source: US Food and Drug Administration, "Use the Nutrition Facts Label to Reduce Your Intake of Sodium in Your Diet," June 8, 2018, https://www.fda.gov/food/nutrition-education -resources-materials/use-nutrition-facts-label-reduce-your-intake-sodium-your-diet (accessed February 16, 2020).

Wheat Bread. Several companies do market totally sodium-free varieties, but their taste (at least for me) leaves a lot to be desired.

- **Soup** was once the quintessential high-sodium food. Now, though, many soups made by Imagine (Light in Sodium), Pacific (Light in Sodium), Amy's (Light in Sodium), Dr. McDougall (Lower Sodium), Campbell (Well Yes! Lightly Salted), and others have around 300 mg of sodium per cup. That's a far cry from the 1980s when canned soups often had 1,000 mg or more per cup and companies said they couldn't produce a tasty version with less. Health Valley markets no-salt-added soups with about 50 to 135 mg of sodium that occurs naturally in the ingredients, but I think they need a dash of salt, lite salt (see brand information below), or other seasonings to taste good.

- **Peanut butter** is not very salty, but why buy Jif, Peter Pan, and other salted brands that have about 140 mg of sodium per 2 tablespoons when numerous brands have 0 mg.

- **Sandwiches**, one of the American Heart Association's Salty Six, are usually big sodium sources. For a cheese sandwich, you could save up to 400 mg by switching from American cheese (470 mg per ounce) to Swiss cheese (50 mg) or Cheddar cheese (180 mg). Using lower-sodium bread could save you another couple of hundred milligrams. If you switched from cheese to an unsalted peanut butter and jelly (or banana) sandwich, you would be left with just the sodium in the bread.

- **Pasta sauces** typically have 350 to 450 mg per half-cup serving, and a few reach 600 mg. *Consumer Reports* rated The Silver Palate Low Sodium Marinara and Victoria Low Sodium Marinara sauces (with 115 and 120 mg, respectively) as the best, though costlier, pasta sauces.[5]

- **Chicken (and red meat)** with added salt have flooded supermarket shelves. Perdue Boneless Skinless Chicken Breast with Rib Meat, for example, has 270 percent more sodium than Perdue Chicken Split Breasts.

- **Deli meats** are often heavily salted. Boar's Head turkey breast products range from 55 mg (no salt added) to 700 mg (Blackened Turkey Breast) per 2-ounce serving. Dietz & Watson offers Turkey Breast with between 50 mg (No Salt Added) and 390 mg (Honey Coated Maple); its Gourmet Lite version uses potassium salt to help lower sodium to 240 mg. Safeway Select Naturally Smoked Thick Sliced Bacon has 45 percent less sodium than the same amount of Smithfield Naturally Hickory Smoked Bacon.

- **Nuts** and **chips** come in reduced-sodium versions that are widely available and have one-third to one-half less sodium than the standard varieties.

Such comparisons indicate that cutting sodium consumption in half may not be so challenging. But sodium levels in some categories, such as cottage cheese, ketchup, and American cheese, are fairly similar across many brands. (Interestingly, in a large survey of adults in New York City, the frequent label readers with hypertension did not consume less sodium than other people, but that behavior need not apply to you.)[6]

If you do not have food labels handy, a new (and free) nutrition resource sponsored by the food industry can be found at www.SmartLabel.org. Many of the largest companies, as well as some smaller ones, contribute to that easy-to-use database, which provides information about nutrition, ingredients, allergens, and more. Some online shopping sites, such as www.Peapod .com and www.Walmart.com, also provide nutrition information for thousands of foods.

The most comprehensive database is the US Department of Agriculture's FoodData Central website (https://fdc.nal.usda.gov/), which provides the nutritional values of thousands of packaged and restaurant foods, as well as produce and other unprocessed foods. When you enter the name of a food category on the home page—"mushrooms," let's say—you'll find that the database lists about 3,000 entries, ranging from plain mushrooms to organic sunflower mushroom stew. Here are some tips to narrow your search within a manageable range: When the first results page comes up, unclick three of the boxes that appear along the left-hand side of your screen (smartphones may have limited options, so best to use a computer), leaving only SR Legacy. Those foods are mostly non-branded. If you're searching for a particular brand or processed food, enter the generic name on the home page (for instance, "hamburger"). Then, on the first results page, type in the brand name or product ("Big Mac") at the top of the left column, check the "Require All Words" right below that, and then check the box for "Branded" as well as "SR Legacy." If you cannot find the exact product you're researching, look for something similar; its nutritional value will likely be fairly similar.

Restaurants are treacherous territory for health-conscious people. First take advantage of the nutrition information posted on the websites of most chain restaurants, or on FoodData Central. Alternatively, chain restaurants are required to provide brochures (or a computer kiosk or other vehicle) listing the same nutrition information that appears on Nutrition Facts labels. You might find some shocking comparisons. One example: Arby's Curly French Fries have more than four times as much sodium as McDonald's French Fries (735 mg vs. 170 mg per 3.5 ounces).

A great online resource for restaurant nutrition is MenuStat (www .menustat.org), which is operated by the New York City health department. It provides periodically updated nutrition information for more than four thousand foods offered by about 100 chain restaurants, from Applebee's to Zaxby's.

Some newer chain restaurants feature meals labeled with "fresh," "sustainable," "vegetarian," or other buzzwords that ad agents put on their websites, so diner beware. Those meals might be better than some standard fare, but sodium is still often a real problem. Consider Seasons 52's Kona-Crusted Lamb Loin with 2,080 mg of sodium or its Open-Face B.L.T.A. with 1,850. Or True Food Kitchen's Cauliflower Polenta has 1,820 mg and its Unbeatable Burger has 1,880. At non-chain restaurants, upscale or down-home, your best lower-salt bet is to order a salad—but guard against salty croutons and olives, and ask for oil and vinegar dressing. Most cooks at such restaurants are probably not aware of how much sodium is in the food they serve, and have little control of it in any case: the salt is built into most sauces, soups, gravies, baked goods, cheeses, processed meats, and other items that restaurants buy from suppliers. So even if you ask that no extra salt be added to your dish, the sodium reduction is likely to be small.

Chefs who pride themselves on cooking from scratch can be more proactive about keeping a lid on sodium. They turn to the vast array of herbs and spices, lemon juice, garlic, and other low-sodium or sodium-free ingredients that can replace—often more deliciously—the flavor obtained from salt. Cooking this way requires an investment, however, in prep time and ingredients, and it may be too expensive for many establishments to avoid the use of all processed foods when they need to maintain a bottom line in the black.

What's the bottom line for us, in restaurants and at the grocery store? It is virtually impossible to rely mostly on processed and restaurant foods and achieve a low- or even moderate-sodium diet. One solution is to reserve processed foods and eating out for special occasions, or for days when you just can't face cooking from scratch. But the best way to lower your sodium intake is to replace processed with unprocessed "whole" foods and prepare low-sodium, delicious meals at home. (I know—easier said than done, especially if you hate cooking!) Make sure you have a good low-salt cookbook, such as the American Heart Association's *Low-Salt Cookbook*. And see the tips in box 11.2 for cooking with less salt.[7]

Fortunately, consuming less salt gradually decreases one's preference for salty foods and increases one's enjoyment of lower-sodium foods. Gary Beauchamp of the Monell Chemical Senses Center, an expert on taste preferences, said that after getting used to less-salty meals, "things that used to taste just right now taste too salty, and things that used to taste not salty enough, taste just right."[8] (Beauchamp was a co-author of the 2010 report from the Institute of Medicine, now the National Academy of Medicine, on how to achieve a lower-sodium food supply.) Beauchamp and others at Monell found that people adjust to less-salty foods within two or three months, and they often end up preferring less-salty foods.[9]

Some critics of reducing sodium contend that if manufacturers and restaurants used less salt, consumers would simply use their handy saltshakers to add back the missing salt—or add back even more. The 2005

Box 11.2
Tips for lower-salt cooking at home

- *Read food labels!* You will usually find a range of sodium levels in different brands of the same food (but also keep an eye on serving sizes, calories, added sugars, and saturated fat). Look for "no salt added" or "low sodium" on labels.

- When cooking from a recipe, try using one-fourth or one-half less salt than the recipe calls for and note that amount on the recipe. If the dish tastes fine, reduce the salt even more the next time you make it. When possible, wait to add salt until you are done cooking, and slowly add it to taste. I find that most recipes recommend more salt than is needed, and some do not need it at all.

- Substitute the same amount of Diamond Crystal Kosher Salt as the recipe lists for regular salt. That would cut sodium by half because of the shape of the crystals. When used in soups, stews, and sauces, the Diamond brand may take a bit longer to dissolve. (But if a recipe calls for the Diamond Crystal Kosher Salt, do not substitute regular kosher salt unless you use half as much.) A side note: despite its name, there's nothing "kosher" about the salt; all salt is kosher. Rather, kosher salt was developed to help draw blood from meat, which is one step in the koshering process.

- Taste before salting. And if you do add salt, add as little as possible, even just a shake or two might be enough. Use a "lite salt" in which half of the ordinary salt has been replaced with potassium salt or try Diamond Crystal Kosher Salt.

- Be aware that garlic salt, onion salt, and similar condiments consist mostly of salt.

- Drain and rinse salted canned vegetables and other foods. That can reduce sodium by around 40 percent—less for green beans, more for tuna.

- Use different seasonings, such as black or cayenne pepper, lemon juice or balsamic vinegar (a great way to add zip to vegetables, chicken, tofu, or fish); or try sodium-free spice mixtures (such as Mrs. Dash, McCormick, or Chef Paul Prudhomme). Or make your own seasoning blend (see box 11.3). Be careful not to zip up the meal with too much cayenne—a mistake I sometimes make—or you'll zap it right into your trash bin! You can add more pepper at the table, but you cannot take out what you used on the stove!

- Take saltshakers off the table to reduce temptation, but still replace the regular salt with reduced-sodium salt for when you do use them.

Box 11.3

Making your own salt-free seasoning mix

You can buy sodium-free seasonings made by McCormick, Mrs. Dash, Trader Joe's, or Lawry's at grocery stores—or you can make your own. When using these recipes (add or subtract ingredients as you wish), make sure to blend well. Place the ingredients in a small jar and *shake well*.

Savory Seasoning

> 1¼ teaspoons celery seed
>
> 2 tablespoons crushed marjoram
>
> 2 tablespoons crushed savory
>
> 2 tablespoons crushed thyme
>
> 1 tablespoon crushed basil
>
> Yield: about ½ cup

Courtesy of Northwest Kidney Centers

https://www.nwkidney.org/recipe/savory-seasoning/

Spicy Seasoning

> 3 tablespoons celery seed
>
> 1 tablespoon onion powder (not onion salt)
>
> 1 teaspoon garlic powder
>
> 2 tablespoons crushed oregano
>
> 1 tablespoon crushed thyme
>
> 1½ teaspoons ground bay leaf
>
> 1½ teaspoons black pepper
>
> 1½ teaspoons ground cloves
>
> Yield: about ½ cup

Courtesy of Center for Science in the Public Interest

"Dietary Guidelines for Americans" laid that concern to rest: "When consumers are offered a lower-sodium product, they typically do not add table salt to compensate for the lower sodium content, even when available."[10] Monell researchers found that after cutting the sodium content of specially prepared meals in half, people added back only 20 percent of what was removed.[11]

One of the pitfalls of cooking from scratch is that countless recipes in newspapers, cooking magazines, cookbooks, and websites are loaded with unnecessary salt. Normally, the Food section of my hometown newspaper offers reasonably healthy recipes, but sometimes it slips up. A cheeseburger sandwich prepared according to a *Washington Post* recipe is packed with 720 calories and 1,220 mg of sodium.[12] A recipe for pizza with 500 calories per slice has 1,010 mg of sodium.[13] But kudos to the *Post* for providing nutrition breakdowns; the *New York Times* and most other sources of recipes do not.

Articles quoting chefs may add to the problem. One extreme example comes from cookbook superstar Samin Nosrat, who confessed to being salt-obsessed in a recent *New York Times* article: "At some point during every cooking class I teach, I do my signature move: dramatically add handful upon handful of salt to a large pot of boiling water, then taste it and add even more."[14] Can you imagine the public outcry if articles encouraged people to smoke cigarettes or spray pesticides in their children's bedrooms?

Fortunately, not all the influences out there preach using salt with abandon. One surprising convert to low-salt cooking was Craig Claiborne, the renowned *New York Times* food editor and self-admitted salt "addict." Perhaps because of his love of salt, according to an article in the *Journal of the American Medical Association*, he suffered from hypertension, edema, and an unquenchable thirst.[15] Motivated by the urgency of his health problems, he co-authored *Craig Claiborne's Gourmet Diet*, a best-selling cookbook featuring low-sodium, low-sugar recipes. In *Time* magazine, Claiborne offered consumers some pithy "secrets":

> If you wish to wean your taste buds away from salt, the object is to find other flavors that will distract your palate. . . . I prefer fresh herbs like parsley, tarragon, finely chopped garlic, and fresh grated horseradish; spices like curry and chili powders, powdered mustard (made into a paste with water), hot pepper flakes, a generous grinding of black pepper and sugar. . . . Use the freshest foods that can be found. There are four vegetables that make an especially fine feast without salt. These are mushrooms, eggplants, really fresh red ripe tomatoes, and good quality onions, white or red.[16]

One easy way to cut sodium when you're cooking from scratch is to use the reduced-sodium salts made with potassium chloride (aka potassium salt). As I discuss in chapter 9, some people say that potassium salt tastes exactly like salt and love sprinkling a little on their food, but others find that using too much results in a terrible bitter or metallic aftertaste. So the best substitutes probably are those with about half of the regular salt replaced with potassium salt. Popular brands include Morton's Lite Salt and Good-Salt from Finland. But don't use twice as much just because they are low in sodium! I have found that the reduced-sodium products work great in just about any food. However, if you have chronic kidney disease or a heart condition, talk to your doctor before using potassium-based seasonings.

Because I'm no professional chef, I asked some experts for their cooking advice. Cary Neff, the vice-president of corporate culinary support for Morrison Healthcare, wrote the *New York Times* best-selling cookbook *Conscious Cuisine*. Echoing Craig Claiborne, he said we should focus not on subtracting sodium but rather on adding flavor, because that should automatically lead to needing less salt. His top tips include:

- Bring out the flavor by roasting or sautéing.
- Toast grains, such as rice and barley, in a dry frying pan for several minutes (stir several times to prevent burning) before adding water and boiling them. Also toast spices, such as mustard seeds and cumin seeds, then grind them to a powder in a small blender. The toasting really accentuates their taste and aroma.
- Save chicken bones in a plastic bag in your freezer. Keep another bag with trimmings from carrots, onions, and other vegetables. When you have time, dump the ingredients into a pot of boiling water and produce your own flavorful chicken or vegetable broth or stock (when you include bones). That's perfect for preparing a soup or grain.

Kate Sherwood, who writes the "Healthy Cook" page for the Center for Science in the Public Interest's (CSPI) *Nutrition Action Healthletter*, trained at the Culinary Institute of America. She is passionate about creating dishes that are both delicious *and* healthful. None of that "salt to taste" stuff for Kate! She told me, "While no ingredient or combination can entirely replace salt, good technique and quality ingredients make cooking with less salt possible." Here are several of her favorite suggestions:

- Taste your food before adding salt. "I like to keep the salt away from the mindless salters in my family (husband and dad) so that they have to *ask* for the salt, and I can make sure they've tasted the food before adding more."
- Use ingredients that are salty (capers, olives, feta cheese, anchovies) sparingly but take advantage of the fact that they add discrete blasts of saltiness to otherwise lightly seasoned dishes.

- Use spices, herbs, and acidic ingredients (citrus juices, vinegars) to enhance flavor.
- Savory dishes, such as salads or grain dishes that include fruit, have a good sweet/tart balance, and so they need less salt to taste good.

Sea Salt: No Health Potion

In a 2013 opinion survey of 1,000 US adults, 59 percent believed that sea salt contained less sodium than regular table salt.[17] In fact, that is rarely the case. Most sea salts—and table salt—are at least 98 percent sodium chloride, with other minerals present in such small amounts that they have no effect on health.[18]

All salt is technically "sea" salt. Even the salt dug out of salt mines, the source of most table salt, is sea salt, having been left by long-dried-out seas. Whether it is derived from the industrial or artisanal dehydration of ocean water a year ago or by nature over millions of years, salt is almost entirely sodium chloride, especially after it is washed and purified. In that sense, creative marketers could call ordinary Morton salt, obtained from mines deep underground, "ancient sea salt untouched by humans for millions of years."

The Culinary Institute of America recommends that chefs use sea salt, not because it is lower in sodium, but because it might improve flavor and is "label friendly."[19] Indeed, stating "a touch of sea salt" on a menu or label might *suggest* to consumers that the product is healthier and allow manufacturers to use a little less salt.

Stephanie L. Drake and MaryAnne Drake, at the Department of Food, Bioprocessing, and Nutrition Sciences at North Carolina State University, compared the mineral content and taste of 38 different sea salts, along with table salts and "lite" salts.[20] Two salts from Hawaii—Haleaka Red salt and Kilauea Black salt—had almost 25 percent less sodium than table salt.

In the taste tests organized by the Drakes, New Zealand organic sea salt, Sonoma salt from California, and numerous others tasted a little different from table salt. But those tests were done with salt crystals and not salt added to foods, which could mask any taste differences. I tried adding fleur de sel, Himalayan pink salt, and a couple of other sea salts to low-sodium vegetable broth and to unseasoned brown rice and could not taste any difference.

But I admit that my palate is not the most refined. *Cook's Illustrated*, considered by many to be the arbiter of all cooking controversies, taste-tested half a dozen salts. It concluded:

> The results were definitive: Tasters couldn't tell one salt from another in cooked applications. Only when the salts were sprinkled over slices of beef tenderloin could tasters detect subtle flavor nuances. . . . Our advice? Save your money and use fancy sea salts only for garnishing.[21]

A Swedish company, Saltwell AB, harvests sea salt in Chile that is naturally high in potassium—about 30 percent—and so contains that much less sodium. Saltwell tells food manufacturers that they can label foods made with that specialty salt simply as "salt" to avoid highlighting the presence of chemical-sounding potassium, but I'm not sure that is consistent with FDA rules.[22] Many kidney patients and people taking certain antihypertensive medications need to avoid too much potassium.

If you flew from Chile to Israel, you could go to the Dead Sea and obtain salt that is even lower in sodium. Salona Low Sodium Sea Salt consists mostly of potassium and magnesium salts and has only one-twentieth as much sodium as table salt.[23] Its manufacturer, a Danish company, says that it can replace up to half the normal amount of salt in foods.[24]

Some marketers make sea salt out to be a panacea for practically every ill. To pick one egregious example, consider Dr. Josh Axe's advice (www.DrAxe .com). Axe, who says he is a certified doctor of natural medicine, doctor of chiropractic, and clinical nutritionist, touts sea salt as an almost magical mineral that regulates blood pressure, increases energy, helps reduce signs of aging, improves brain function, eliminates mucus buildup, supports libido, and much more. Axe and others often assert that sea salt contains dozens of minerals that regular salt does not have. That is often true, but the amounts of those minerals are typically trivial and have a trivial effect on health.

If you are surprised that most sea salts are just as unhealthy as table salt, you may be shocked by their prices. For example, SaltWorks (www.seasalt .com) sells a 6-ounce package of Fleur de Sel (obtained for hundreds of years from the Rhône river delta west of Marseille, France) for $10.99, or $29.30 per pound. Or you could spend $7.99 for 1.5 ounces of Icelandic Flake Sea Salt or Kala Namak Sulphur Salt ($85.23 per pound). Or, at Salt Cellar (www .salt-cellar.com), you could spend $15 for 1.5 ounces of Black Truffle Sea

Salt ($160 per pound). Maybe those high prices encourage people to use less salt, or maybe they contribute to a mystique around sea salt. In any case, you could buy a 26-ounce canister of table salt for about 60 cents per pound, roughly one-hundredth to one-fiftieth the price of some fancy artisanal salts.

My bottom line on sea salt: use a little, especially as a garnish, if you like its taste more than regular salt, but do not believe any of the hogwash about its health benefits.

Healthy Diets Are More Than Just Low in Salt

I have focused almost totally on salt, because I think it is causing more harm to our health than just about anything else in our diet. But there is more to eating healthfully than just keeping sodium in check. It is worth paying special attention to another mineral, potassium, because it is an essential nutrient and a powerful antidote to the effects of too much sodium. Most of the best sources of potassium are also all-around healthy foods, as I indicate in table 11.2. Build several of the foods high in the table into your diet every day, and you will easily consume at least 3,000 mg of potassium.

For optimal health, people need to focus on numerous nutrients in their diets, not on just one or two. The "Dietary Guidelines for Americans" and other reliable sources of nutrition information generally recommend—and I know I have said this before!—consuming mostly fruits, vegetables, nuts, whole grains, non-fried seafood, low-fat animal products, and polyunsaturated vegetable oil (such as soy and canola) . . . while limiting intakes of refined sugars and starches (soft drinks, candy, cake, cookies, white bread), saturated fat (meat and full-fat dairy foods), and sodium (packaged and restaurant foods).

Bonnie Liebman, CSPI's nutrition director, has translated the DASH–sodium type of diet, widely accepted as being super-healthy, into an eating plan (see table 11.3). Use the number and size of servings as a guide and aim roughly to average over a week the numbers of daily servings shown. If that is too complicated, just incorporate the "Dietary Guidelines" principles into your life. The trick is to find healthy foods and recipes that you love and keep those foods around the house. With the right ingredients handy, you should be able to whip up healthy, delicious salads, hearty soups and stews, sandwiches, and stir-fry meals in short order. (And, yes, it's OK to cheat

Table 11.2

Potassium content of selected foods (mg)

Baked potato with skin, medium	925
Acorn squash, baked, 1 cup	895
Salmon, farmed, raw, 6 oz.	650
Sweet potato with skin, baked, medium	540
Cantaloupe, large, ¼	540
Orange juice, 1 cup	495
Spinach, cooked, ½ cup	420
Banana, medium	420
Yogurt, plain, low-fat, 6 oz.	400
McDonald's Quarter Pounder sandwich	385
Black beans, canned, ½ cup	370
Milk, low-fat (1%), 1 cup	365
Chicken breast, boneless, 5 oz. cooked	345
Pizza, cheese, Pizza Hut 14″ Thin 'N Crispy, 2 slices	310
Lettuce, romaine, 2 cups loosely packed	230
Tomato, small, whole, 4 oz.	215
Apple, medium, 3-inch diameter	195
Cheerios, 1 oz.	180
Ice cream, vanilla, ⅔ cup	175
Whole wheat bread, 2 slices, 64 g	160
Pasta, dry, 2 oz.	125
Shrimp, jumbo, cooked, 6	60
Tortilla chips, 1 oz.	60

Source: US Department of Agriculture. USDA Food Composition Databases. https://fdc.nal.usda.gov/ (accessed December 8, 2018).

Table 11.3

A healthy eating plan for a 2,100-calorie diet*

Food Group	Daily Servings	1 Serving is
Vegetables and Fruit	11	½ cup vegetables, 1 cup greens, 1 piece fruit
Grains	4	½ cup cooked pasta or rice or 1 slice of mostly whole-grain bread
Low-Fat Dairy	2	1 cup milk or yogurt or 1½ oz. hard cheese
Legumes or Nuts	2	½ cup beans, ¼ cup nuts, or 4 oz. tofu
Poultry, Fish, Lean Meat	1	¼ lb. cooked (not fried)
Oils and Fat	2	1 tablespoon vegetable oil or margarine
Desserts, Sweets	2	1 teaspoon sugar, 1 small cookie
Wild Card	1	Poultry, fish, meat, oils/fat, grains, desserts, or sweets

* Adjust the numbers of servings for diets higher or lower in calories.
Source: *Nutrition Action Healthletter*, November 2017.

Box 11.4

Tips from people who cut the salt and improved their health

I have heard from many people who changed their lifestyle after being diagnosed with high blood pressure. Some people focused on reducing their sodium intake, but most took a broader approach: eating more produce, going vegetarian or vegan, avoiding added sugars and fats/oils, exercising more, and losing weight. Most of the people I heard from (admittedly not a random sample) say they experienced benefits. For many that meant reducing the dosages of their blood pressure meds, or even getting off them altogether. But some people's bodies just did not cooperate, and they continued to need just as much medication as before. Consider these (lightly edited) tips for cutting salt.

Susan F., Paso Robles, California: I believe my blood pressure responded when I lowered salt intake significantly and increased consumption of fruit and vegetables. I didn't lose weight or eat less as I am already on the thin side (5'6" and 122 lbs., age 73). I exercise regularly and have done so for years.

About 6 months ago, my nurse practitioner noticed my BP was elevated (145 over 90-something.) As my BP was usually low (110 over 70-something was common) my doc suggested testing at home and reporting back daily for a while. I did that and started salt restriction and the deliberate addition of

Box 11.4 (continued)

potassium-rich foods to my diet. After a month or so, I was seeing 120 over 80 +/-. Last visit to the doc, 110 over 80. I'm still pretty careful but the fear of god has abated somewhat so I cheat a bit when eating away from home. One of my brilliant observations is that eating commercially prepared food is probably not good for my health.

Douglas F., Newton, New Jersey: I was able to avoid having to take blood pressure drugs altogether. My blood pressure readings were getting high in the 150 to 160 range. Now they are down to 130. I was able to achieve this by changing to a low-sodium diet. I carefully read the nutrition labels in the supermarket and avoid foods that are notorious for being high in sodium. Other changes included eating more fruits and vegetables—up to 10 servings per day—exercising regularly, and focusing on reduction of stress.

Cameron McL., Pensacola, Florida: I am a 60-year-old female with a strong family history of cardiovascular disease. I went from a low-salt diet to an almost no-salt one and have been eating an exclusively plant-based diet for 20 years. My daily sodium intake was probably between 2,000 and 4,000 milligrams. After the change it is probably about 2,000. Even that modest change plus exercise lowered my BP over three months from 130/80 to about 110/70 on an average day. I have never taken meds for high blood pressure but had another medical problem that made it important to lower my BP. As a control, I did not change my diet or exercise habits and so credit the change with lowering sodium intake.

Eileen F., Los Angeles, California: I have been a vegetarian for decades. About a year ago I became vegan and within 5 months my blood pressure went from borderline high (I was on meds for it) to borderline low. I actually had to go in to get my BP checked three times because they wanted to make sure it wasn't a fluke. I think a more plant-based diet (more vegetables and beans and tofu) made a big difference. My doctor took me off the meds.

When I went vegan, I started to cook more, thus reducing processed food from my diet. I definitely stopped eating as much cookie and chip and cracker type food, which I know has a lot of sodium. Also, I have noticed that I don't need my food to be as salty. I used to use much more to flavor food.

Fred G., Richfield, Ohio: For 40 years I have dealt with high blood pressure and reduced my salt intake over those years. I have been on a limited salt (but not very low-salt) diet for the past 20 years. . . . I have taken two medications for many years—one always being a beta blocker. My blood pressure has been controlled satisfactorily with this combination of diet and medications, but diet alone has not come close to working.

Box 11.4 (continued)

Daniel B., Honolulu, Hawaii: Not only do I feel better, I have noticed a decreased swelling in my lower legs at the end of the day as a result of NO added salt to my diet. . . . I have not needed to wear compression socks and have reduced my Losartan [blood pressure medicine] to 25 from 50mg. I try to go back to the web pages of all the processed foods that I eat and drink [and check the nutrition numbers]. I work with general rules and have no absolute "don't buys":

Rule 1: If I know it has salt, I eat less of it (latkes, bagels, pretzels, nuts).

Rule 2: I use salt substitutes like Trader Joe's "21 Seasoning Salute" or "Mrs. Dash." I NEVER add any salt to foods.

Rule 3: At restaurants, I order all sauces and gravies on the side, tasting them first for salt. For my favorite Japanese restaurants, I have "gifted" them a can of "lower salt" soy sauce.

Rule 4: For fast foods, when necessary, I eat at restaurants like Subway that have online nutrition calculators. That alerts me to salt in each one of their ingredients so I can avoid/limit/use less processed meats and cheeses. Their breads are loaded with salt.

Rule 5: We have no saltshaker on our table. If I don't see it, I won't consume it.

Elinor G., Sarasota, Florida: My doctor took me off blood pressure medication after only three weeks of being on a plant-based, whole-food diet!!!! Just avoiding processed food did it!

John H., Silver Spring, Maryland: For well over a decade, we have deliberately avoided large intakes of salt. Our main tool is reading the nutrition labels when shopping and not eating unlabeled foods [such as at parties] that are notoriously high in salt (and usually also in fat), such as chips. One of our biggest surprises was how many soups contain large amounts of salt. Owing to our long-term reduction in salt content, common salty foods taste too salty to us. We are also near-vegetarians (pescatarians, to be specific), and neither of us has high blood pressure (we are 77 and 83 years old).

Jeanne W., Grand Rapids, Minnesota: Funny you should ask! My doctor just reduced my blood pressure meds in half. I exercise at the "Y" for 2 or 3 hours Monday through Friday. My goal is a whole-food, plant-based diet but mess up at times. I have reduced salt intake, and staying away from processed foods is huge. I am also not pre-diabetic anymore.

from time to time with less healthy packaged and restaurant foods—we all do!) For some personal stories from people who opted for lower-salt diets and were—usually—rewarded with better health, see box 11.4.

So with the scientific facts in the first few chapters of this book and the tips and personal stories in this chapter, I hope you will be well on your way not only to delicious, less salty meals but also to better health. In the epilogue I put the salt–health issue in the context of other science policy controversies fanning the fires of salt wars, and examine the lessons we have learned on the battlefield.

Epilogue: Salt's Lesson on Industry and Public Health

"The War Over Salt, It's the Food Industry vs. an Army of Medical Experts."
—title of Melanie Warner's *New York Times* article, 2008[1]

The great bulk of scientific research has demonstrated that diets high in sodium increase blood pressure, which in turn increases the risk of cardiovascular and kidney diseases. Salty diets may also contribute to mild cognitive impairment, erectile dysfunction, obesity, osteoporosis, headaches, impaired vision, and edema. On the other hand, some studies, which were deeply flawed, indicated that reducing sodium consumption is unnecessary and even dangerous. The sharp disagreement between two warring camps of scientists has led to decades of confusion and delay in reducing Americans' consumption of sodium—and in improving their health. Where have we seen that movie before?

In fact, similar scenarios have occurred in numerous other spheres of science and science policy. Powerful industries, aided and abetted by a handful of contrarian studies and sympathetic journalists, have "manufactured doubt," arguing that the current scientific evidence was not sufficient to prove that asbestos and cigarettes caused cancer, that lead poisoned workers and children, that the burning of fossil fuels is changing our planet's climate, and that certain pesticides and antibiotics harmed the environment, farmworkers, and the public.

But the salt situation is not entirely analogous. In those other science and policy battles, powerful industries sought to protect their profits by fending off government regulation. The salt industry is nothing compared to an ExxonMobil, Dow, or Philip Morris (and their respective industries) in terms of size and political clout. Moreover, food-grade salt represents only a minor portion of the sales of Morton Salt Co., North America's largest salt producer, let alone the German mining company that now owns Morton. Cargill, another major salt manufacturer, also sells shiploads of soybean meal to China and truckloads of Shady Brook Farms turkeys to American supermarkets. Rather, salt is a cheap, minor ingredient in tens of thousands of processed foods manufactured by thousands of companies. Although the salt industry's trade association, the Salt Institute, roared loudly over the years, its demise was barely noticed. It is the mainstream food industry that uses salt and has had the power to stymy effective government action.

Much of the food industry (buttressed by some academic researchers) has denied that the 100-plus randomized controlled trials (RCTs) proving that high-sodium diets increase blood pressure provide a sufficient basis on which to take regulatory action—even though no one doubts that high blood pressure causes heart attacks, strokes, and kidney disease. Taking a cue from other industries that have fought off public health actions, food companies have exaggerated the imperfections in the case against salt and demanded ever more proof that their products were harmful. To that end, one of the sodium skeptics' key, if subtle, achievements was managing over the years to move the goal posts.

Health experts had long ago come to a consensus that high-sodium diets were a major cause of hypertension, and that was reason enough to lower sodium intakes. Half a century ago the White House Conference on Food, Nutrition, and Health felt there was enough evidence to reduce sodium levels to prevent or ameliorate hypertension. Forty years ago the first "Dietary Guidelines for Americans" advised Americans to consume less sodium. More than a quarter-century ago the National High Blood Pressure Education Program of the National Institutes of Health said that the "data clearly show" that high salt intake is "one of the important mass exposures that accounts for the generally unfavorable blood pressure distribution."[2]

But beginning around 30 years ago opponents of sodium reduction began demanding further proof that lowering sodium would improve health, and not impair it. In particular, they wanted proof that lowering sodium would not just reduce blood pressure but also the risk of heart attacks and strokes. They demanded new RCTs on sodium and cardiovascular disease, which happen to be time-consuming, prohibitively costly—and not necessarily conclusive. Lawrence J. Appel, the hypertension expert at Johns Hopkins, says that their strategy seems to be "to raise the bar for evidence to a point where the evidence just will never be there."[3] Conducting more research to better understand the causes of health problems, and to find treatments for them, is certainly a good thing, and sometimes an RCT overturns long-held beliefs. But in the case of salt and health, many different strands of strong evidence have persuaded experts around the world that the costs of inaction far outweigh the chances that more research would overturn the consensus and demonstrate conclusively that lowering sodium intakes resulted in health risks. And waiting for that new research would greatly delay the adoption of life-saving programs and regulations.

The opponents of lowering sodium nevertheless amassed enough political influence to get anti-regulatory Congresses to fund the 2013 Institute of Medicine (IOM) and 2019 National Academy of Medicine (NAM) reviews. Those reviews based their recommendations almost exclusively on the relatively few studies that looked at direct links between salt and cardiovascular disease, downplaying the much richer body of evidence that salty diets cause hypertension, which in turn causes heart attacks, strokes, and kidney disease. Then, perhaps to the chagrin of those who demanded both reports, the IOM and NAM committees found that a national goal of 2,300 mg of sodium per day was safe and would lower disease rates. But the continuing controversy confused the public, and conducting those reviews delayed limiting sodium in school foods and implementing the Food and Drug Administration's sodium-reduction plan. Also, because the committees relied primarily on RCTs, and there were no RCTs involving sodium intakes of under 2,300 mg per day, they could not endorse the sodium intakes under 2,300 mg that had been recommended especially for people over about 50, people with elevated or high blood pressure, and African Americans, all of whom have a higher risk of cardiovascular disease than the average adult.

Jeremiah Stamler, of the Northwestern University Feinberg School of Medicine, is considered by some to be the global dean of cardiovascular research, having conducted research about risk factors and prevention since 1948. (He has also been celebrated for standing up to, and ultimately suing, the communist-hunting House Committee on Un-American Activities in 1965.[4]) Back in 2002, Stamler and his co-author Paul Elliott published a rebuttal of a paper that lent support to those who were demanding ever-more evidence before agreeing that people should consume less sodium. Stamler and Elliot summed up that position this way:

The proponents of the "do nothing" approach have no case for the status quo as the preferred public health option. In fact, the body of scientific knowledge affords no basis for valid debate; efforts to promote the idea that there is a scientifically grounded "controversy" in this area—as in the area of tobacco and disease—are scientifically unsound and detrimental to health.[5]

Aside from contending that the evidence is not sufficient to warrant policy change, companies play the hardship card by claiming they would suffer economic catastrophe if they had to reformulate their products or adopt new production methods. "Costs would go through the roof!" But time and time again, new regulations have proven to be "technology forcing." That is, when confronted by new legal requirements, companies are often able to develop new technologies or manufacturing processes to meet or exceed the tougher limits—and sometimes even save money. (When it comes to lowering sodium intake, the "technology" might be as simple as using less salt.) Henry Waxman (D–CA), who for decades was a leading champion in the House of Representatives for protecting public health and the environment, observed:

> In fact, automakers met with relative ease the ambitious [air pollution] standards they once claimed would destroy jobs and cast the economy into recession. . . . While industry claims often frame the debate, they are usually exaggerated, not accurate descriptions of the truth but tactics to stop unwanted measures, regardless of need or merit.[6]

Trade associations are among the most formidable lobbying entities in Washington; the most powerful food industry organization was the Grocery Manufacturers Association (GMA), but it had many allies representing the snack food, meat, poultry, restaurant, baked-goods, and other segments of the food industry. Waxman explained why trade associations typically oppose life-saving health and environmental legislation:

> Because trade groups exist to represent the interests of an entire industry, their main concern is maintaining the happiness of all their members. Trade groups always push to weaken a bill to the point where none of their members object to it, which is why they are often such a negative force in the legislative process.[7]

I was pleased, if a bit surprised, that in 2007 and 2013, the GMA partnered with the Center for Science in the Public Interest on conferences aimed at "Getting to 2,300." Our goal was to gently encourage companies to lower sodium to safer levels. But the GMA became increasingly reluctant to support sodium reductions the closer the FDA got to recommending a formal plan for achieving them. Developments in 2019, however, suggest that there will be less organized opposition to lowering sodium: the GMA transformed into the Consumer Brands Association and stopped lobbying against sodium reductions, and the Salt Institute closed its doors.

John Dement, a professor in Duke University's Division of Occupational and Environmental Medicine, made the following comment about corporate-funded asbestos risk assessments, but it applies as well to the food and salt industries: "All they've accomplished is to try to generate doubt where, really, little doubt existed."[8]

Echoing that is David Michaels, who was Assistant Secretary of Labor for Occupational Safety and Health in the Obama administration. In his book *Doubt Is Their Product*, he details how product-defense specialists manufacture doubt about second-hand smoke, workplace pollutants, and other health hazards. More broadly he explains how industry has institutionalized doubt, uncertainty, and delay by advocating a raft of bureaucratic hurdles that impede or permanently derail health and environmental protections.[9] He reports that the Salt Institute had tried to use an obscure federal law, the Data Quality Act, to effectively "censor" the National Heart, Lung, and Blood Institute. Michaels called that law "a wonderful new weapon in the arsenal of all those who oppose public health and workplace regulations, as well as independent, serious science."

A tactic parallel to "doubt" for opposing public health and environmental laws is to hold high the twin banners of "nanny state" and "personal freedom." Those slogans have been invoked by libertarians and industries to characterize reform efforts related to everything from salt to soft drinks to tobacco to guns to class-action litigation, and they are intended to resonate with our inner beings as freedom-loving Americans. Example: the *New York Post* headline proclaiming, "The Nanny State's War on Salt Won't Make Us Healthier."[10]

The ultimate practitioner of this tactic is the Center for Consumer Freedom (CCF). It pretends to be a "nonprofit organization devoted to promoting personal responsibility and protecting consumer choices."[11] In fact, its well-funded activities are apparently underwritten by the various industries—soft drink, meat, restaurant—that it defends with nasty full-page ads and angry websites. Almost everyone and everything is a nanny (the word is used 408 times on the group's website): environmental and animal-welfare activists, the states of California and Mississippi, the Center for Science in the Public Interest, and most especially former New York City mayor Michael Bloomberg, who was depicted in a full-page newspaper ad wearing a dress, for advocating smaller soft drink containers and requiring calories on menus of chain restaurants. the CCF claims to be "devoted to protecting consumer choices," but don't expect the center to satisfy your choice to know who sponsors its campaigns—that is a closely held secret. All it admits to is support from "restaurants, food companies and thousands of individual consumers." I'm skeptical of the latter, but we are not about to get any further information.

An important factor that aids and abets industry efforts to postpone, weaken, or kill corrective action is that products like salt and asbestos are not like airplane or automobile crashes. When the causes of injury, sickness, or death are obvious, society may take relatively quick remedial action. The problem is when substances plant seeds in childhood or early adulthood that do not blossom into heart attacks or cancer until decades later. That leaves plenty of room for arguments over the severity and causes of the harm. In many cases—lead, tobacco, asbestos, pesticides, greenhouse gases, and, indeed, salt—there were (and always will be) gaps in the knowledge about their health impacts. More studies were conducted, but critics pointed to more gaps. Finally, though, after decades of research, activism, argument, and delay, policy makers acknowledged that the evidence of harm was overwhelming and began instituting public health protections.

And so it is with salt, arguably the most harmful substance in our food supply. The overwhelming preponderance of evidence supports the near certainty that reducing sodium in the food supply would prevent tens of thousands of illnesses and deaths each year and save many billions of dollars. The time has come to end the indecision and delays, to stop waiting for that ever-elusive perfect proof. The time has come to declare the salt wars over, and for policy makers in the United States and around the world to act decisively to protect consumers from overly salty diets.

Acknowledgments

As every author knows, books don't just spring fully formed from one person's mind, but are guided by experiences enriched by numerous people. I would especially like to recognize my colleagues at the Center for Science in the Public Interest on whom I have relied for years. First and foremost, Bonnie F. Liebman, CSPI's director of nutrition, has worked alongside me since 1977 on salt and many other issues. In particular, she cut her advocacy teeth on CSPI's salt petitions to the US Food and Drug Administration in 1978 and 1981 and has followed the issue ever since. Margo G. Wootan, vice-president of nutrition policy, was instrumental in getting the US Department of Agriculture to greatly improve nutrition standards, including sodium, for school meals. Peter G. Lurie, who took over from me as CSPI's president in 2017, provided valuable detailed comments on drafts of this book. Caitlin Dow provided invaluable research advice. Over the years, several CSPI attorneys, especially Bruce Silverglade, Benjamin Cohen, and Laura MacCleery, crafted groundbreaking petitions, lawsuits, and other measures to encourage the Food and Drug Administration to fulfill its responsibility to the public on salt and other issues. Helping in a different way, attorneys Lisa Mankofsky and Matthew Simon carefully reviewed a draft and helped expunge possible problems. And thank you, senior nutritionist Lindsay Moyer for imparting to me some of your amazing knowledge of the composition of packaged and restaurant foods.

I also would like to thank numerous scientists for their perspective on the research on salt and health, including Michael H. Alderman, Lawrence J. Appel, Gary K. Beauchamp, Norm R. C. Campbell, Nancy R. Cook, Stephen Havas, Feng J. He, Graham A. MacGregor, Frank M. Sacks, and Paul K. Whelton. But I must claim responsibility for any errors or for misinterpretations of their and others' research.

Conversations with former officials at the Food and Drug Administration, the White House, and elsewhere helped me understand what was happening behind the scenes as the Obama administration developed a scientifically supportable and politically viable plan to reduce sodium in the food supply. Those people include Sam Kass, Michael M. Landa, Jessica Leighton, and Michael R. Taylor, as well as others who preferred not to be named. I also greatly appreciated conversations with several current or former industry officials, including Lisa Thorsten, Richard L. Hanneman, and Morton Satin, who helped me understand what was happening behind their scenes; others requested anonymity. On a different front, attorney Marshall L. Matz provided his insights into the forces influencing school foods.

A special shout-out to Max Sinsheimer, my literary agent who connected me to the terrific folks at MIT Press. And another one to my editor, Mary Bagg, who is a living incarnation of the *Chicago Manual of Style* and who had endless patience in helping make *Salt Wars* both accurate and literate . . . but the buck stops with me for any remaining errors or inartful language.

Finally, I thank Donna Lenhoff, my dear spouse of 30 years, for her love, for putting up with my foibles, and for relieving me of some of my household duties when I was in the throes of writing this book.

Appendix A

List of Information Boxes, Figures, and Tables

Chapter 5: The Mouse That Roared: The Salt Institute
Figure 5.1   The salt institute's going-out-of-business notice

Chapter 7: Less-Salty Diets around the Globe
Figure 7.1   Sid the Slug was a key spokescharacter in the UK's salt-
              awareness campaign
Figure 7.2   Front-of-package warning labels
Table 7.1   International actions to limit sodium

Chapter 8: Policy Paralysis in the United States
Box 8.1   Timeline of policy activities related to salt

Chapter 9: Progress at Last!
Box 9.1   Salt hero—American Heart Association
Figure 9.1   Saltshaker warning icons
Table 9.1   Company commitments to lowering sodium

Chapter 11: Protecting Your Own Health
Box 11.1   FDA definitions of sodium-related terms on food labels
Box 11.2   Tips for lower-salt cooking at home
Box 11.3   Making your own salt-free seasoning mix
Box 11.4   Tips from people who cut the salt and improved their health
Table 11.1   My sodium intake form
Table 11.2   Potassium content of selected foods (mg)
Table 11.3   A healthy eating plan for a 2,100-calorie diet

Appendix B

Abbreviations

ACE	angiotensin converting enzyme
AHA	American Heart Association
AMA	American Medical Association
AND	Academy of Nutrition and Dietetics
APHA	American Public Health Association
ARBs	angiotensin II receptor blockers
CCF	Center for Consumer Freedom
CDC	Centers for Disease Control and Prevention
CEO	Chief Executive Officer
CIA	Culinary Institute of America
CKD	chronic kidney disease
CSPI	Center for Science in the Public Interest
DASH	Dietary Approaches to Stop Hypertension
ED	erectile dysfunction
ENaC	epithelial sodium channel
FDA	US Food and Drug Administration
FSA	United Kingdom's Food Standards Agency
GMA	Grocery Manufacturers Association (renamed Consumer Brands Association)
GRAS	generally recognized as safe
HHS	US Department of Health and Human Services
ILSI	International Life Sciences Institute
INSERM	French National Institute of Health and Medical Research
IOM	Institute of Medicine (renamed National Academy of Medicine)

MCI	mild cognitive impairment
MSG	monosodium glutamate
NAM	National Academy of Medicine
NIH	National Institutes of Health
NHANES	National Health and Nutrition Examination Survey
NHLBI	National Heart, Lung, and Blood Institute
NSRI	National Salt Reduction Initiative
PHRI	Public Health Research Institute
PURE	Prospective Urban Rural Epidemiology study
SCOGS	Select Committee on GRAS Substances
SNA	School Nutrition Association
TIA	transient ischemic attack
TOHP	Trials of Hypertension Prevention
TONE	Trial of Nonpharmacologic Interventions in the Elderly
UK	United Kingdom
USDA	US Department of Agriculture
WHO	World Health Organization

Notes

Chapter 1

1. K. Y. Masibay, "Salt Makes Everything Taste Better," *Fine Cooking* 91, https://www.finecooking.com/article/salt-makes-everything-taste-better (accessed November 4, 2019).

2. S. Nosrat and W. MacNaughton, *Salt, Fat, Acid, Heat: Mastering the Elements of Good Cooking* (New York: Simon and Schuster, 2017).

3. R. Bayless, interview with E. Lewine, "Midwest Mex," *New York Times Magazine*, February 17, 2008, https://www.nytimes.com/2008/02/17/magazine/17wwln-domains-t.html.

4. Label Insight database, https://www.labelinsight.com/, August 6, 2019.

5. L. Layton, "FDA Plans to Limit Amount of Salt Allowed in Processed Foods for Health Reasons," *Washington Post*, April 20, 2010, http://www.washingtonpost.com/wp-dyn/content/article/2010/04/19/AR2010041905049.html?hpid=topnews.

6. Exploratorium, "The Race of Microorganisms," https://www.exploratorium.edu/cooking/pickles/salt.html (accessed September 11, 2018).

7. M. D. Hoffman, K. J. Stuempfle, and T. Valentino, "Sodium Intake during an Ultramarathon Does Not Prevent Muscle Cramping, Dehydration, Hyponatremia, or Nausea," *Sports Medicine—Open* 1, no. 1 (2015): 39.

8. Healthline, "Low Blood Sodium (Hyponatremia)," https://www.healthline.com/health/hyponatremia#prevention (accessed February 6, 2020).

9. R. Horton, "Have the Salt Sellers Got Their Hearts in the Right Place?" *Observer of London*, June 22, 1997, 43.

10. T. G. Pickering, "The History and Politics of Salt," *Journal of Clinical Hypertension* 4, no. 3 (2002): 226–228.

11. US Department of Agriculture, "Questions and Answers on Descriptive Designation for Raw Meat and Poultry Products with Added Solutions," December 24, 2015, https://www.fsis.usda.gov/wps/wcm/connect/70c4707c-d4cf-4845-b97f-ad8dc23e4c 46/Q-A-Added-Solutions-122415.pdf?MOD=AJPERES (accessed October 29, 2019).

12. Press conference, Washington, DC, February 24, 2010.

13. US Department of Agriculture, "Final Rule: Descriptive Designation for Raw Meat and Poultry Products Containing Added Solutions," 79 Fed. Reg. 79043, December 31, 2014, https://www.federalregister.gov/documents/2014/12/31/2014-30472/ descriptive-designation-for-raw-meat-and-poultry-products-containing-added -solutions#h-14 (accessed August 22, 2018).

14. US Department of Agriculture, Food Safety and Inspection Service, "Common or Usual Name for Raw Meat and Poultry Products Containing Added Solutions," *Federal Register* 79, no. 144 (July 27, 2011): 44855–44865.

15. S. S. Franklin, L. Thijs, T. W. Hansen, et al., "White-Coat Hypertension: New Insights from Recent Studies," *Hypertension* 62, no. 6 (Dec. 2013): 982–987.

16. American Heart Association, "Salt vs. Sodium: Are They the Same?" *AHA Healthy for Good* (blog), July 22, 2014, https://sodiumbreakup.heart.org/salt-vs-sodium (accessed September 4, 2018).

17. S. B. Eaton, S. B. Eaton III, and M. J. Konner, "Paleolithic Nutrition Revisited: A Twelve-Year Retrospective on Its Nature and Implications," *European Journal of Clinical Nutrition* 51 (1997): 207–216.

18. J. Stamler, "Dietary Salt and Blood Pressure," *Annals of the New York Academy of Sciences* 676, no. 1 (1993): 122–156.

19. American Heart Association News, "Retired? Hardly—at 99, this Pioneering Heart Doctor is Still Leading the Way," October 18, 2019, https://www.heart.org/ en/news/2019/10/18/retired-hardly-at-99-this-pioneering-heart-doctor-is-still-leading -the-way? (accessed October 23, 2019).

20. H. Karppanen and E. Mervaala, "Sodium Intake and Hypertension," *Progress in Cardiovascular Diseases* 49, no. 2 (2006): 59–75.

21. J. L. Anderson, "Blood Gold," *New Yorker*, November 11, 2019.

22. W. J. Oliver, E. L. Cohen, and J. V. Neel, "Blood Pressure, Sodium Intake, and Sodium Related Hormones in the Yanomamo Indians, a 'No-Salt' Culture," *Circulation* 52 (1975): 146–151.

23. National Academy of Sciences, *Dietary Reference Intakes for Water, Potassium, Sodium, Chloride, and Sulfate* (Washington, DC: The National Academies Press, 2005), https://www.nap.edu/read/10925/chapter/1.

24. H. Nakagawa and K. Miura, "Salt Reduction in a Population for the Prevention of Hypertension," *Environmental Health and Preventive Medicine* 9 (2004): 123–129.

25. National Academies of Sciences, Engineering, and Medicine, *Dietary Reference Intakes for Sodium and Potassium* (Washington, DC: The National Academies Press, 2019), https://doi.org/10.17226/25353.

26. American Heart Association, "Recommended Dietary Pattern to Achieve Adherence to the American Heart Association/American College of Cardiology (AHA/ACC) Guidelines," *Circulation* 134 (2016): e505–e529.

27. World Health Organization, "Salt Reduction," June 30, 2016, http://www.who.int/news-room/fact-sheets/detail/salt-reduction (accessed September 3, 2018).

28. National Institute for Health and Care Excellence, *Prevention of Cardiovascular Disease at the Population Level* (London: National Institute for Health and Care Excellence, 2010); NICE PH25 (public health guidance 25), https://www.nice.org.uk/guidance/ph25/resources/cardiovascular-disease-prevention-pdf-1996238687173.

29. A. Carriquiry, A. J. Moshfegh, L. C. Steinfeldt, et al., "Trends in the Prevalence of Excess Dietary Sodium Intake—United States, 2003–2010," *Morbidity and Mortality Weekly Report* 62 (2013): 1021–1025.

30. National Academies of Sciences, Engineering, and Medicine, *Dietary Reference Intakes for Sodium and Potassium* (Washington, DC: The National Academies Press, 2019), https://doi.org/10.17226/25353 (accessed March 11, 2019).

31. J. K. Ahuja, S. Wasswa-Kintu, D. B. Haytowitz, et al., "Sodium Content of Popular Commercially Processed and Restaurant Foods in the United States," *Prevention Medicine Reports* 2 (2015): 962–967.

32. A. J. Moran, M. Ramirez, and J. P. Block, "Consumer Underestimation of Sodium in Fast Food Restaurant Meals: Results from a Cross-Sectional Observational Study," *Appetite* 113 (June 1, 2017): 155–161.

33. US Department of Agriculture, Agricultural Research Service, "FoodData Central," USDA food composition databases, https://fdc.nal.usda.gov/ (accessed October 31, 2019).

34. US Department of Agriculture, Agriculture Research Service, "What We Eat in America," https://www.ars.usda.gov/northeast-area/beltsville-md-bhnrc/beltsville-human-nutrition-research-center/food-surveys-research-group/docs/wweia-data-tables/ (accessed August 8, 2019); Center for Science in the Public Interest, "Reducing Sodium: A Look at State Savings in Health Care Costs," May 21, 2015, https://cspinet.org/sites/default/files/attachment/Sodium%20Report%20Final%205%20 20%2015.pdf (accessed August 8, 2019).

35. Centers for Disease Control and Prevention, "Usual Sodium Intakes Compared with Current Dietary Guidelines—United States, 2005–2008," *Morbidity and Mortality Weekly Report* 60 (2011): 1413–1417.

36. E. Decker, speaking at a public meeting of the Dietary Guidelines Advisory Committee. March 29, 2019. https://www.youtube.com/watch?v=HJQqDl7M-wU (accessed November 24, 2019).

37. R. L. Bailey, D. J. Catellier, S. Jun, et al., "Total Usual Nutrient Intakes of US Children (under 48 months): Findings from the Feeding Infants and Toddlers Study (FITS) 2016," *Journal of Nutrition* 148, no. 9S (2018): 1557S–1566S; S. Jun, D. J. Catellier, A. L. Eldridge, et al., "Usual Nutrient Intakes from the Diets of US Children by WIC Participation and Income: Findings from the Feeding Infants and Toddlers Study (FITS) 2016," *Journal of Nutrition* 148, no. 9S (2018): 1567S–1574S.

38. K. J. Overwyk, L. Zhao, Z. Zhang, et al., "Trends in Blood Pressure and Usual Dietary Sodium Intake among Children and Adolescents, National Health and Nutrition Examination Survey 2003 to 2016," *Hypertension* 74, no. 2 (2019): 260–266.

39. M. E. Cogswell, C. M. Loria, A. L. Terry, et al., "Estimated 24-Hour Urinary Sodium and Potassium Excretion in US Adults," *JAMA* 319, no. 12 (March 27, 2018): 1209–1220.

40. US Department of Agriculture, "Both at Home and Away, Americans Are Choosing More Lower Fat Foods Than They Did 35 Years Ago," October 1, 2018, https://www.ers.usda.gov/amber-waves/2018/october/both-at-home-and-away-americans-are-choosing-more-lower-fat-foods-than-they-did-35-years-ago/ (accessed March 20, 2019).

41. US Department of Agriculture, Economic Research Service, "Food Consumption and Nutrient Intakes, 2007–2010," August 20, 2019, https://www.ers.usda.gov/data-products/food-consumption-and-nutrient-intakes/food-consumption-and-nutrient-intakes/#Nutrient%20Intake%20Estimates (accessed September 7, 2019).

42. M. F. Jacobson and J. G. Hurley, *Restaurant Confidential* (New York: Workman Publishing, 2002).

43. M. A. McCrory, A. G. Harbaugh, S. Appeadu, et al., "Fast-Food Offerings in the United States In 1986, 1991, and 2016 Show Large Increases in Food Variety, Portion Size, Dietary Energy, and Selected Micronutrients," *Journal of the Academy of Nutrition and Dietetics* 119, no. 6 (2019): 923–933.

44. "Chili's Nutrition," September 30, 2019, https://brinker-chilis.cdn.prismic.io/brinker-chilis%2F5f27a96d-e996-4465-a91e-54f52bbf037f_chilis-nutrition-menu-generic.pdf (accessed October 29, 2019).

45. D. Prasad, T. A. Mezzacca, A. V. Anekwe, et al., "Sodium, Calorie, and Sugary Drink Purchasing Patterns in Chain Restaurants: Findings from NYC," *Preventive Medicine Reports* 17 (2020), https://doi.org/10.1016/j.pmedr.2019.101040.

46. International Food Information Council, "2019 Food & Health Survey," https:// foodinsight.org/wp-content/uploads/2019/05/IFIC-Foundation-2019-Food-and -Health-Report-FINAL.pdf (accessed September 4, 2019).

47. Pew Research Center, "Public Perspectives on Food Risks," November 19, 2018, http://www.pewinternet.org/2018/11/19/public-perspectives-on-food-risks/ (accessed September 4, 2019).

48. Food Marketing Institute, US Grocery Shopper Trends reports.

49. L. J. Harnack, M. E. Cogswell, J. M. Shikany, et al., "Sources of Sodium in US Adults from 3 Geographic Regions," *Circulation* 135 (2017): 1775–1783.

50. American Heart Association, "Most Americans Don't Understand the Health Effects of Wine and Sea Salt, Survey Finds," April 25, 2011, https://www.prnewswire .com/news-releases/most-americans-dont-understand-health-effects-of-wine-and -sea-salt-survey-finds-120595304.html.

51. US Department of Agriculture, USDA food composition databases, https://fdc .nal.usda.gov/ (accessed September 10, 2018).

52. Peapod by Giant, https://www.peapod.com/product-search/whole%2520chicken (accessed March 11, 2019).

53. KFC, "Interactive Nutrition Menu," April 19, 2018, https://www.kfc.com/ nutrition/full-nutrition-guide (accessed September 10, 2018).

54. City of El Paso, "Chemical Analysis—City Water," https://www.epwater.org/ UserFiles/Servers/Server_6843404/File/Our%20Water/Water%20Quality/chemanalysis .pdf (accessed February 23, 2019).

55. University of Maryland Extension, "Sodium in Your Well Water: A Health Concern," June 2019, https://extension.umd.edu/sites/extension.umd.edu/files/_docs/ publications/Sodium%20in%20well%20water%20FS%201084%20%281%29.pdf (accessed September 5, 2019).

56. Alka-Seltzer Extra Strength, drug facts, https://dailymed.nlm.nih.gov/dailymed/ fda/fdaDrugXsl.cfm?setid=49b73bd5-6465-05eb-e054-00144ff88e88&type=display (accessed February 23, 2019).

57. International Food Information Council, "Consumer Sodium Research," 2011, https://foodinsight.org/wp-content/uploads/2011/10/Sodium-2011_Final-Report _0916.pdf (accessed June 3, 2019).

58. Goop.com (blog), "Don't Blame the Saltshaker: Hidden Sodium and Our Hypertension Problem," https://goop.com/wellness/health/dont-blame-the-salt-shaker-hidden -sodium-and-our-hypertension-problem/ (accessed November 3, 2018).

59. US Department of Agriculture, "Added Sugars in Adults' Diet: What We Eat in America, NHANES 2015–2016," Food Surveys Research Group Dietary Data Brief

No. 24, October 2019, https://www.ars.usda.gov/ARSUserFiles/80400530/pdf/DBrief/ 24_Sources_of_Added_Sugars_in_Adults'_Diet_2015-2016.pdf (accessed January 18, 2020).

Chapter 2

1. Institute of Medicine, *Strategies to Reduce Sodium Intake in the United States* (Washington, DC: The National Academies Press, 2010).

2. Centers for Disease Control and Prevention, "Heart Attack," August 18, 2017, https://www.cdc.gov/heartdisease/heart_attack.htm (accessed October 26, 2019); Centers for Disease Control and Prevention, "Heart Disease Fact Sheet," August 23, 2017, https://www.cdc.gov/dhdsp/data_statistics/fact_sheets/fs_heart_disease.htm (accessed October 26, 2019).

3. Centers for Disease Control and Prevention, "Stroke Fact Sheet," September 1, 2017, https://www.cdc.gov/dhdsp/data_statistics/fact_sheets/fs_stroke.htm (accessed January 20, 2020).

4. Centers for Disease Control and Prevention, "Stroke Facts," January 31, 2020, https://www.cdc.gov/stroke/facts.htm (accessed February 23, 2020).

5. J. B. Taylor, "My Stroke of Insight," TED (video), February 2008, https://www .ted.com/talks/jill_bolte_taylor_s_powerful_stroke_of_insight (accessed October 27, 2019).

6. Harvard Women's Health Watch, "Mini-stroke: What Should You Do?" March 2014, https://www.health.harvard.edu/heart-health/mini-stroke-what-should-you-do (accessed October 26, 2019).

7. Q. Yang, X. Tong, L. Schieb, et al., "Vital Signs: Recent Trends in Stroke Death Rates—United States, 2000–2015," *Morbidity and Mortality Weekly Report* 66 (2017): 933–399.

8. L. Ambard and E. Beaujard, "Causes de'l hypertension arterielle," *Archives générales de Médecine de Paris* 1 (1904): 520–533.

9. "The Use of Salt," *JAMA* 293 (2005): 100.

10. F. M. Allen and J. W. Sherrill, "The Treatment of Arterial Hypertension," *Journal of Metabolic Research* 2 (1922): 429–545.

11. Sources for box 2.1: "Among adults, 54 percent of African Americans have hypertension": Centers for Disease Control and Prevention, "High Blood Pressure, Facts about Hypertension," January 28, 2020, https://www.cdc.gov/bloodpressure/ facts.htm?CDC_AA_refVal=https%3A%2F%2Fwww.cdc.gov%2Fdhdsp%2Fdata _statistics%2Ffact_sheets%2Ffs_bloodpressure.htm (accessed February 6, 2020). "80

to 90 percent of adults will develop hypertension": P. Muntner, R. M. Carey, S. Gidding, et al., "Potential US Population Impact of the 2017 ACC/AHA High Blood Pressure Guideline," *Circulation* 137 (2018): 109–118; R. S. Vasan, A. Beiser, S. Seshadri, et al., "Residual Lifetime Risk for Developing Hypertension in Middle-Aged Women and Men," *JAMA* 287 (2002): 1003–1010. "Hypertension is responsible for over \$131 billion in annual healthcare costs": E. B. Kirkland, "Trends in Healthcare Expenditures among US Adults with Hypertension: National Estimates, 2003–2014," *Journal of the American Heart Association* 7 (2018): e008731. "Together, coronary heart disease and stroke kill about 500,000 people annually": E. J. Benjamin, M. J. Blaha, S. E. Chiuve, et al., "Heart Disease and Stroke Statistics—2017 Update: A Report from the American Heart Association," *Circulation* 135 (2017): e146–e603. "High blood pressure is a primary or contributing cause of 472,000 deaths per year," "About 7 of every 10 people suffering a first heart attack have high blood pressure": Centers for Disease Control and Prevention, "High Blood Pressure, Facts about Hypertension," January 28, 2020, https://www.cdc.gov/bloodpressure/ facts.htm?CDC_AA_refVal=https%3A%2F%2Fwww.cdc.gov%2Fdhdsp%2Fdata _statistics%2Ffact_sheets%2Ffs_bloodpressure.htm (accessed February 6, 2020). "The average adult should consume no more than 2,300 mg of sodium per day": US Department of Health and Human Services and US Department of Agriculture, *Dietary Guidelines for Americans 2015–2020, 8th Edition* (December 2015), http:// health.gov/dietaryguidelines/2015/guidelines/. "Average sodium intake of sodium for everyone 2 and older is 3,400 mg per day": L. J. Harnack, M. E. Cogswell, J. M. Shikany, et al., "Sources of Sodium in US Adults from 3 Geographic Regions," *Circulation* 135 (2017): 1775–1183. "For children, the recommended sodium limits are 1,200 mg for ages 1 to 3": National Academies of Sciences, Engineering, and Medicine, *Dietary Reference Intakes for Sodium and Potassium* (Washington, DC: The National Academies Press, 2019), https://www.nap.edu/download/25353. "Children 6 to 10 years old actually consume 2,900 mg of sodium per day": US Food and Drug Administration, "You May Be Surprised by How Much Salt You're Eating," January 23, 2018, https://www.fda.gov/ForConsumers/ConsumerUpdates/ucm327369.htm (accessed March 11, 2018). "Worldwide, reducing sodium intakes to an average of 2,000 mg per day could prevent about 2.5 million deaths": World Health Organization, "Salt Reduction," June 30, 2016, http://www.who.int/mediacentre/factsheets/ fs393/en/ (accessed October 20, 2019).

12. G. A Porter, "Chronology of the Sodium Hypothesis and Hypertension," *Annals of Internal Medicine* 98, no. 2 (1983): 720–723.

13. "The Therapeutic Role of the Kempner Diet," *New England Journal of Medicine* 240 (February 10, 1949): 236.

14. E. H. Estes and L. Kerivan, "An Archaeologic Dig: A Rice-Fruit Diet Reverses ECG Changes in Hypertension," *Journal of Electrocardiology* 47, no. 5 (September–October 2014): 599–607.

15. Estes and Kerivan, "An Archaeologic Dig."

16. "Report: Rice Doctor Admitted to Whippings in Depositions," Associated Press, October 19, 1997, https://apnews.com/c89424d1d36a4f42d7ef87a0c95e9248.

17. P. Klemmer, C. E. Grim, and F. C. Luft, "Who and What Drove Walter Kempner? The Rice Diet Revisited," *Hypertension* 64 (2014): 684–688.

18. D. M. Watkin, H. F. Froeb, F. T. Hatch, et al., "Effects of Diet in Essential Hypertension: II. Results with Unmodified Kempner Rice Diet in Fifty Hospitalized Patients," *American Journal of Medicine* 9, no. 4 (October 1950): 441–493.

19. G. R. Meneely and C. O. T. Ball, "Experimental Epidemiology of Chronic Sodium Chloride Toxicity and the Protective Effect of Potassium Chloride," *American Journal of Medicine* 25 (1958): 713–725.

20. L. K. Dahl and M. Heine, "Primary Role of Renal Homografts in Setting Chronic Blood Pressure Levels in Rats," *Circulation Research* 36 (1975): 692–696.

21. F. Elijovich, M. H. Weinberger, C. A. Anderson, et al., "Salt Sensitivity of Blood Pressure: a Scientific Statement from the American Heart Association," *Hypertension* 68, no. 3 (September 2016): e7–e46.

22. D. Denton, R. Weisinger, N. I. Mundy, et al., "The Effect of Increased Salt Intake on Blood Pressure of Chimpanzees," *Nature Medicine* 10, no. 1 (October 1995): 1009–1016.

23. O. M. Dong, "Excessive Dietary Sodium Intake and Elevated Blood Pressure: A Review of Current Prevention and Management Strategies and the Emerging Role of Pharmaconutrigenetics," *BMJ Nutrition, Prevention and Health* 1, no. 1 (2018): 7–16, http://dx.doi.org/10.1136/bmjnph-2018-000004.

24. D. Denton, R. Weisinger, N. I. Mundy, et al., "The Effect of Increased Salt Intake on Blood Pressure of Chimpanzees," *Nature Medicine* 10, no. 1 (October 1995): 1009–1016.

25. Denton et al., "The Effect of Increased Salt Intake."

26. W. J. Oliver, E. L. Cohen, and J. V. Neel, "Blood Pressure, Sodium Intake, and Sodium Related Hormones in the Yanomamo Indians, a 'No-Salt' Culture," *Circulation* 52 (1975): 146–151.

27. N. T. Mueller, O. Noya-Alarcon, M. Contreras, et al., "Association of Age with Blood Pressure across the Lifespan in Isolated Yanomami and Yekwana Villages," *JAMA Cardiology* 3 (2018): 1247–1249; S. A. E. Peters, P. Muntner, and M. Woodward, "Sex Differences in the Prevalence of, and Trends in, Cardiovascular Risk Factors, Treatment, and Control in the United States, 2001 to 2016," *Circulation* 139 (2019):

1025–1035; supplemental data, https://www.ahajournals.org/doi/suppl/10.1161/
CIRCULATIONAHA.118.035550 (accessed February 27, 2020).

28. Sources for box 2.2: "Prehistoric animals developed powerful physiological processes"; G. MacGregor, "Dietary Sodium and Potassium Intake and Blood Pressure,"
Lancet 321, no. 8327 (April 2, 1983): 750–753. • "Almost everyone consumes less
potassium than they should": "Salt and Your Health, Part I: The Sodium Connection," *Harvard Men's Health Watch*, October 2010, https://www.health.harvard.edu/
newsletter_article/salt-and-your-health (accessed August 18, 2019). • "When compared with the BP of wild animals or of primitive man, BP levels considered to be
'normal' in civilized countries may actually be hypertensive": H. Nakagawa and K.
Miura, "Salt Reduction in a Population for the Prevention of Hypertension," *Environmental Health and Preventive Medicine* 9 (2004): 123–129. Figure 2.1: American Heart
Association. • "What Is High Blood Pressure?" 2017, https://www.heart.org/en/
health-topics/high-blood-pressure/understanding-blood-pressure-readings (accessed
October 13, 2019). • "President FDR long had a blood pressure problem": T. Bishop
and V. M. Figueredo, "Hypertensive Therapy: Attacking the Renin-Angiotensin
System," *Western Journal of Medicine* 175, no. 2 (August 2001): 119–124; A. B.
Sobocinski, "The President's Vital Signs: A Look Back at FDR's Heart Health," Navy
Medicine Live, Official blog of the US Navy Bureau of Medicine and Surgery, http://
navymedicine.navylive.dodlive.mil/archives/8066 (accessed July 8, 2018). • "Sadly,
few physicians knew at the time": R. A. Pizzi, "Developing Diuretics," *Modern Drug
Discovery* 6 (February 2003): 19–20. • "The relationship between blood pressure level
and risk of developing cardiovascular disease is strong, continuous, graded, consistent, independent, and etiologically significant": S. Havas, E. J.Roccella, and C.
Lenfant, "Reducing the Public Health Burden from Elevated Blood Pressure Levels in
the United States by Lowering Intake of Dietary Sodium, *American Journal of Public
Health* 94 (2004): 19–22. • "in 2017 the threshold for stage 1 hypertension was low-
ered again": P. K. Whelton, R. M. Carey, W. S. Aronow, et al., "2017 ACC/AHA/
AAPA/ABC/ACPM/AGS/APhA/ASH/ASPC/NMA/PCNA Guideline for the Prevention,
Detection, Evaluation, and Management of High Blood Pressure in Adults: Executive
Summary. A Report of the American College of Cardiology/American Heart Association Task Force on Clinical Practice Guidelines," *Journal of the American College of
Cardiology* 71, no. 19 (May 15, 2018): e127–e248. Correction: *Journal of the American
College of Cardiology* 71, no. 19 (2018): 2275–2279. • "That lower threshold for concern": P. Muntner, R. M. Carey, S. Gidding, et al., "Potential US Population Impact
of the 2017 ACC/AHA High Blood Pressure Guideline," *Circulation* 137, no. 2 (January 9, 2018): 109–118. • "Rises in blood pressure strike blacks earlier, hypertension
is often more severe": American Heart Association, "African Americans and Heart
Disease, Stroke," July 31, 2015, https://www.heart.org/en/health-topics/consumer
-healthcare/what-is-cardiovascular-disease/african-americans-and-heart-disease
-stroke (accessed October 16, 2019). • "And some medications are less effective":

American Heart Association, "What about African Americans and High Blood Pressure?" 2017, https://www.heart.org/-/media/data-import/downloadables/2/8/a/pe-abh-what-about-african-americans-and-high-blood-pressure-ucm_300463 (accessed October 16, 2019). • "African Americans may carry a gene that makes them more salt sensitive": American Heart Association. "High Blood Pressure and African Americans," October 31, 2016. https://www.heart.org/en/health-topics/high-blood-pressure/why-high-blood-pressure-is-a-silent-killer/high-blood-pressure-and-african-americans (accessed October 16, 2019). • "Blacks consume slightly less sodium than whites": National Academies of Sciences, Engineering, and Medicine, *Dietary Reference Intakes for Sodium and Potassium* (Washington, DC: The National Academies Press, 2019), table 11-2 https://doi.org/10.17226/25353. • "That's roughly the same benefit": P. K. Whelton, R. M. Carey, W. S. Aronow, et al., "2017 ACC/AHA/AAPA/ABC/ACPM/AGS/APhA/ASH/ASPC/NMA/PCNA Guideline"; "Correction."

29. E. D. Freis, "The Role of Salt in Hypertension," *Blood Pressure* 1 (1992): 196–200; E. D. Freis, "Salt, Volume, and the Prevention of Hypertension," *Circulation* 53 (1976): 589–595.

30. P. F. Sinnet and H. M. Shyte, "Epidemiological Studies in a Total Highland Population, Tukisenta New Guinea: Cardiovascular Disease and Relevant Clinical, Electrocardiographic, Radiological and Biochemical Findings," *Journal of Chronic Diseases* 26 (1973): 265–290.

31. M. Gurven, A. D. Blackwell, D. E. Rodríguez, et al., "Does Blood Pressure Inevitably Rise with Age? Longitudinal Evidence among Forager-Horticulturalists," *Hypertension* 60 (2012): 25–33.

32. American Heart Association, "Statistical Fact Sheet 2013 Update, High Blood Pressure," 2013. https://www.heart.org/idc/groups/heart-public/@wcm/@sop/@smd/documents/downloadable/ucm_319587.pdf (accessed March 4, 2019).

33. J. Swales, "Dietary Salt and Hypertension," *Lancet* 315, no. 8179 (1980): 1177–1179.

34. F. J. He and G. A. MacGregor, "A Comprehensive Review on Salt and Health and Current Experience of Worldwide Salt Reduction Programmes," *Journal of Human Hypertension* 23 (2009): 363–384.

35. L. B. Page, A. Damon, and R. J. Moellering Jr., "Antecedents of Cardiovascular Disease in Six Solomon Island Societies," *Circulation* 49 (1974): 1132–1146.

36. G. A. MacGregor, N. D. Markandu, G. A. Sagnella, D. R. G. Singer, and F. P. Cappuccio, "Double-blind Study of Three Sodium Intakes and Long-term Effects of Sodium Restriction in Essential Hypertension," *The Lancet* 2 (1989): 1244–1247.

37. F. M. Sacks, L. P. Svetkey, W. M. Vollmer, et al., "Effects on Blood Pressure of Reduced Dietary Sodium and the Dietary Approaches to Stop Hypertension (DASH) Diet," *New England Journal of Medicine* 344 (2001): 3–10.

38. F. M. Sacks, B. Rosner, and E. H. Kass, "Blood Pressure in Vegetarians," *American Journal of Epidemiology* 100 (1974): 390–398.

39. F. M. Sacks, email correspondence with the author, August 28, 2019.

40. W. M. Vollmer, F. M. Sacks, J. Ard, et al., "Effects of Diet and Sodium Intake on Blood Pressure: Subgroup Analysis of the DASH–sodium Trial," *Annals of Internal Medicine* 135 (2001): 1019–1028.

41. R. Cooper, "Cardiovascular Prevention through Precision," Speech at the scientific symposium to celebrate the 100th birthday of Jeremiah Stamler, MD, October 25, 2019.

42. National Heart, Lung, and Blood Institute, "DASH Eating Plan," NIH Publication No. 06–4082, April 2006. https://www.nhlbi.nih.gov/files/docs/public/heart/new_dash.pdf (accessed September 8, 2019)

43. N. Karanja, K. J. Lancaster, W. M. Vollmer, et al., "Acceptability of Sodium-reduced Research Diets, including the Dietary Approaches To Stop Hypertension Diet, among Adults with Prehypertension and Stage 1 Hypertension," *Journal of the American Dietetic Association* 107, no. 9 (2007): 1530–1538.

44. F. J. He and G. A. MacGregor, "Effect of Modest Salt Reduction on Blood Pressure: a Meta-Analysis of Randomized Trials: Implications for Public Health," *Journal of Human Hypertension* 16 (2002): 761–70.

45. F. J. He, personal communication with the author, September 5, 2018.

46. L. Huang, K. Trieu, S. Yoshimura, et al., "Effect of Dose and Duration of Reduction in Dietary Sodium on Blood Pressure Levels: Systematic Review and Meta-analysis of Randomised Trials," *BMJ* 368 (2020): m315, http://dx.doi.org/10.1136/bmj.m315 (accessed February 27, 2020).

47. N. R. Cook, J. Cohen, P. R. Hebert, et al., "Implications of Small Reductions in Diastolic Blood Pressure for Primary Prevention," *Archives of Internal Medicine* 155 (1995): 701–709.

48. L. J. Appel, M. A. Espeland, L. Easter, et al., "Effects of Reduced Sodium Intake on Hypertension Control in Older Individuals: Results from the Trial of Nonpharmacologic Interventions in the Elderly (TONE)," *Archives of Internal Medicine* 161 (2001): 685–693.

49. E. D. Freis, "Salt, Volume, and the Prevention of Hypertension," *Circulation* 53 (1976): 589–95.

50. G. A. MacGregor, "Dietary Sodium and Potassium Intake and Blood Pressure," *The Lancet* 321, no. 8327 (April 2, 1983): 750–753.

51. J. Henney, Press conference for 2010 Institute of Medicine report on lowering sodium intakes, April 20, 2010, http://www.nationalacademies.org/podcast/042110SodiumStrategies.mp3 (accessed September 15, 2018).

52. S. L. Jackson, Z. Zhang, J. L. Wiltz, et al., "Hypertension among Youths—United States, 2001–2016," *Morbidity and Mortality Weekly Report* 67 (2018): 758–762.

53. R. M. Lauer, W. R. Clarke, L. T. Mahoney, et al., "Childhood Predictors for High Adult Blood Pressure: the Muscatine Study," *Childhood Hypertension* 93, no. 1 (February 1993): 23–40.

54. S. L. Jackson, Z. Zhang, J. L. Wiltz, et al., "Hypertension among Youths—United States, 2001–2016," *Morbidity and Mortality Weekly Report* 67 (2018): 758–762.

55. A. Hofman, A. Hazebroek, and H. A. Valkenburg, "A Randomized Trial of Sodium Intake and Blood Pressure in Newborn Infants," *JAMA* 250, no. 3 (July 15, 1983): 370–373.

56. J. M. Geleijnse, A. Hofman, J. C. Witteman, et al., "Long-term Effects of Neonatal Sodium Restriction on Blood Pressure," *Hypertension* 29 (1997): 913–917.

57. J. Maalouf, M. E. Cogswell, M. Bates, et al., "Sodium, Sugar, and Fat Content of Complementary Infant and Toddler Foods Sold in the United States, 2015," *American Journal of Clinical Nutrition* 105 (June 2017): 1443–1452.

58. R. C. Ellison, A. L. Capper, W. P. Stephenson, et al., "Effects on Blood Pressure of a Decrease in Sodium Use in Institutional Food Preparation: the Exeter-Andover Project," *Journal of Clinical Epidemiology* 42, no. 3 (1989): 201–208.

59. S. S. Franklin and N. D. Wong, "Hypertension and Cardiovascular Disease: Contributions of the Framingham Heart Study," *Global Heart* 8, no. 1 (March 2013): 49–57; S. Lewington, R. Clarke, N. Qizilbash, et al., "Age-Specific Relevance of Usual Blood Pressure to Vascular Mortality: A Meta Analysis of Individual Data for One Million Adults in 61 Prospective Studies," *Lancet* 360 (2002): 1903–1913.

60. P. Strazzullo, L. D'Elia, N. B. Kandala, et al., "Salt Intake, Stroke, and Cardiovascular Disease: Meta-analysis of Prospective Studies," *BMJ* 339 (2009): b4567.

61. Currency Conversion Calculator, Investing.com, https://www.investing.com/currencies/gbp-usd-converter (accessed September 8, 2019).

62. National Institute for Health and Care Excellence, "Cardiovascular Disease Prevention," June 2010, https://www.nice.org.uk/guidance/ph25/chapter/3-Considerations (accessed August 19, 2018).

63. UK Department of Health, "National Diet and Nutrition Survey—Assessment of Dietary Sodium in Adults (Aged 19 to 64 Years) in England, 2011," June 21 2012, https://assets.publishing.service.gov.uk/government/uploads/system/uploads/attachment_data/file/213420/Sodium-Survey-England-2011_Text_to-DH_FINAL1

.pdf (accessed October 16, 2019); L. Hyseni, A. Elliot-Green, F. Lloyd-Williams, et al., "Systematic Review of Dietary Salt Reduction Policies: Evidence for an Effectiveness Hierarchy?" *PLoS ONE* 12, no. 5 (2017): e0177535, http://journals.plos.org/plosone/article/file?id=10.1371/journal.pone.0177535&type=printable.

64. Public Health England, "Salt Targets 2017: Progress Report—A Report on the Food Industry's Progress towards Meeting the 2017 Salt Targets," December 2018, https://publichealthengland.exposure.co/salt-reduction-programme.

65. F. J. He, H. C. Brinsden, and G. A. MacGregor. "Salt Reduction in the United Kingdom: A Successful Experiment in Public Health," *Journal of Human Hypertension* 28, no. 6 (2014): 345–352.

66. National Institute for Health and Care Excellence, "Cardiovascular Disease Prevention," June 2010, https://www.nice.org.uk/guidance/ph25/chapter/3-Considerations (accessed August 19, 2018).

67. H. Y. Chang, Y. W. Hu, C. S. Yue, et al., "Effect of Potassium-Enriched Salt on Cardiovascular Mortality and Medical Expenses of Elderly Men," *American Journal of Clinical Nutrition* 83, no. 6 (2006): 1289–1296.

68. Institute of Medicine (US) Committee on Strategies to Reduce Sodium Intake; J. E. Henney, C. L. Taylor, C. S. Boon, eds., *Strategies to Reduce Sodium Intake in the United States* (Washington DC: The National Academies Press, 2010).

69. The Trials of Hypertension Prevention Collaborative Research Group, "The Effects of Nonpharmacologic Interventions on Blood Pressure of Persons with High Normal Levels: Results of the Trials of Hypertension Prevention, Phase I," *JAMA* 267 (1992): 1213–1220; The Trials of Hypertension Prevention Collaborative Research Group, "Effects of Weight Loss and Sodium Reduction Intervention on Blood Pressure and Hypertension Incidence in Overweight People with High-Normal Blood Pressure: The Trials of Hypertension Prevention, Phase II," *Archives of Internal Medicine* 157, no. 1 (March 24, 1997): 65–67.

70. N. R. Cook, J. A. Cutler, E. Obarzanek, et al., "Long Term Effects of Dietary Sodium Reduction on Cardiovascular Disease Outcomes: Observational Follow-Up of the Trials of Hypertension Prevention (TOHP)," *BMJ* 334, no. 7599 (April 28, 2007): 885–888.

71. Cook et al. "Long Term Effects of Dietary Sodium Reduction."

72. F. Godlee, "Time to Talk Salt," *BMJ* 334 (April 28, 2007), https://www.bmj.com/content/334/7599/0.1.

73. National Academies of Sciences, Engineering, and Medicine, *Dietary Reference Intakes for Sodium and Potassium* (Washington, DC: The National Academies Press, 2019), https://doi.org/10.17226/25353 (accessed April 22, 2019).

74. F. J. He, M. Tan, Y. Ma, et al., "Salt Reduction to Prevent Hypertension and Cardiovascular Disease: *JACC* State of the Art Review," *Journal of the American College of Cardiology* 75, no. 6 (February 2020): 632–647.

75. S. Havas, E. J. Roccella, and C. Lenfant, "Reducing the Public Health Burden from Elevated Blood Pressure Levels in the United States by Lowering Intake of Dietary Sodium," *American Journal of Public Health* 94 (2004): 19–22.

76. K. Palar and R. Sturm, "Potential Societal Savings from Reduced Sodium Consumption in the US Adult Population," *American Journal of Health Promotion* 24 (2009): 49–57.

77. G. Danaei, E. L. Ding, D. Mozaffarian, et al., "The Preventable Causes of Death in the United States: Comparative Risk Assessment of Dietary, Lifestyle, and Metabolic Risk Factors," *PLoS Medicine* 6, no.4 (2009): e1000058.

78. C. M. Smith-Spangler, J. L. Juusola, E. A. Enns, et al., "Population Strategies to Decrease Sodium Intake and the Burden of Cardiovascular Disease," *Annals of Internal Medicine* 152 (2010): 481–487.

79. K. Bibbins-Domingo, G. M. Chertow, P. G. Coxson, et al., "Projected Effect of Dietary Salt Reductions on Future Cardiovascular Disease," *New England Journal of Medicine* 362 (2010): 590–599.

80. P. G. Coxson, N. R. Cook, M. Joffres, et al., "Mortality Benefits from US Population-Wide Reduction in Sodium Consumption: Projections from 3 Modeling Approaches," *Hypertension* 61, no. 3 (March 2013): 564–570.

81. D. Mozaffarian, S. Fahimi, G. M. Singh, et al., Global Burden of Diseases Nutrition and Chronic Diseases Expert Group, "Global Sodium Consumption and Death from Cardiovascular Causes," *New England Journal of Medicine* 371 (2014): 624–634.

82. J. Pearson-Stuttard, C. Kypridemos, B. Collins, et al., "Estimating the Health and Economic Effects of the Proposed US Food and Drug Administration Voluntary Sodium Reformulation: Microsimulation Cost-Effectiveness Analysis," *PLoS Medicine* 15, no. 4 (April 10 2018): e1002551.

83. A. Jessup and D. Wilmoth, US Department of Health and Human Services, "The Value of a National Reduction in Dietary Sodium from Processed and Restaurant Foods," preliminary draft, October 22, 2013 (in the author's files).

84. N. Graudal, G. Jürgens, B. Baslund, et al., "Compared with Usual Sodium Intake, Low- and Excessive-Sodium Diets are Associated with Increased Mortality: A Meta-Analysis," *American Journal of Hypertension* 27 (2014): 1129–1137.

85. National Institute of Alcohol Abuse and Alcoholism, "Alcohol Facts and Statistics," August 2018, https://www.niaaa.nih.gov/alcohol-health/overview-alcohol -consumption/alcohol-facts-and-statistics (accessed October 20, 2018).

86. N. Bomey, "US Vehicle Deaths Topped 40,000 in 2017, National Safety Council Estimates," *USA Today*, February 15, 2018, https://www.usatoday.com/story/money/cars/2018/02/15/national-safety-council-traffic-deaths/340012002/.

87. T. R. Frieden and P. A. Briss, "We Can Reduce Dietary Sodium, Save Money, and Save Lives," *Annals of Internal Medicine* 152, no. 8 (2010): 526–527.

88. Centers for Disease Control and Prevention, "Preventing Stroke Deaths," September 6, 2017, https://www.cdc.gov/vitalsigns/stroke/infographic.html#graphic (accessed February 23, 2020); Centers for Disease Control and Prevention, "Achievements in Public Health, 1900–1999: Decline in Deaths from Heart Disease and Stroke—United States, 1900–1999, *MMWR Weekly* 48, no. 30 (August 6, 1999): 649–656, https://www.cdc.gov/mmwr/preview/mmwrhtml/mm4830a1.htm (accessed February 23, 2020).

89. J. V. Joosens, H. Kesteloot, and A. Amery, *New England Journal of Medicine* 300 (1979): 1396.

90. M. Burnier, "Medication Adherence and Persistence as the Cornerstone of Effective Antihypertensive Therapy," *American Journal of Hypertension* 19, no. 11 (2006): 1190–1196.

91. B. Vrijens, S. Antoniou, M. Burnier, et al., "Current Situation of Medication Adherence in Hypertension," *Frontiers in Pharmacology* 8 (2017): 100, doi:10.3389/fphar.2017.00100.

92. J. B. Byrd, G. M. Chertow, and V. Bhalla, "Hypertension Hot Potato—Anatomy of the Angiotensin-Receptor Blocker Recalls," *New England Journal of Medicine* 380 (2019): 1589–1591.

93. A. Soni and E. Mitchell, "Agency for Healthcare Research and Quality: Expenditures for Commonly Treated Conditions among Adults Age 18 and Older in the US Civilian Noninstitutionalized Population," Statistical brief 487, 2013, https://meps.ahrq.gov/data_files/publications/st487/stat487.pdf (accessed February 25, 2019).

94. Department of Health and Human Services, FY 2020 budget, https://www.nhlbi.nih.gov/sites/default/files/media/docs/FY_2020_NHLBI_CJ.pdf (accessed September 8, 2019).

95. E. Judd and D. A. Calhoun, "Apparent and True Resistant Hypertension: Definition, Prevalence and Outcomes," *Journal of Human Hypertension* 4, no. 28 (2014): 463–468.

96. E. Pimenta, K. K. Gaddam, M. N. Pratt-Ubunama, et al., "Relation of Dietary Salt and Aldosterone to Urinary Protein Excretion in Subjects with Resistant Hypertension," *Hypertension* 51, no. 2 (2008): 339–344.

97. R. M. Carey, D. A. Calhoun, G. L. Bakris, et al.; American Heart Association Professional/Public Education and Publications Committee of the Council on

Hypertension; Council on Cardiovascular and Stroke Nursing; Council on Clinical Cardiology; Council on Genomic and Precision Medicine; Council on Peripheral Vascular Disease; Council on Quality of Care and Outcomes Research; and Stroke Council, "Resistant Hypertension: Detection, Evaluation, and Management: A Scientific Statement from the American Heart Association," *Hypertension* 72 (2018): e53–e90.

98. Centers for Disease Control and Prevention, "Chronic Kidney Disease Basics," December 6, 2018. https://www.cdc.gov/kidneydisease/basics.html (accessed October 24, 2019).

99. V. A. Luyckx, M. Tonelli, and J. W. Stanifer, "The Global Burden of Kidney Disease and the Sustainable Development Goals," *Bulletin of the World Health Organization* 96 (2018): 414–422D.

100. National Kidney Foundation, "Kidney Disease: The Basics," https://www.kidney.org/news/newsroom/factsheets/KidneyDiseaseBasics (accessed October 24, 2019).

101. R. Boero, A. Pignataro, and F. Quarello, "Salt Intake and Kidney Disease," *Journal of Nephrology* 15 (2002): 225–229; American Kidney Fund, "Kidney Failure/ ESRD Diet," https://www.kidneyfund.org/kidney-disease/kidney-failure/esrd-diet/ (accessed February 8, 2020).

102. C. Garofalo, S. Borrelli, M. Provenzano, et al., "Dietary Salt Restriction in Chronic Kidney Disease: a Meta-Analysis of Randomized Clinical Trials," *Nutrients* 10, no. 6 (2018): E732, http://dx.doi.org/10.3390/nu10060732.

103. K. T. Mills, J. Chen, W. Yang, et al., Chronic Renal Insufficiency Cohort (CRIC) Study Investigators, "Sodium Excretion and the Risk of Cardiovascular Disease in Patients with Chronic Kidney Disease," *JAMA* 315 (2016): 2200–2210.

104. K. Boyd, "What Is Ischemic Optic Neuropathy?" *American Academy of Ophthalmology*, May 31, 2019, https://www.aao.org/eye-health/diseases/what-is-ischemic-optic-neuropathy (accessed November 5, 2019).

105. A. Biggers, "Everything You Should Know about Eye Stroke," *Medical News Today*, June 12, 2017. https://www.medicalnewstoday.com/articles/317877.php (accessed November 5, 2019).

106. The SPRINT MIND Investigators for the SPRINT Research Group, "Effect of Intensive vs Standard Blood Pressure Control on Probable Dementia: A Randomized Clinical Trial," *JAMA* 321, no. 6 (2019): 553–561.

107. K. Yaffe, "Prevention of Cognitive Impairment with Intensive Systolic Blood Pressure Control," *JAMA* 321, no. 6 (2019): 548–549.

108. Alzheimer's Association, "Study Shows Intensive Blood Pressure Control Reduces Risk of Mild Cognitive Impairment (MCI) and the Combined Risk of MCI

and Dementia," news release, July 25, 2018, https://www.alz.org/aaic/releases_2018/ AAIC18-Wed-developing-topics.asp (accessed May 13, 2019).

109. G. Faraco, K. Hochrainer, S. G. Segarra, et al., "Dietary Salt Promotes Cognitive Impairment through Tau Phosphorylation," *Nature* 574 (2019), http://dx.doi .org/10.1038/s41586-019-1688-z.

110. Weill Cornell Medical, "A High-Salt Diet Produces Dementia in Mice," news release, January 16, 2018, https://news.weill.cornell.edu/news/2018/01/a-high-salt -diet-produces-dementia-in-mice (accessed October 29, 2019).

111. M. Amer, M. Woodward, and L. J. Appel, "Effects of Dietary Sodium and the DASH Diet on the Occurrence of Headaches: Results from Randomised Multicentre DASH–Sodium Clinical Trial," *BMJ Open* 4 (2014): 4:e006671; L. Chen, Z. Zhang, W. Chen, et al., "Lower Sodium Intake and Risk of Headaches: Results from the Trial of Nonpharmacologic Interventions in the Elderly," *American Journal of Public Health* 106 (July 2016): 1270–1275.

112. N. P. Shah, M. Cainzos-Achirica, D. I. Feldman, et al., "Cardiovascular Disease Prevention in Men with Vascular Erectile Dysfunction: The View of the Preventive Cardiologist," *American Journal of Medicine* 129, no. 3 (March 2016): 251–259.

113. H. A. Feldman, I. Goldstein, D. G. Hatzichristou, et al., "Impotence and Its Medical and Psychosocial Correlates: Results of the Massachusetts Male Aging Study," *Journal of Urology* 151 (1994): 54–61.

114. Mayo Clinic Staff, "High Blood Pressure and Sex: Overcome the Challenges," January 9, 2019. https://www.mayoclinic.org/diseases-conditions/high-blood-pressure/ in-depth/high-blood-pressure-and-sex/art-20044209 (accessed November 4, 2019).

115. S. B. Eaton, S. B. Eaton III, and M. J. Konner, "Paleolithic Nutrition Revisited: A Twelve-Year Retrospective on its Nature and Implications," *European Journal of Clinical Nutrition* 51 (1997): 207–216.

116. "WHO Guideline: Potassium Intake for Adults and Children," Geneva, World Health Organization (WHO), 2012.

117. N. J. Aburto, S. Hanson, H. Gutierrez, et al., "Effect of Increased Potassium Intake on Cardiovascular Risk Factors and Disease: Systematic Review and Meta-Analyses," *BMJ* 346 (April 3, 2013): f1378.

118. Y. G. Peng, W. Li, X. X. Wen, et al., "Effects of Salt Substitutes on Blood Pressure: A Meta-Analysis of Randomized Controlled Trials," *American Journal of Clinical Nutrition* 100 (2014): 1448–1454.

119. L. D'Elia, C. Iannotta, P. Sabino, et al., "Potassium-Rich Diet and Risk of Stroke: Updated Meta-Analysis," *Nutrition, Metabolism, and Cardiovascular Diseases* 24 (2014): 585–587.

120. Q. Yang, T. Liu, E. V. Kuklina, et al., "Sodium and Potassium Intake and Mortality among US Adults: Prospective Data from the Third National Health and Nutrition Examination Survey," *Archives of Internal Medicine* 171 (2011): 1183–1191; N. R. Cook, E. Obarzanek, J. A. Cutler, et al., for the Trials of Hypertension Prevention Collaborative Research Group, "Joint Effects of Sodium and Potassium Intake on Subsequent Cardiovascular Disease: The Trials of Hypertension Prevention (TOHP) Follow-Up Study," *Archives of Internal Medicine* 169 (2009): 32–40; "ACC/AHA/ AAPA/ABC/ACPM/AGS/APhA/ASH/ASPC/NMA/PCNA Guideline for the Prevention, Detection, Evaluation, and Management of High Blood Pressure in Adults: A Report of the American College of Cardiology/American Heart Association Task Force on Clinical Practice Guidelines," *Journal of the American College of Cardiology* 71 (2018): e127–e248.

121. World Health Organization, "Guideline: Potassium Intake for Adults and Children," Geneva, World Health Organization (WHO), 2012.

122. National Academies of Sciences, Engineering, and Medicine, *Dietary Reference Intakes for Sodium and Potassium* (Washington, DC: The National Academies Press, 2019).

123. National Academies of Sciences, Engineering, and Medicine, *Dietary Reference Intakes for Sodium and Potassium.*

124. World Health Organization, "Guideline: Potassium Intake for adults and Children," Geneva, World Health Organization (WHO), 2012.

125. D. K. Arnett, R. S. Blumenthal, M. A. Albert, et al., "2019 ACC/AHA Guideline on the Primary Prevention of Cardiovascular Disease: Executive Summary: A Report of the American College of Cardiology/American Heart Association Task Force on Clinical Practice Guidelines," *Journal of the American College of Cardiology* 74, no. 10 (2019): 1376–1414.

126. R. L. Bailey, E. A. Parker, D. G. Rhodes, et al., "Estimating Sodium and Potassium Intakes and their Ratio in the American Diet: Data from the 2011–2012 NHANES," *Journal of Nutrition* 146 (2016): 745–750.

127. National Institutes of Health, Office of Dietary Supplements, "Potassium: Fact Sheet for Health Professionals," July 9, 2019, https://ods.od.nih.gov/factsheets/ Potassium-HealthProfessional/#en21 (accessed February 23, 2020).

128. Harvard Women's Health Watch, "Avoiding the Pain of Kidney Stones," July 2018, https://www.health.harvard.edu/diseases-and-conditions/avoiding-the-pain-of -kidney-stones (accessed October 24, 2019).

129. Institute of Medicine, *Dietary Reference Intakes for Calcium and Vitamin D* (Washington, DC: The National Academies Press, 2011).

130. F. J. He and G. A. MacGregor, "A Comprehensive Review on Salt and Health and Current Experience of Worldwide Salt Reduction Programmes," *Journal of Human Hypertension* 23 (2009): 363–384.

131. A. Devine, R. A. Criddle, I. M. Dick, et al., "A Longitudinal Study of the Effect of Sodium and Calcium Intakes on Regional Bone Density in Postmenopausal Women," *American Journal of Clinical Nutrition* 62 (1995): 740–745.

132. J. Z. Ilich, R. A. Brownbill, and D. C. Coster, "Higher Habitual Sodium Intake Is Not Detrimental for Bones in Older Women with Adequate Calcium Intake," *European Journal of Applied Physiology* 109 (2010): 745–755.

133. B. Dawson-Hughes, email correspondence with the author, October 22, 2019.

134. F. J. He, N. M. Marrero, and G. A. MacGregor, "Salt Intake Is Related to Soft Drink Consumption in Children and Adolescents: A Link to Obesity?" *Hypertension* 51 (2008): 629–634.

135. R. Horton, "Health: Have the Salt Sellers Got Their Hearts in the Right Place?" Observer, *Life Magazine* (June 22, 1997): 43.

136. L. Zhao, M. E. Cogswell, Q. Yang, et al., "Association of Usual 24-h Sodium Excretion with Measures of Adiposity among Adults in the United States: NHANES, 2014," *American Journal of Clinical Nutrition* 109 (2019): 139–147.

137. L. Zhou, J. Stamler, Q. Chan, et al., and INTERMAP Research Group, "Salt Intake and Prevalence of Overweight/Obesity in Japan, China, the United Kingdom, and the United States: The INTERMAP Study," *American Journal of Clinical Nutrition* 110 (2019): 34–40.

138. Cleveland Clinic, "Feel Bloated? 5 Odd Reasons for Your Stomach Pain," https://health.clevelandclinic.org/feel-bloated-5-odd-reasons-stomach-pain/ (accessed August 29, 2018).

139. A. W. Peng, S. P. Juraschek, L. J. Appel, et al., "Effects of the DASH Diet and Sodium Intake on Bloating: Results from the DASH–Sodium Trial," *American Journal of Gastroenterology* 114 (2019): 1109–1115.

140. World Cancer Research Fund International/American Institute for Cancer Research, *Continuous Update Project Report: Diet, Nutrition, Physical Activity and Stomach Cancer*, 2016, http://wcrf.org/stomach-cancer-2016 (accessed August 28, 2018).

141. National Academies of Sciences, Engineering, and Medicine, *Dietary Reference Intakes for Sodium and Potassium* (Washington, DC: The National Academies Press, 2019), https://doi.org/10.17226/25353.

142. B. Stetka, "Has Salt Gotten an Unfair Shake?" *National Public Radio*, September 3, 2017, https://www.npr.org/sections/health-shots/2017/09/03/547827356/has-salt -gotten-an-unfair-shake-sodium-partisans-say-yes (accessed August 15, 2018).

Chapter 3

1. M. H. Alderman, "Dietary Sodium: Where Science and Policy Diverge," *American Journal of Hypertension* 29 (2016): 424–427.

2. J. D. Swales, "Dietary Salt and Hypertension," *Lancet* 1, no. 8179 (May 31, 1980): 1177–1179.

3. G. A. MacGregor and H. E. de Wardener, "Salt, Diet, and Health," *Lancet* 353, no. 9165 (1999): 1709–1710.

4. J. J. Brown, A. F. Lever, J. I. S. Robertson, et al., "Salt and Hypertension," *Lancet* 324, no. 8400 (August 25, 1984): 456.

5. *White House Conference on Food, Nutrition, and Health: Final Report,* US Government Printing Office, 1970. https://babel.hathitrust.org/cgi/pt?id=umn.31951d0298 7449r;view=1up;seq=61 (accessed November 15, 2018).

6. B. Stetka, "Has Salt Gotten an Unfair Shake?" National Public Radio, September 3, 2017. https://www.npr.org/sections/health-shots/2017/09/03/547827356/has-salt -gotten-an-unfair-shake-sodium-partisans-say-yes (accessed August 15, 2018). (Author converted measurements given in grams to milligrams.)

7. D. A. McCarron and M. H. Alderman, "Reducing Sodium Intake in the Population," *JAMA* 316 (2016): 2550.

8. M. H. Alderman, telephone interview with the author, August 14, 2019.

9. M. H. Alderman and D. A. McCarron, "Are You Getting Too Much Salt in Your Diet? Probably Not," *Wall Street Journal,* June 3, 2019.

10. L. Husten, "Reducing Salt to Very Low Levels May Be Dangerous," *Forbes*, August 9, 2018. https://www.forbes.com/sites/larryhusten/2018/08/09/new-study-adds-to -evidence-that-reducing-salt-to-very-low-levels-may-be-dangerous/.

11. N. Bakalar, "A Low-Salt Diet May Be Bad for the Heart," *New York Times*, May 25, 2016.

12. P. Whoriskey, "Could 95 Percent of the World's People Be Wrong about Salt?" *Washington Post*, May 26, 2015, https://www.washingtonpost.com/news/wonk/wp/ 2015/05/26/could-95-percent-of-the-worlds-people-be-wrong-about-salt/.

13. M. Zaraska, "Pass the Salt, Please: It's Good for You," *Washington Post*, May 4, 2015, https://www.washingtonpost.com/national/health-science/we-eat-a-lot-of -salt-but-scientists-say-there-are-good-reasons-for-that/2015/05/04/69ff7058-c806 -11e4-a199-6cb5e63819d2.

14. P. Whoriskey, "Is the American Diet Too Salty? Scientists Challenge the Long-standing Government Warning," *Washington Post*, April 6, 2015, https://www

.washingtonpost.com/news/wonk/wp/2015/04/06/more-scientists-doubt-salt-is-as
-bad-for-you-as-the-government-says/.

15. Editorial Board, "Doubts about Restricting Salt," *New York Times*, May 14, 2013, https://www.nytimes.com/2013/05/15/opinion/doubts-about-restricting-salt.html.

16. G. Taubes, "Salt, We Misjudged You," *New York Times*, June 3, 2012, https://www.nytimes.com/2012/06/03/opinion/sunday/we-only-think-we-know-the-truth-about-salt.html.

17. "Now Salt Is Safe to Eat: Health Fascists Proved Wrong after Lecturing Us All for Years," *Tabloid Watch* (blog), July 6, 2011, http://tabloid-watch.blogspot.com/2011/07/express-takes-on-health-fascists-over.html (accessed November 21, 2018); J. Willey, "Now Salt Is Safe to Eat," *Daily Express*, July 6, 2011, https://www.express.co.uk/news/uk/257048/Now-salt-is-safe-to-eat.

18. J. Stamler, from letter (not intended to be published) to the publisher, executive editor, and science editor of the *New York Times*, January 20, 1992 (copy letter sent to the author for his files).

19. National Research Council, *Diet and Health: Implications for Reducing Chronic Disease Risk* (Washington, DC: The National Academies Press, 1989), https://www.ncbi.nlm.nih.gov/pubmed/25032333.

20. N. Graudal, T. Hubeck-Graudal, G. Jürgens, et al., "Dose-Response Relation Between Dietary Sodium and Blood Pressure: A Meta-Regression Analysis of 133 Randomized Controlled Trials," *American Journal of Clinical Nutrition* 109, no. 5 (2019): 1273–1278.

21. L. Huang, K. Trieu, S. Yoshimura, et al., "Effect of Dose and Duration of Reduction in Dietary Sodium on Blood Pressure Levels: Systematic Review and Meta-Analysis of Randomised Trials," *BMJ* 368 (2020): m315, doi:10.1136/bmj.m315 (accessed February 27, 2020).

22. IOM (Institute of Medicine), *Sodium Intake in Populations: Assessment of Evidence* (Washington, DC: The National Academies Press, 2013).

23. G. Kolata, "No Benefit Seen in Sharp Limits on Salt in Diet," *New York Times*, May 14, 2013.

24. Centers for Disease Control and Prevention, "Sodium and the National Academies of Science (NAS) Health and Medical Division (HMD)," October 18, 2017, https://www.cdc.gov/salt/sodium_iom.htm (accessed March 21, 2019).

25. J. J. DiNicolantonio, P. Di Pasquale, R. S. Taylor, et al., "Low Sodium Versus Normal Sodium Diets in Systolic Heart Failure: Systematic Review and Meta-Analysis," Retraction notice, *Heart* 2013; published online March 12, http://dx.doi.org/10.1136/heartjnl-2012–302337.

26. P. K. Whelton, L. J. Appel, R. L. Sacco, et al., "Sodium, Blood Pressure, and Cardiovascular Disease: Further Evidence Supporting the American Heart Association Sodium Reduction Recommendations," *Circulation* 126, no. 24 (December 11, 2012): 2880–2889.

27. J. J. DiNicolantonio, P. Di Pasquale, R. S. Taylor, et al., "Low Sodium Versus Normal Sodium Diets in Systolic Heart Failure," Retraction notice.

28. Taubes, "Salt, We Misjudged You."

29. D. Mozaffarian, October 19, 2016. Docket No. FDA-2014-D-0055. (Author has converted measurements given in grams to milligrams.)

30. G. Mancia, S. Oparil, P. K. Whelton, et al., "The Technical Report on Sodium Intake and Cardiovascular Disease in Low- and Middle-Income Countries by the Joint Working Group of the World Heart Federation, the European Society of Hypertension and the European Public Health Association," *European Heart Journal* 38 (2017): 712–719.

31. H. W. Cohen, S. M. Hailpern, et al., "Sodium Intake and Mortality in the NHANES II Follow-Up Study," *American Journal of Medicine* 119, no. 275 (2006): e7–e14.

32. F. J. He, H. E. de Wardener, and G. A. MacGregor, "Sodium Intake and Mortality in the NHANES II Follow-Up Study," *American Journal of Medicine* 120, no. 1 (January 2007): e5.

33. M. H. Alderman, "Salt, Blood Pressure and Health: A Cautionary Tale," *International Journal of Epidemiology* 31 (2002): 311–315.

34. M. H. Alderman, telephone interview with the author, August 14, 2019.

35. H. Karppanen and E. Mervaala, "Sodium Intake and Mortality," *Lancet* 351 (1998): 1509.

36. M. E. Cogswell, K. Mugavero, et al., "Dietary Sodium and Cardiovascular Disease Risk—Measurement Matters," *New England Journal of Medicine* 375, no. 6 (August 11, 2016): 580–586.

37. P. Singer, H. Cohen, and M. Alderman, "Assessing the Associations of Sodium Intake with Long-Term All-Cause and Cardiovascular Mortality in a Hypertensive Cohort," *American Journal of Hypertension* 28 (2015): 335–342.

38. N. Graudal, G. Jürgens, B. Baslund, et al., "Compared with Usual Sodium Intake, Low- and Excessive-Sodium Diets are Associated with Increased Mortality: A Meta-Analysis," *American Journal of Hypertension* 27 (September 2014): 1129–1137, http://dx.doi.org/10.1093/ajh/hpu028.

39. F. J. He and G. A. MacGregor, "Salt Intake and Mortality," *American Journal of Hypertension* 27, no. 11 (November 2014): 1424, http://dx.doi.org/10.1093/ajh/hpu095.

40. F. J. He, M. Tan, Y. Ma, et al., "Salt Reduction to Prevent Hypertension and Cardiovascular Disease: *JACC* State of the Art Review," *Journal of the American College of Cardiology* 75, no. 6 (Feb. 2020): 632–647.

41. L. K. Cobb, C. A. M. Anderson, P. Elliott, et al., "Methodological Issues in Cohort Studies That Relate Sodium Intake to Cardiovascular Disease Outcomes: A Science Advisory from the American Heart Association," *Circulation* 129 (2014): 1173–1186.

42. M. O'Donnell, A. Mente, S. Rangarajan, et al., "Urinary Sodium and Potassium Excretion, Mortality, and Cardiovascular Events," *New England Journal of Medicine* 371 (2014): 612–623. (Erratum, *New England Journal of Medicine* 371 [2014]: 1267.)

43. A. Mente, M. O'Donnell, S. Rangarajan, et al., "Associations of Urinary Sodium Excretion with Cardiovascular Events in Individuals with and without Hypertension: A Pooled Analysis of Data from Four Studies," *Lancet* 388, no. 10043 (July 30, 2016): 465–475.

44. L. Husten, "Top Cardiologist Blasts Nutrition Guidelines," *CardioBrief*, February 27, 2017, http://www.cardiobrief.org/2017/02/27/top-cardiologist-blasts-nutrition-guidelines/.

45. I. Johnston, "*Lancet* Attacked for Publishing Study Claiming Low-Salt Diet Could Kill You," *Independent*, May 21, 2016, https://www.independent.co.uk/news/science/salt-diet-heart-disease-death-lancet-a7040546.html.

46. N. Graudal, "Sodium and Cardiovascular Disease," *New England Journal of Medicine* 371, no. 22 (November 27, 2014): 2136–2137.

47. Johnston, "*Lancet* Attacked for Publishing Study."

48. N. R. Cook, "Correspondence: Sodium and Cardiovascular Disease," *New England Journal of Medicine* 371 (2014): 2134–2139.

49. Cobb et al., "Methodological Issues in Cohort Studies."

50. L. Huang, M. Crino, J. H. Wu, et al., "Mean Population Salt Intake Estimated from 24-h Urine Samples and Spot Urine Samples: A Systematic Review and Meta-Analysis," *International Journal of Epidemiology* 45 (2016): 239–250.

51. R. H. G. Olde Engberink, T. C. van den Hoek, N. D. van Noordenne, et al., "Use of a Single Baseline Versus Multiyear 24-hour Urine Collection for Estimation of Long-Term Sodium Intake and Associated Cardiovascular and Renal Risk," *Circulation* 136, no. 10 (2017): 917–926.

52. R. H. G. Olde Engberink, B.-J. H. van den Born, H. Peters-Sengers, et al., "Response by Olde Engberink et al. to Letter Regarding Article, 'Use of a Single Baseline Versus Multiyear 24-Hour Urine Collection for Estimation of Long-Term Sodium Intake and Associated Cardiovascular and Renal Risk,'" *Circulation* 137, no. 14 (2018): 1538–1539.

53. F. J. He, N. R. C. Campbell, et al., "Errors in Estimating Usual Sodium Intake by the Kawasaki Formula Alter Its Relationship with Mortality: Implications for Public Health," *International Journal of Epidemiology* 47 (2018): 1784–1795, http://dx.doi .org/10.1093/ije/dyy114.

54. N. R. Cook, L. J. Appel, and P. K. Whelton, "Lower Levels of Sodium Intake and Reduced Cardiovascular Risk," *Circulation* 129 (2014): 981–989.

55. N. R. Cook, email to the author, October 9, 2019.

56. T. Neale, "Is It Time to Loosen Restrictions on Saturated Fats and Salt?" *tctMD*, December 14, 2018, https://www.tctmd.com/news/it-time-loosen-restrictions -saturated-fats-and-salt.

57. S. Yusuf, quoted during a discussion at NAM regarding a public workshop to review the dietary reference intakes for sodium and potassium, March 7, 2018.

58. N. R. C. Campbell, "Dissidents and Dietary Sodium: Concerns about the Commentary by O'Donnell et al.," *International Journal of Epidemiology* 46 (2017): 362–366.

59. M. Tan, F. J. He, and G. A. MacGregor, "Salt and Cardiovascular Disease in PURE: A Large Sample Size Cannot Make Up for Erroneous Estimations," *Journal of the Renin-Angiotensin-Aldosterone System* 19, no. 4 (Oct.–Dec. 2018), http://dx.doi .org/10.1177/1470320318810015.

60. American Heart Association, "American Heart Association Comment Strongly Refutes Study Findings on Sodium Consumption," May 21, 2016, https://newsroom .heart.org/news/american-heart-association-strongly-refutes-study-findings-on -sodium-consumption (accessed September 10, 2019).

61. D. A. McCarron, A. G. Kazaks, J. C. Geerling, et al., "Normal Range of Human Dietary Sodium Intake: A Perspective Based on 24-Hour Urinary Sodium Excretion Worldwide," *American Journal of Hypertension* 26 (2013): 1218–1223.

62. D. A. McCarron, J. C. Geerling, A. G. Kazaks, et al., "Can Dietary Sodium Intake Be Modified by Public Policy?" *Clinical Journal of the American Society of Nephrology* 4 (2009): 1878–1882.

63. Rebuttal by F. P. Cappuccio, S. Capewell, F. J. He, and G. A. MacGregor, "Salt: The Dying Echoes of the Food Industry," *American Journal of Hypertension* 27 (2014): 279–281.

64. J. G. Forte, J. M. Miguel, J. Miguel, et al., "Salt and Blood Pressure: A Community Trial," *Journal of Human Hypertension* 3 (1989): 179–184.

65. M. Maillot and A. Drewnowski, "A Conflict between Nutritionally Adequate Diets and Meeting the 2010 Dietary Guidelines for Sodium," *American Journal of Preventive Medicine* 42 (2012): 174–179.

66. P. Britten, L. E. Cleveland, K. L. Koegel, et al., "Updated US Department of Agriculture Food Patterns Meet Goals of the 2010 Dietary Guidelines," *Journal of the Academy of Nutrition and Dietetics* 112 (2012): 1648–1655.

67. M. H. Alderman, "Dietary Sodium: Where Science and Policy Diverge," *American Journal of Hypertension* 29 (2016): 424–427.

68. F. J. He and G. A. MacGregor, "Reducing Population Salt Intake Worldwide: From Evidence to Implementation," *Progress in Cardiovascular Disease* 52 (2010): 363–382.

69. B. Stetka, "Has Salt Gotten an Unfair Shake?" National Public Radio, September 3, 2017, https://www.npr.org/sections/health-shots/2017/09/03/547827356/has-salt -gotten-an-unfair-shake-sodium-partisans-say-yes (accessed August 15, 2018).

70. B. H. Scribner, "Salt and Hypertension," *JAMA* 250 (1983): 388–389.

71. M. Wijkman, "Diuretics and Cerebrovascular Outcomes—Beyond Traditional Endpoints," *Journal of Clinical Hypertension* 17 (2005): 273–274.

72. Institute of Medicine, *Strategies to Reduce Sodium Intake in the United States* (Washington, DC: The National Academies Press, 2010).

73. M. H. Alderman, letter, *JAMA* 303, no. 19 (2010): 1917–1918.

74. P. Elliott and J. Stamler, "Commentary: Evidence on Salt and Blood Pressure Is Consistent and Persuasive," *International Journal of Epidemiology* 31 (2002): 316–319.

75. L. J. Appel, "Salt Reduction in the United States," *BMJ* 333, no. 7568 (2006): 561–562.

76. G. A. MacGregor, email to the author, October 25, 2019.

77. P. Strazzullo, "Benefit Assessment of Dietary Salt Reduction: While the Doctors Study, Should More People Die?" *Journal of Hypertension* 29 (2011): 829–831.

78. D. W. Jones, F. C. Luft, P. K. Whelton, M. H. Alderman, et al., "Can We End the Salt Wars with a Randomized Clinical Trial in a Controlled Environment?" *Hypertension* 72, no. 1 (2018): 10–11.

79. University of Pittsburgh, Human Research Protection Office, *Research Involving Prisoners*, Chapter 26. https://www.irb.pitt.edu/book/export/html/366 (accessed November 11, 2019).

80. S. Y. Angell, "A Diet Study on Prisoners? Wrong on Many Levels [letter]," *New York Times*, June 11, 2018.

81. L. J. Appel, interview with the author, November 25, 2019.

82. M. H. Alderman, interview with the author, August 14, 2019.

83. J. Morris, "Ford Spent $40 Million to Reshape Asbestos Science," The Center for Public Integrity, February 16, 2016, https://www.publicintegrity.org/2016/02/16/19297/ford-spent-40-million-reshape-asbestos-science (accessed July 9, 2018).

Chapter 4

1. F. J. He and G. A. MacGregor, "A Comprehensive Review on Salt and Health and Current Experience of Worldwide Salt Reduction Programmes," *Journal of Human Hypertension* 23 (2009): 363–384.

2. National Academies of Sciences, Engineering, and Medicine, *Dietary Reference Intakes for Sodium and Potassium* (Washington, DC: The National Academies Press, 2019), https://www.nap.edu/download/25353.

3. H. B. Evich, "Obama Takes Aim at Salt," *Politico*, June 1, 2016, https://www.politico.com/story/2016/06/obama-salt-reduction-fda-223769 (accessed October 17, 2019).

4. D. Owen, "Is Noise Pollution the Next Big Public-Health Crisis?" *New Yorker*, May 13, 2019, https://www.newyorker.com/magazine/2019/05/13/is-noise-pollution-the-next-big-public-health-crisis?.

5. J. Majkut, "John Chafee's 1986 Climate Hearings," June 15, 2016, Niskanen Center website, https://niskanencenter.org/blog/john-chafees-1986-climate-hearings/ (accessed September 11, 2018).

Chapter 5

1. L. Roman, quoted in L. Petrecca, "Chinese Takeout Has So Much Salt It Should Carry a 'Health Warning,' UK Advocacy Group Says." *USA Today*, March 15, 2018, https://www.usatoday.com/story/news/2018/03/15/salt-gets-some-stinging-criticism-well-strong-defense-during-salt-awareness-week/423903002/; L. Roman, quoted in N. Hellmich, "Keeping a Lid on Salt: Not So Easy," *USA Today*, April 28, 2010.

2. Salt Institute, Form 990, December 2015, http://990s.foundationcenter.org/990_pdf_archive/362/362235413/362235413_201512_990O.pdf (accessed July 28, 2018).

3. Salt Institute, "Everything's Better with a Little Salt," http://www.saltinstitute.org/. Link no longer active.

4. Salt Institute, "Who Is the Salt Guru" (video), http://www.saltinstitute.org/salt-101/ask-the-salt-guru/ (accessed August 22, 2018).

5. Salt Institute, "Food Salt Essential for Life, Health," September 29, 2011 (in author's files).

6. Salt Institute, "World Food Day: Celebrating the Role of Salt," October 16, 2018. http://saltinstitute.org/press_releases/world-food-day-celebrating-role-salt/ (accessed February 16, 2019).

7. Salt Institute, "Food Salt Essential for Life, Health," September 29, 2011 (in author's files).

8. V. Wong, "New York Will Require Salt Warnings on Menus, Outraging the Lobby," *Buzzfeed*, September 9, 2015, https://www.buzzfeednews.com/article/venessawong/new-york-warning-label-for-salt.

9. P. K. Whelton, M. H. Weinberger, et al., "Junk Science or Junk Journalism—Whose Interests Are the Media Really Serving?" *PRNewswire*, January 15, 1997.

10. ProPublica (website), "Salt Institute," nonprofit tax code designation, https://projects.propublica.org/nonprofits/organizations/362235413 (accessed March 13, 2018).

11. Salt Institute statement on CSPI lawsuit, October 8, 2015, http://www.saltinstitute.org/press_releases/salt-institute-statement-on-cspi-lawsuit/ (accessed July 28, 2018).

12. T. M. Andrews, "The Great Salt Debate: So Bad?" *Atlantic*, May 16, 2013. https://www.theatlantic.com/health/archive/2013/05/the-great-salt-debate-so-bad/275888/.

13. "FDA Salt Regulation—Lori Roman & Michael Jacobson," *The Colbert Report* (video clip), May 3, 2010, http://www.cc.com/video-clips/i2zwg4/the-colbert-report-fda-salt-regulation---lori-roman---michael-jacobson (accessed March 13, 2018).

14. Salt Institute, Form 990, December 2015, http://990s.foundationcenter.org/990_pdf_archive/362/362235413/362235413_201512_990O.pdf (accessed July 28, 2018).

15. The Center for Media and Democracy, "Education Action Group," *Sourcewatch* (website), https://www.sourcewatch.org/index.php/Education_Action_Group (accessed July 28, 2018).

16. J. Gunlock, "It's Time to #BanBossy School Lunch Ladies," Independent Women's Forum (website), September 5, 2014. https://www.iwf.org/2014/09/11/time-to-ban-bossy-school-lunch-ladies-%e2%80%a2-cam-company/ (accessed July 28, 2018).

17. J. Gunlock, "Political Agendas versus Sound Nutrition," Independent Women's Forum's *Policy Focus* 4, no. 6 (June 2014), http://c1355372.cdn.cloudfiles.rackspacecloud.com/6c2eb28f-2403-48ea-a7c2-56152bba721e/PolicyFocus14_June_p2-3.pdf (accessed July 28, 2018).

18. ProPublica (website), "Salt Institute Form 990, 2018," https://projects.propublica
.org/nonprofits/organizations/362235413/201910919349300526/IRS990   (accessed
November 8, 2019).

19. W. P. Bolen, US Geological Survey. "Salt. Mineral Commodity Summaries," January
2018,   https://s3-us-west-2.amazonaws.com/prd-wret/assets/palladium/production/
mineral-pubs/salt/mcs-2018-salt.pdf (accessed December 22, 2018).

20. R. Hanneman, interview with the author, August 21, 2019.

21. Salt Institute, "Salt & Health Newsletter," 2011, http://www.saltinstitute.org/
wp-content/uploads/2013/11/SH-4th-qtr-2011.pdf (accessed August 22, 2018).

22. C. Wallis, "Salt: A New Villain?" *Time*, March 15, 1982.

23. Dummies B2B, https://www.dummies.com/biz.html (accessed August 1, 2018).
Salt for Dummies is not available online—not even on Amazon or through its used
book sellers—now that the Salt Institute is out of business.

24. Salt Institute, "Salt Shocker—CDC Shifts from Ebola to Cottage Cheese!!" You-
Tube (video), March 31, 2011, https://www.youtube.com/watch?v=8xxA1ZTMsnI
(accessed February 16, 2019).

25. US Department of Health, Education, and Welfare, *Healthy People: The Surgeon
General's Report on Health Promotion and Disease Prevention* (1979) DHEW publication
no. (PHS) 79-55071.

26. Salt Institute, Letter to the secretaries of the US Department of Agriculture and
US Department of Health and Human Services, April 11, 2016. http://saltinstitute.
org/wp-content/uploads/2016/04/Salt-Institute-USDA-HHS-Letter-4-11-16.pdf
(accessed November 10, 2018).

27. Salt Institute, "Salt Institute Asks Government Panel for a Fair Review of
Sodium," press release, March 7, 2018. http://saltinstitute.org/press_releases/salt
-institute-asks-government-panel-fair-review-sodium/ (accessed November 11, 2018).

28. "NYC Considers High-Sodium Warning on Chain Restaurant Menus," CBS
News, June 10, 2015, https://www.cbsnews.com/news/nyc-considers-high-sodium
-warning-on-chain-restaurant-menus/ (accessed March 14, 2018); Salt Institute,
http://www.saltinstitute.org/press_releases/nyc-health-department-wrong-on-high
-sodium-warnings/ (accessed March 14, 2018).

29. M. B. Quirk, "Restaurant Group Sues NYC over New Salt Warning Labels," *Con-
sumerist*, December 4, 2015, https://consumerist.com/2015/12/04/restaurant-group
-sues-nyc-over-new-salt-warning-labels/.

30. Open Secrets, Lobbying database, https://www.opensecrets.org/lobby/ (accessed
September 19, 2018); Lobbying Report, https://soprweb.senate.gov/index.cfm?event
=getFilingDetails&filingID=BD214631-661D-4085-9238-4F4DACE1F106&filing

TypeID=69; Lobbying Report, https://soprweb.senate.gov/index.cfm?event=getFilin gDetails&filingID=E216BF65-AE4C-47E2-85D2-6D55FF292A8A&filingTypeID=60.

31. US Department of Health and Human Services, *Healthy People 2000: Consortium Action* (1992 edition), https://archive.org/stream/healthypeopl20000publ/healthypeopl 20000publ_djvu.txt (accessed September 27, 2018).

32. E. Halsey, "Is Salt Bad or Not?" *CNN*, September 19, 1996.

33. R. Rowen and C. Schrader, *Control High Blood Pressure Without Drugs: A Complete Hypertension Handbook.* (New York: Atria Books, 2001).

34. M. Warner, "The War over Salt," *New York Times*, September 13, 2006, http:// www.nytimes.com/2006/09/13/business/13salt.html.

35. M. Chase, "Do New Data Dash Advice to Cut Salt?" *Wall Street Journal*, August 24, 1998, https://www.wsj.com/articles/SB903904851697789000; M. Satin, interview with the author, August 22, 2019.

36. D. W. Jones, F. C. Luft, P. K. Whelton, M. H. Alderman, et al., "Can We End the Salt Wars with a Randomized Clinical Trial in a Controlled Environment?" *Hypertension* 72, no. 1 (2018): 10–11.

37. Salt Institute, Form 990 for 2016, http://990s.foundationcenter.org/990_pdf_arc hive/362/362235413/362235413_201612_990O.pdf (accessed August 1, 2018).

38. P. Babjak, email to the author, July 26, 2018.

39. L. Roman, email to the author, August 29, 2019.

40. P. Cattan, "Sel, le vice caché," *TOC*, no. 18 (March 2006).

41. C. Labbé and O. Recasens, "Un scientifique sous surveillance," *Le Point*, no. 1530, January 11, 2002.

42. "Scientist Treated like a Terrorist for His Damning Report on Salt," *Scotsman*, January 14, 2002, https://www.scotsman.com/news/world/scientist-treated-like-a -terrorist-for-his-damning-report-on-salt-1-594725.

43. "Un cherheer de l'Inserm sur ecoute [An Inserm researcher bugged]" *L'Obs*, January 11, 2002, https://www.nouvelobs.com/societe/20020110.OBS2181/un-chercheur -de-l-inserm-sur-ecoute.html; C. Labbé and O. Recasens, "Un scientifique sous surveillance," *Le Point*, no. 1530, January 11, 2002.

44. S. Coignard, *La vendetta française* (The French vendetta) (Paris: Albin Michel, 2003).

45. V. Olivier, "Pierre Meneton, l'obstiné," *L'Express*, January 26, 2011, https://www .lexpress.fr/actualite/societe/sante/pierre-meneton-l-obstine_956016.html.

46. B. Moinier, Comité des Salines de France, letter to Christian Brechot, Director General, Inserm, April 6, 2006 (translated from the French; letter in author's files).

47. Olivier, "Pierre Meneton, l'obstiné."

48. Cattan, "Sel, le vice cache."

49. G. A. MacGregor and H. E. deWardener, "The French Salt Industry in Court," *Lancet* 373 (2009): 990–992, https://scihub.bban.top/https://www.thelancet.com/journals/lancet/article/PIIS0140673609605894/fulltext?rss=yes.

50. "The Salt Lobby Loses Its Case against an Inserm Researcher," *Libération*, March 13, 2008, https://www.liberation.fr/societe/2008/03/13/le-lobby-du-sel-perd-son-proces-contre-un-chercheur-de-l-inserm_22384.

51. Salt Association, "Position Statement," undated, http://www.saltassociation.co.uk/salt-the-facts/salt-position-statement/ (accessed February 28, 2020).

52. BBC News, "Watchdog Rejects Salt Complaint," April 19, 2005, http://news.bbc.co.uk/2/hi/health/4461673.stm (accessed February 18, 2020).

Chapter 6

1. M. Nestle, *Unsavory Truth* (New York: Basic Books, 2018).

2. L. I. Lesser, C. B. Ebbeling, M. Goozner, et al., "Relationship between Funding Source and Conclusion among Nutrition-Related Scientific Articles," *PLoS Medicine* 4, no. 1 (January 2007): e5, https://www.ncbi.nlm.nih.gov/pmc/articles/PMC1764435/; M. Nestle, *Unsavory Truth: How Food Companies Skew the Science of What We Eat* (New York: Basic Books, 2018).

3. B. I-San Lin, interview with the author, October 12, 2018.

4. D. Michaels, *The Triumph of Doubt* (New York: Oxford University Press, 2020).

5. M. Chase, "Do New Data Dash Advice to Cut Salt?" *Wall Street Journal*, August 24, 1998, https://www.wsj.com/articles/SB903904851697789000.

6. P. Kincaid-Smith and M. H. Alderman, "Universal Recommendations for Sodium Intake Should Be Avoided [letter]," *Medical Journal of Australia* 170 (1999): 174–175.

7. M. H. Alderman, *Medical Journal of Australia* 170 (1999): 163, 171.

8. H. W. Cohen, S. M. Hailpern, J. Fang, and M. H. Alderman, "Sodium Intake and Mortality in the NHANES II Follow-Up Study," *American Journal of Medicine* 119, no. 3 (2006): 275, e7–e14.

9. G. Kolata, "Low-Salt Diet Ineffective, Study Finds, Disagreement Abounds," *New York Times*, May 4, 2011, https://www.nytimes.com/2011/05/04/health/research/04salt.html (accessed September 1, 2019).

10. M. H. Alderman and H. Cohen, *Lancet* 378 (2011): 1993–1994.

11. M. H. Alderman, curriculum vitae, https://www.einstein.yu.edu/images/faculty/experts/profiles/29/alderman%20cv%2010.6.11.pdf (accessed March 28, 2019).

12. F. J. He and G. A. MacGregor, "Salt Intake and Mortality," *American Journal of Hypertension* 26 (2014): 1424.

13. M. H. Alderman, interview with author, August 14, 2019, and email, September 2, 2019.

14. Portland Pet Food Company, "Meet the Team," https://portlandpetfoodcompany.com/pages/meet-the-team (accessed February 18, 2020); The McCarron Group, http://www.mccarrongroup.com/ (accessed August 20, 2019).

15. The McCarron Group, "Testimonials," http://www.mccarrongroup.com/?page_id=22 (accessed September 10, 2019).

16. D. A. McCarron, "The Dietary Guideline for Sodium: Should We Shake It Up? Yes!" *American Journal of Clinical Nutrition* 71 (2000): 1013–1019.

17. McCarron, "The Dietary Guideline for Sodium."

18. E. Rosenthal, "Hypertension Research Challenges Role of Salt," *New York Times*, December 31, 1991.

19. G. Taubes, "The (Political) Science of Salt," *Science* 281 (1998): 898–907.

20. K. Doheny, "Americans Still Reaching for the Salt," WebMD.com, October 20, 2010, https://www.webmd.com/hypertension-high-blood-pressure/news/20101020/americans-still-reaching-for-the-salt-shaker#1 (accessed January 28, 2020).

21. Salt Institute, Form 990 for 2016; P. Babjak, CEO, Academy of Nutrition and Dietetics, email correspondence with the author, July 26, 2018.

22. D. W. Jones, F. C. Luft, P. K. Whelton, M. H. Alderman, et al., "Can We End the Salt Wars with a Randomized Clinical Trial in a Controlled Environment?" *Hypertension* 72, no. 1 (2018): 10–11.

23. "Correction to: Can We End the Salt Wars with a Randomized Clinical Trial in a Controlled Environment?" *Hypertension* 72 (2018): e35, https://www.ahajournals.org/doi/10.1161/HYP.0000000000000082.

24. D. A. McCarron, National Academy of Medicine, *Workshop for the Committee to Review the Dietary Reference Intakes for Sodium and Potassium,*" http://www.nationalacademies.org/hmd/~/media/Files/Activity%20Files/Nutrition/ReviewDRIforSodiumandPotassium/March%20Public%20Workshop/Powerpoints/42%20David%20McCarron.pdf (after his presentation the website was corrected to disclose conflicts of interest; accessed September 3, 2019).

25. S. M. Lee, "A Prison Study Aims to End the 'Salt Wars.' It Turns Out the Salt Industry Wants to Help Fund It," buzzfeednews.com, September 18, 2018, https:// www.buzzfeednews.com/article/stephaniemlee/salt-institute-sodium-study-prison -funding.

26. *Consensus Conference on Nutrition*, May 14–16, 2014, https://web.archive .org/web/20160328032900/http://nutritioncvd2014.com/body.cfm?id=19 (accessed October 18, 2019).

27. Public Health Research Institute, *Tackling Global Health Challenges*, 2019 research report (accessed October 20, 2019); Clinical Trials Ontario, "Pharmaceuticals," August 16, 2019. https://www.investinontario.com/pharmaceuticals#intro (accessed October 21, 2019); Faculty of Health Sciences, "$40-Million Investment Launches International Hypertension Study," June 15, 2011, https://dailynews .mcmaster.ca/articles/40-million-investment-launches-international-hypertension -study/ (accessed October 21, 2019).

28. F. Fickweiler, W. Fickweiler, and E. Urbach, "Interactions between Physicians and the Pharmaceutical Industry Generally and Sales Representatives Specifically and Their Association with Physicians' Attitudes and Prescribing Habits: A Systematic Review," *BMJ Open* 7 (2017): e016408.

29. Nestle, *Unsavory Truth*.

Chapter 7

1. D. Mozaffarian, S. Fahimi, G. M. Singh, et al. "Global Sodium Consumption and Death from Cardiovascular Causes," *New England Journal of Medicine* 371 (2014): 624–634. (The author converted the measurements given in grams to milligrams.)

2. World Health Organization, *Hypertension*, May 16, 2019, https://www.who.int/ news-room/fact-sheets/detail/hypertension (accessed September 11, 2019).

3. World Health Organization, "Global NCD Target—Reduce High Blood Pressure," September 2016, https://www.who.int/beat-ncds/take-action/policy-brief-reduce-high -blood-pressure.pdf (accessed January 9, 2020); GBD 2013 Risk Factors Collaborators, "Global, Regional, and National Comparative Risk Assessment of 79 Behavioural, Environmental and Occupational, and Metabolic Risks or Clusters of Risks in 188 Countries, 1990–2013: A Systematic Analysis for the Global Burden of Disease Study 2013," *Lancet* 386 (2015): 2287–2323.

4. GBD 2017 Diet Collaborators. "Health Effects of Dietary Risks in 195 Countries, 1990–2017: A Systematic Analysis for the Global Burden of Disease Study 2017," *Lancet*, April 3, 2019, https://doi.org/10.1016/S0140-6736(19)30041-8.

5. D. Mozaffarian, S. Fahimi, G. M. Singh, et al., for the Global Burden of Diseases Nutrition and Chronic Diseases Expert Group (NUTRICODE), "Global Sodium

Consumption and Death from Cardiovascular Causes," *New England Journal of Medicine* 371 (August 14, 2014): 624–634 (suppl. appendix table S7).

6. "Salt Reduction Can Save Many Lives at Low Cost," Resolve to Save Lives (website), https://www.resolvetosavelives.org/sodium/ (accessed November 10, 2019).

7. H. Karppanen and E. Mervaala, "Sodium Intake and Hypertension," *Progress in Cardiovascular Diseases* 49, no. 2 (2006): 59–75.

8. L. Hyseni, A. Elliot-Green, F. Lloyd-Williams, et al., "Systematic Review of Dietary Salt Reduction Policies: Evidence for an Effectiveness Hierarchy?" *PLoS ONE* 12, no. 5 (2017): e0177535, http://journals.plos.org/plosone/article/file?id=10.1371/journal.pone.0177535&type=printable; Institute of Medicine, *Strategies to Reduce Sodium Intake in the United States* (Washington, DC: The National Academies Press, 2010).

9. L. Hyseni, A. Elliot-Green, F. Lloyd-Williams, et al., "Systematic Review of Dietary Salt Reduction Policies: Evidence for an Effectiveness Hierarchy?" *PLoS ONE* 12, no. 5 (2017): e0177535, http://journals.plos.org/plosone/article/file?id=10.1371/journal.pone.0177535&type=printable.

10. World Health Organization (WHO), "Community-Based Efforts to Reduce Blood Pressure and Stroke in Japan, March 2013," https://www.who.int/features/2013/japan_blood_pressure/en/ (accessed August 10, 2019).

11. US Food and Drug Administration, "Voluntary Sodium Reduction Goals: Target Mean and Upper Bound Concentrations for Sodium in Commercially Processed, Packaged, and Prepared Foods; Draft Guidance for Industry," June 2, 2016, 81 Fed. Reg. (35363) 35363–35367, https://www.federalregister.gov/documents/2016/06/02/2016-12950/voluntary-sodium-reduction-goals-target-mean-and-upper-bound-concentrations-for-sodium-in (accessed September 23, 2018).

12. World Health Organization (WHO), "Progress in Reducing Salt Consumption in Turkey," April 8, 2013, http://www.euro.who.int/en/countries/turkey/news/news/2013/04/progress-in-reducing-salt-consumption-in-turkey (accessed April 4, 2019).

13. Overview: K. Trieu, B. Neal, C. Hawkes, et al., "Salt Reduction Initiatives around the World—A Systematic Review of Progress towards the Global Target," *PLoS ONE* 10, no. 7: e0130247, https://doi.org/10.1371/journal.pone.0130247 (accessed February 17, 2020). Selected sources for table 7.1: **Argentina:** The World Bank, *Prevention of Health Risk Factors in Latin America and the Caribbean: Governance of Five Multisectoral Efforts* (Washington, DC: World Bank, 2014); J. Konfino, T. A. Mekonnen, P. G. Coxson, et al., "Projected Impact of a Sodium Consumption Reduction Initiative in Argentina: An Analysis from the CVD Policy Model—Argentina," *PLoS ONE* 8, no. 9 (2013): e73824, doi:10.1371/journal.pone.0073824; **Australia:** R. Lindberg, T. Nichols, and C. Yam. "The Healthy Eating Agenda in Australia: Is Salt a Priority for Manufacturers?" *Nutrients* 9, no. 8 (2017): 881, doi:10.3390/nu9080881; **Austria:** Bundesministerium Für Gesundheit, Austrian Salt Initiative, 2014, http://www.bmgf

.gv.at/cms/site2/attachments/7/1/0/CH1396/CMS1385031886552/who_conference _factsheet_oesi_final.pdf; **Bahrain:** G. Y. Lim, "Slashing Salt: Bahrain Follows Kuwait and Qatar in Move to Reduce Levels in Baked Goods," FoodNavigator-Asia.com, September 11, 2019, https://www.foodnavigator-asia.com/Article/2019/09/11/Slashing -salt-Bahrain-follows-Kuwait-and-Qatar-in-move-to-reduce-levels-in-baked-goods#; **Belgium:** European Commission, "National Salt Initiatives: Implementing the EU Framework for Salt Reduction Initiatives," 2009, http://bit.ly/1FTKE4A; Health, Food Chain Safety and Environment, 2013, *Moins de sel dans l'alimentation des Belges*, http://www.health.belgium.be/eportal/19088825_FR?backNode=9735#.U5s6j_ ldWIM; **Brazil:** M. Brown, World Action on Salt and Health, "Brazil's Salt Reduction Program," October 4, 2017, http://www.worldactiononsalt.com/blog/2017/brazils -salt-reduction-program.html (accessed February 17, 2020); **Bulgaria:** European Commission, Survey on Members States' Implementation of the Salt Reduction Framework, 2012, http://ec.europa.eu/health/nutrition_physical_activity/docs/salt _report1_en.pdf; **Canada:** Government of Canada, "Toward Front-of-Package Nutri- tion Labels for Canadians," https://www.canada.ca/en/health-canada/programs/ front-of-package-nutrition-labelling/consultation-document.html; **Chile:** C. Corva- lán, M. Reyes, M. L. Garmendia, et al., "Structural Responses to the Obesity and Non-communicable Diseases Epidemic: Update on the Chilean Law of food Label- ling and Advertising," *Obesity Reviews* 20, no. 3 (2018): doi:10.1111/obr.12802. **Ecuador:** A. A. Díaz, P. M. Veliz, G. Rivas-Mariño, "Food Labeling in Ecuador: Imple- mentation, Results, and Pending Actions," *Pan American Journal of Public Health* 41 (2017): 41, e54, https://translate.google.com/translate?hl=en&sl=es&u=https://www .researchgate.net/publication/325226975_Food_labeling_in_Ecuador_implementation _results_and_pending_actions&prev=search (accessed February 18, 2020); **Finland:** H. Karppanen and E. Mervaala, "Sodium Intake and Hypertension," *Progress in Car- diovascular Diseases* 49, no. 2 (2006): 59–75; **Greece:** European Commission, Survey on Members States' Implementation of the Salt Reduction Framework, 2012, http:// ec.europa.eu/health/nutrition_physical_activity/docs/salt_report1_en.pdf; **Hungary:** "Assessment of the Impact of a Public Health Product Tax," http://www.euro.who .int/data/assets/pdf_file/0008/332882/assessment-impact-PH-tax-report.pdf; **Israel:** State of Israel, Ministry of Health, "Food Label and Nutrition Label," 2018, https:// www.health.gov.il/English/Topics/FoodAndNutrition/Nutrition/Adequate_nutrition/ Pages/labeling.aspx and other sources; **Kuwait:** World Health Organization, "Kuwaitis Lower Blood Pressure by Reducing Salt in Bread," September 2014, https:// www.who.int/features/2014/kuwait-blood-pressure/en/; **Mexico:** F. Cortez, "Mexico Front of Pack Labeling Warning Signs," USDA Foreign Agricultural Service, August 23, 2019, https://apps.fas.usda.gov/newgainapi/api/report/downloadreportbyfilena me?filename=Mexico%20Front%20of%20Pack%20Labeling%20Warning%20Signs _Mexico%20ATO_Mexico_8-23-2019.pdf; **Netherlands:** E. H. M. Temme, M. A. H. Hendriksen, I. E. J. Milder, et al., "Salt Reductions in Some Foods in the Netherlands: Monitoring of Food Composition and Salt Intake," *Nutrients* 9 (2017): 791; **Para- guay:** Consensus Action on Salt & Health, 2013 annual report, http://apps

.charitycommission.gov.uk/Accounts/Ends18/0001098818_ AC_20130430_E_C.pdf; **Peru:** N. Michail, "Peru: Nutrition Warning Labels Become Mandatory," FoodNavigator-latam, https://www.foodnavigator-latam.com/Article/2019/06/17/Peru-Nutrition-warning-labels-become-mandatory#; **South Africa:** S. A. E. Peters, E. Dunford, L. J. Ware et al., "The Sodium Content of Processed Foods in South Africa during the Introduction of Mandatory Sodium Limits," *Nutrients* 9, no. 4 (2017): 404–419; South Africa Department of Health, Government notice no. R. 214, "Regulations Relating to the Reduction of Sodium in Certain Foodstuffs and Related Matters, March 20, 2013, and May 31, 2019, https://www.foodfocus.co.za/assets/documents/UPDATED_Notice%20214%20-Regulations%20relating%20reduction%20of%20sodium.pdf; **Turkey:** World Health Organization, "Progress in Reducing Salt Consumption in Turkey," August 4, 2013, http://www.euro.who.int/en/countries/turkey/news/news/2013/04/progress-in-reducing-salt-consumption-in-turkey (accessed February 17, 2020); Y. Erdem, T. Akpolat, Ü. Derici, et al., "Dietary Sources of High Sodium intake in Turkey: SALTURK II," *Nutrients* 9, no. 9 (2017): 933, doi:10.3390/nu9090933; **United States:** see details of US efforts in chapter 9; **United Kingdom:** Public Health England, "Salt Targets 2017: Progress Report—A Report on the Food Industry's Progress towards Meeting the 2017 Salt Targets," December 2018, https://assets.publishing.service.gov.uk/government/uploads/system/uploads/attachment_data/file/765571/Salt_targets_2017_progress_report.pdf; **Uruguay:** Global Advertising Lawyers Association, "New Front- of-Package Labeling Regulation in Uruguay," *Gala Gazette* 13, no. 4.

14. F. Godlee, "The Food Industry Fights for Salt," Editorial, *BMJ* 312 (1996): 1239–1240.

15. "Order of the British Empire," *Gazette*, June 8, 2019, https://www.thegazette.co.uk/notice/3294142.

16. Action on Salt, "About Us," http://www.actiononsalt.org.uk/about/#targetText =Action%20on%20Salt%20is%20successfully,to%20cooking%2C%20and%20 the%20table (accessed September 2, 2019).

17. G. A. MacGregor, email to the author, October 25, 2019.

18. F. J. He, H. C. Brinsden, and G. A. MacGregor, "Salt Reduction in the United Kingdom: A Successful Experiment in Public Health," *Journal of Human Hypertension* 28, no. 6 (2014): 345–352.

19. Public Health England, "Salt Reduction Targets for 2017," March 2017, https://assets.publishing.service.gov.uk/government/uploads/system/uploads/attachment_data/file/604338/Salt_reduction_targets_for_2017.pdf (accessed September 12, 2019).

20. "PHE Starts Next Stage of New Salt Reduction Targets for Everyday Foods," *F&D Technology*, February 6, 2020, https://www.foodanddrinktechnology.com/news/31024/phe-engages-with-food-industry-on-new-salt-reduction-targets-for-everyday

-foods/ (accessed February 28, 2020); Public Health England, "Draft Proposals: 2023 Salt Reduction Targets," February 2020. In the author's files.

21. UK Food Standards Agency, August 25, 2016, "Public Information Film," https://www.youtube.com/watch?v=ti_JN2yFYPw (accessed December 22, 2018).

22. F. J. He, H. C. Brinsden, and G. A. MacGregor, "Salt Reduction in the United Kingdom: A Successful Experiment in Public Health," *Journal of Human Hypertension* 28, no. 6 (2014): 345–352.

23. G. A. MacGregor, F. J. He, and S. Pombo-Rodrigues, "Food and the Responsibility Deal: How the Salt Reduction Strategy Was Derailed," *BMJ* 350 (2015): h1936.

24. A. A. Laverty, C. Kypridemos, P. Seferidi, et al., "Quantifying the Impact of the Public Health Responsibility Deal on Salt Intake, Cardiovascular Disease and Gastric Cancer Burdens: Interrupted Time Series and Microsimulation Study," *Journal of Epidemiology and Community Health*, 73 (2019): 881-887. Public Health England, Assessment of salt intake (2020), https://bit.ly/3cVGj6z.

25. E. Dunford, J. Webster, M. Woodward, et al., "The Variability of Reported Salt Levels in Fast Foods Across Six Countries: Opportunities for Salt Reduction," *Canadian Medical Association Journal* 184, no. 9 (2012): 1023–1028.

26. McDonald's, Burger King, and Subway (UK and US websites), September 12, 2019.

27. T. R. Frieden, "Sodium Reduction—Saving Lives by Putting Choice into Consumers' Hands," *JAMA* 316, no. 6 (2016): 579–580; F. J. He, M. Tan, Y. Ma, et al., "Salt Reduction to Prevent Hypertension and Cardiovascular Disease: *JACC* State of the Art Review," *Journal of the American College of Cardiology* 75, no. 6 (February 2020): 632–647.

28. Individual sources for figure 7.2: (top) L. Rodriguez, Chilean Ministry of Health, "The Implementation of New Regulations on Nutritional Labelling in Chile," https://www.wto.org/english/tratop_e/tbt_e/8_Chile_e.pdf (accessed August 1, 2018); (middle) Courtesy of Israel Ministry of Health; (bottom) © All Rights Reserved. Health Canada, *Consultation on Proposed Front-of-Package Labelling* (adapted and reproduced with permission from the Minister of Health, 2019).

29. M. Shoup, "Brazil: Front of Package Warning Labels Found to Be an 'Important Addition' to Nutrition Facts," FoodNavigator–latam.com, July 15, 2019, https://www.foodnavigator-latam.com/Article/2019/07/15/Brazil-Front-of-package-warning -labels-found-to-be-an-important-addition-to-nutrition-facts (accessed September 12, 2019); Vital Strategies, "Brazilians Call for New Food Warning Label System," news release, November 13, 2018, http://www.vitalstrategies.org/press/brazilians-call -for-new-food-warning-label-system/ (accessed April 4, 2019).

30. M. Mora-Plazas, L. F. Gómez, D. R. Miles, et al., "Nutrition Quality of Packaged Foods in Bogotá, Colombia: A Comparison of Two Nutrient Profile Models," *Nutrients* 11, no. 5 (2019): 1011, https://www.mdpi.com/2072-6643/11/5/1011.

31. Pan American Health Organization, "Ecuador, Chile and Bolivia Defend Labeling of Processed Foods at PAHO Meeting," September 29, 2016, https://www.paho .org/hq/index.php?option=com_content&view=article&id=12542%3Aecuador -chile-bolivia-defienden-etiquetado-alimentos-procesados-&catid=8883%3A55-dc -events&Itemid=42100&lang=en (accessed August 1, 2018).

32. L. S. Taillie, M. Reyes, M. A. Colchero, et al., "An Evaluation of Chile's Law of Food Labeling and Advertising on Sugar-sweetened Beverage Purchases from 2015 to 2017: A Before-and-After Study." *PLoS Medicine* 17, no. 2 (2020): e1003015, https:// doi.org/10.1371/journal.pmed.1003015.

33. J. Jacobs, "Chile's Sugary Food Fight Echoes around the World," *Financial Times*, March 11, 2020, https://www.ft.com/content/d481cf02-1e47-11e9-a46f -08f9738d6b2b.

34. C. Johnson, J.A. Santos, E Sparks, et al., "Sources of Dietary Salt in North and South India Estimated from 24 hour Dietary Recall," *Nutrients* 11, no. 2 (2019): 318.

Chapter 8

1. M. F. Jacobson, B. F. Liebman, and G. Moyer, *Salt: The Brand Name Guide to Sodium Content* (New York: Warner Books, 1983), 63.

2. Institute of Medicine, *Strategies to Reduce Sodium Intake in the United States* (Washington, DC: The National Academies Press, 2010).

3. *White House Conference on Food, Nutrition, and Health: Final Report* (US Government Printing Office, 1970), https://babel.hathitrust.org/cgi/pt?id=umn.31951d029 87449r;view=1up;seq=61 (accessed November 15, 2018).

4. National Institutes of Health, *Hypertension*, report no. 1714 (Washington, DC, Government Printing Office, 1969).

5. P. H. Wiggins, "Nestlé to Acquire Beech-Nut Baby Foods," *New York Times*, November 21, 1979.

6. M. Burros, "Baby Foods: Taking a Closer Look," *New York Times*, February 10, 1977.

7. US Senate, Select Committee on Nutrition and Human Needs, *Dietary Goals for the United States* (February 1977), https://ia800505.us.archive.org/13/items/ CAT10527234/CAT10527234.pdf (accessed March 12, 2020).

8. E. D. Freis, "Salt, Volume, and the Prevention of Hypertension," *Circulation* 53 (1976): 589–595.

9. *Congressional Record—Senate*, September 10, 1979, 23910, https://www.govinfo
.gov/content/pkg/GPO-CRECB-1979-pt18/pdf/GPO-CRECB-1979-pt18-4-2.pdf
(accessed February 25, 2020).

10. Center for Science in the Public Interest, *Petition to FDA for a Rule to Label the Sodium Content of Foods*, July 10, 1978.

11. Center for Science in the Public Interest, *Petition to FDA for a Rule to Regulate the Sodium Content of Processed Foods*, July 10, 1978.

12. Center for Science in the Public Interest, *Petition to FDA for a Rule Requiring Health Notices on Salt Packages*, December 28, 1981.

13. M. Jacobson, "The Deadly White Powder," *Mother Jones* (July 1978): 12–20.

14. S. A. Miller, interview with the author, March 24, 1978.

15. US Food and Drug Administration, "FDA's Approach to the GRAS Provision: A History of Processes," April 2006, https://www.fda.gov/food/ingredientspackagingla
beling/gras/ucm094040.htm (accessed September 21, 2018).

16. Life Sciences Research Office, Federation of American Societies for Experimen-tal Biology, "SCOGS-102. Evaluation of the Health Effects of Sodium Chloride and Potassium Chloride as Food Ingredients," 1979, http://wayback.archive-it.org/
7993/20171031064319/https://www.fda.gov/Food/IngredientsPackagingLabeling/
GRAS/SCOGS/ucm260741.htm (accessed April 6, 2019).

17. S. A. Miller, letter to CSPI, September 3, 1980.

18. "Retired Frito-Lay Executive Dies of Heart Attack," Associated Press, August 15, 1985, https://apnews.com/d83900be7efe188f0877d071054745ee (accessed February 25, 2020).

19. "Experts Testify on Salt's Value," *Bandwagon* (a Frito-Lay periodical), undated (in author's files).

20. R. Lin, interview with the author, October 11, 2018.

21. R. Lin, interview with the author; also R. Lin, memo to R. Hilton and A. Wohl-man in preparation for the GRAS meeting, "Position Paper on Salt," August 31, 1978.

22. US Food and Drug Administration, "Status of FDA Sodium Activities," June 1983.

23. C. Wallis, "Salt: a New Villain?" *Time*, March 15, 1982.

24. B. F. Liebman, M. Jacobson, and G. Moyer, *Salt: The Brand Name Guide to Sodium Content* (New York: Warner Books, 1983), 58–60.

25. A. H. Hayes, Testimony, House Subcommittee on Health and the Environment, September 25, 1981.

26. US Food and Drug Administration, *Report on the Food and Drug Administration's activities on Sodium Labeling*, January 26, 1985.

27. B. F. Liebman, M. Jacobson, and G. Moyer, *Salt: The Brand Name Guide to Sodium Content*. (New York: Warner Books, 1983), 60–61.

28. C. Wallis, "Salt: A New Villain?" *Time*, March 15, 1982.

29. B. F. Liebman, M. Jacobson, and G. Moyer, *Salt: The Brand Name Guide to Sodium Content* (New York: Warner Books, 1983), 63.

30. US Food and Drug Administration, *Safety Review of Sodium Chloride; Policy Notice; Solicitation of Views*, Fed. Reg. 47, no. 118: 26590-5, June 18, 1982.

31. J. P. Hile, US Food and Drug Administration, letter to CSPI, August 18, 1982.

32. US Food and Drug Administration, Fed Reg. 49(76); April 18, 1984, 15510–15535, http://cdn.loc.gov/service/ll/fedreg/fr049/fr049076/fr049076.pdf (accessed October 6, 2018).

33. R. Lin, memo to Dennis Heard, Calcium Antihypertension Campaign, January 28, 1982 (in the author's files).

34. R. Lin, memo to Dennis Heard.

35. R. Lin, email to the author, January 30, 2020.

36. N. Karanja and D. A. McCarron, "Calcium and Hypertension," *Annual Review of Nutrition* 6 (1986): 475–496.

37. R. Lin, email to the author, January 29, 2020.

38. L. S. Sims, *The Politics of Fat: Food and Nutrition Policy in America* (New York: M. E. Sharpe, 1998).

39. M. Jacobson, "Salt: The Forgotten Killer," Center for Science in the Public Interest, February 1, 2005, https://cspinet.org/resource/salt-forgotten-killer-feb-2005 (accessed August 21, 2018).

40. Center for Science in the Public Interest, *Petition for a Writ of Mandamus*, February 24, 2018, https://cspinet.org/sites/default/files/attachment/salt_lawsuit.pdf (accessed August 21, 2018).

41. *Center for Science in the Public Interest et al. v. Dr. Mark Novitch et al.*, United States District Court for the District of Columbia, Memorandum Opinion, June 11, 1984.

42. Center for Science in the Public Interest, "Group asks FDA to Limit Salt in Processed Foods," November 8, 2005, https://cspinet.org/news/group-asks-fda-limit-salt -processed-foods-20051108 (August 21, 2018).

43. Supplemental statement of the Salt Institute to the Food and Drug Administration public hearing on petition to revise the regulatory status of salt and establish food labeling requirements regarding salt and sodium. March 3, 2008. FDA Docket No. 2005P-0450. 2007.

44. D. Q. Haney, "For 90 Percent of Americans, Salt Doesn't Matter Much," Associated Press, November 13, 1990.

45. Meeting with FDA, October 19, 2005.

Chapter 9

1. T. R. Frieden, "Reducing Sodium Intake in the Population," *JAMA* 316 (2016): 2550–2551.

2. S. Havas and B. D. Dickinson, "Reducing the Population Burden of Cardiovascular Disease by Reducing Sodium Intake, A Report of the Council on Science and Health, American Medical Association," *Archives of Internal Medicine* 167, no. 4 (2007): 1460–1468.

3. American Public Health Association, "Implementing Effective Strategies to Reduce Sodium in the Food Supply," November 1, 2011, https://www.apha.org/policies-and -advocacy/public-health-policy-statements/policy-database/2014/07/21/11/ 36/implementing-effective-strategies-to-reduce-sodium-in-the-food-supply (accessed September 6, 2019).

4. New York City Department of Health and Mental Hygiene, "National Salt Reduction Initiative: Packaged and Restaurant Food," https://www1.nyc.gov/site/doh/ health/health-topics/national-salt-reduction-initiative-packaged-food.page (accessed January 12, 2019); "National Salt and Sugar Reduction Initiative," https://www1 .nyc.gov/assets/doh/downloads/pdf/cardio/nsri-partners.pdf (accessed September 13, 2019).

5. C. J. Curtis, J. Clapp, S. A. Niederman, et al., "US Food Industry Progress during the National Salt Reduction Initiative: 2009–2014," *American Journal of Public Health* 106, no. 10 (2016): 1815–1819, doi:10.2105/AJPH.2016.303397.

6. Grocery Manufacturers Association, Comment (appendix C), Docket No FDA-2011-N-0400, January 27, 2012.

7. Curtis et al., "US Food Industry Progress."

8. Institute of Medicine, *Strategies to Reduce Sodium Intake in the United States* (Washington, DC: The National Academies Press, 2010).

9. Institute of Medicine, "FDA Should Set Standards for Salt Added to Processed Foods, Prepared Meals," April 20, 2010, http://www8.nationalacademies.org/onpinews/ newsitem.aspx?RecordID=12818 (accessed September 15, 2018).

10. W. Neuman, "F.D.A. Is Urged to Set Limits for Levels of Salt in Food," *New York Times*, April 20, 2010, https://www.nytimes.com/2010/04/21/us/21salt.html.

11. Institute of Medicine, *Strategies to Reduce Sodium Intake in the United States* (Washington, DC: The National Academies Press, 2010).

12. R. Kahn, "FDA Public Hearing on Salt and Sodium," November 29, 2007, https://www.regulations.gov/document?D=FDA-2007-0545-0018 (accessed February 10, 2020).

13. Media Matters for America, "With a Grain of Salt: Right-Wing Media Claim Government Is Coming for Your Shaker," April 22, 2010, https://www.mediamatters .org/research/2010/04/22/with-a-grain-of-salt-right-wing-media-claim-gov/163659 (accessed July 11, 2019).

14. Neuman, "F.D.A. Is Urged to Set Limits."

15. Salt Institute, "Comment," December 3, 2011. https://www.regulations.gov/ document?D=FSIS-2011-0014-0001 (accessed October 14, 2018).

16. National Frozen Pizza Institute, "Comment," January 27, 2012, https://www .regulations.gov/document?D=FSIS-2011-0014-0285 (accessed December 4, 2019).

17. S. M. Patel, J. P. Gunn, X. Tong, et al., "Consumer Sentiment on Actions Reducing Sodium in Processed and Restaurant Foods," Consumer Styles 2010, *American Journal of Preventive Medicine* 46 (2014): 516–524.

18. L. Layton, "FDA Plans to Limit Amount of Salt Allowed in Processed Foods for Health Reasons, *Washington Post*, April 20, 2010, http://www.washingtonpost.com/ wp-dyn/content/article/2010/04/19/AR2010041905049.html

19. A. H. Hayes, Testimony, House Subcommittee on Health and the Environment, September 25, 1981.

20. J. Anderer, "Startling Study Reveals Majority of US Packaged Food Is Ultra-Processed," StudyFinds.org, July 29, 2019, https://www.studyfinds.org/startling-study -reveals-majority-packaged-food-is-ultra-processed/ (accessed September 13, 2019).

21. US Food and Drug Administration, "FDA Issues Draft Guidance to Food Industry for Voluntarily Reducing Sodium in Processed and Commercially Prepared Food," May 31, 2016, https://www.fda.gov/news-events/press-announcements/fda-issues-draft -guidance-food-industry-voluntarily-reducing-sodium-processed-and-commercially (accessed February 25, 2020).

22. H. B. Evich, "Obama's Latest Food Crackdown: Salt," *Politico*, April 3, 2016, https://www.politico.com/story/2016/04/the-salt-wars-221490.

23. M. Landa, Comment to docket, October 20, 2015, https://www.regulations.gov/ document?D=FDA-2005-P-0196-0050 (accessed October 1, 2018).

24. "Editorial: The First Congressional District and Election 2018," *Talbot Spy*, May 21, 2018, https://talbotspy.org/editorial-the-first-congressional-district-and-election -2018/.

25. Rep. Andy Harris, March 4, 2015, House Agriculture Appropriations Subcommittee Hearing, https://www.youtube.com/watch?v=KDyuxCfJYMU&list=UUvUuV7FiJf Ji1yux4qozgMg&index=16 (accessed August 19, 2019).

26. Center for Science in the Public Interest, *United States District Court for the District of Columbia, Civil Action No. 15-1651*, October 8, 2015, https://cspinet.org/sites/ default/files/attachment/sodium-complaint-final-10-8-15.pdf (accessed August 18, 2018).

27. US Food and Drug Administration, "FDA Food Categories and Voluntary Targets," https://www.fda.gov/downloads/Food/GuidanceRegulation/GuidanceDocuments RegulatoryInformation/UCM504014.pdf (accessed March 17, 2020).

28. US Food and Drug Administration, "Draft Guidance for Industry: Voluntary Sodium Reduction Goals: Target Mean and Upper Bound Concentrations for Sodium in Commercially Processed, Packaged, and Prepared Foods," June 2016, https://www .fda.gov/Food/GuidanceRegulation/GuidanceDocumentsRegulatoryInformation/ ucm494732.htm (accessed October 7, 2019).

29. A. Jessup and D. Wilmoth, US Department of Health and Human Services, "The Value of a National Reduction in Dietary Sodium from Processed and Restaurant Foods," preliminary draft, October 22, 2013 (in the authors' files).

30. US Food and Drug Administration, "FDA Food Categories and Voluntary Targets," https://www.fda.gov/downloads/Food/GuidanceRegulation/GuidanceDocuments RegulatoryInformation/UCM504014.pdf (accessed March 17, 2020).

31. T. R. Frieden, "Sodium Reduction—Saving Lives by Putting Choice into Consumers' Hands," *JAMA* 316, no. 6 (2016): 579–580.

32. Source for box 9.1: American Heart Association, "Heart-Check Food Certification Program Nutrition Requirements," https://www.heart.org/en/healthy-living/ company-collaboration/heart-check-certification/heart-check-in-the-grocery-store/ heart-check-food-certification-program-nutrition-requirements (accessed August 26, 2019).

33. American Heart Association, "FDA Proposes Voluntary Targets for Food Producers to Lower Sodium," June 1, 2016, https://newsarchive.heart.org/fda-proposes -voluntary-targets-for-food-producers-to-lower-sodium/ (accessed February 25, 2020).

34. Center for Science in the Public Interest, "FDA Issues Voluntary Sodium Reduction Targets," June 1, 2016, https://cspinet.org/news/fda-issues-voluntary-sodium -reduction-targets&20160601 (accessed February 25, 2020).

35. U.S. Food and Drug Administration, "FDA Food Categories and Voluntary Targets," https://www.fda.gov/downloads/Food/GuidanceRegulation/GuidanceDocuments RegulatoryInformation/UCM504014.pdf (accessed March 17, 2020).

36. Public Health England, "Salt Targets 2017: Progress Report—A Report on the Food Industry's Progress towards Meeting the 2017 Salt Targets," December 2018, https://assets.publishing.service.gov.uk/government/uploads/system/uploads/attachment_data/file/765571/Salt_targets_2017_progress_report.pdf (accessed October 11, 2019).

37. Salt Institute, "Government's War on Salt Is Malpractice," June 1, 2016, http://www.saltinstitute.org/press_releases/governments-war-on-salt-is-malpractice/ (accessed August 16, 2018).

38. L. Roman, letter to the Secretaries of Agriculture and Health and Human Services, April 11, 2016.

39. SNAC International, "Statement from SNAC International CEO Regarding FDA Release of Sodium Targets per Food Category," June 1, 2016, http://web.archive.org/web/20160611165335/http://snacintl.org/news/latest-headlines/story/statement-from-snac-international-ceo-regarding-fda-release-of-sodium-targets-per-food-category (accessed February 25, 2020).

40. SNAC International, Comment to FDA, October 17, 2016, https://www.regulations.gov/document?D=FDA-2014-D-0055-0429 (accessed January 19, 2020).

41. SNAC International, January 14, 2020, Statement from SNAC (in the author's files).

42. L. Bruner, Grocery Manufacturers Association, "GMA Statement on Sodium Reduction Guidelines," June 1, 2016, https://www.gmaonline.org/news-events/newsroom/gma-statement-on-sodium-reduction-guidelines/. Link no longer active.

43. Grocery Manufacturers Association, October 17, 2016, Docket No. FDA-2014-D-0055; Grocery Manufacturers Association, December 2, 2016, Docket No. FDA-2014-D-0055.

44. FDA Docket No. FDA-2014-D-0055.

45. Mars, "Mars' Position on the Release of the FDA's Draft Voluntary Guidance on Sodium," June 9, 2016, https://www.mars.com/global/our-news/our-stories/press-release/mars-position-release-fda-draft-voluntary-guidelines-sodium (accessed August 19, 2018).

46. "Letter from Food Manufacturers and Health Groups to the Senate Agriculture Appropriations Subcommittee," May 16, 2016, https://foodpolitics.com/wp-content/uploads/senate-ag-approps-sodium-letter-final-5.16.16.pdf (accessed November 13, 2018); E. Crawford, "Stakeholders Laud FDA's Potentially Life-Saving Draft

Voluntary Sodium Reduction Guidance," *FoodNavigator*, June 1, 2016, https://www
.foodnavigator-usa.com/Article/2016/06/01/Stakeholders-laud-FDA-s-draft-voluntary
-sodium-reduction-guidance.

47. Sustainable Food Policy Alliance, "SFPA Supports the National Academies' Findings on the Need to Reduce Dietary Sodium," March 6, 2019, https://foodpolicyalliance
.org/news/sfpa-supports-the-national-academies-findings-on-the-need-to-reduce
-dietary-sodium/ (accessed April 7, 2019).

48. M. R. L'Abbé, interview with the author, October 11, 2018.

49. National Hispanic Medical Association, November 22, 2016, Docket No.
FDA-2014-D-0055.

50. National Medical Association, October 17, 2016, Docket No. FDA-2014-D-0055.

51. S. Gottlieb, US Food and Drug Administration, "Reducing the Burden of Chronic
Disease," March 29, 2018, https://www.fda.gov/NewsEvents/Speeches/ucm603057
.htm (accessed August 17, 2018).

52. H. B. Evich, "Trump Push to Finish Obama Crackdown on Salt Prompts Stealth
Lobbying," *Politico*, April 12, 2019, https://www.politico.com/story/2019/04/12/
fda-sodium-targets-lobbying-1341016.

53. L. MacCleery, quoted in Evich, "Trump Push to Finish Obama Crackdown on
Salt."

54. IOM Strategies to Reduce Sodium Intake Meeting, March 30, 2009.

55. M. Taylor, interview with the author, September 12, 2018; email to the author,
November 6, 2018.

56. M. Taylor, emails to the author, November 6, 2019.

57. M. Landa, interviews with the author, September 27, 2018, and February 15,
2020.

58. H.R. 244, *Consolidated Appropriations Act*, 2017, Section 766, https://www.congress
.gov/bill/115th-congress/house-bill/244 (accessed September 15, 2019).

59. J. Fasano, email to Philip C. Spiller (FDA staffers), July 22, 2013.

60. M. Landa, interview with the author, September 27, 2018.

61. S. Kass, telephone call with the author, November 11, 2019.

62. M. Poos, email to P. Trumbo (both are FDA staff members), July 22, 2013.

63. S. Kass, telephone call with the author, November 11, 2019.

64. M. Hamburg, email to the author, October 29, 2019.

65. S. Kass, telephone call with the author, November 11, 2019.

66. S. Kass, telephone call with the author, November 11, 2019.

67. US Department of Agriculture, "National School Lunch Program," August 20, 2019, https://www.ers.usda.gov/topics/food-nutrition-assistance/child-nutrition-programs/national-school-lunch-program.aspx (accessed October 30, 2019); US Department of Agriculture, "School Breakfast Program," August 20, 2019, https://www.ers.usda.gov/topics/food-nutrition-assistance/child-nutrition-programs/school-breakfast-program/ (accessed October 30, 2019).

68. Food and Nutrition Service, US Department of Agriculture, "Fact Sheet: Healthy, Hunger-Free Kids Act School Meals Implementation," June 1, 2017, https://www.fns.usda.gov/pressrelease/2014/009814 (accessed October 27, 2018), act is available at https://www.congress.gov/111/plaws/publ296/PLAW-111publ296.pdf (accessed October 29, 2018).

69. US Department of Agriculture, Food and Nutrition Service, "Nutrition Standards in the National School Lunch and School Breakfast Programs; Final Rule," *Federal Register* 77, no. 17 (January 26, 2012): 4088–4167.

70. H. B. Evich, "Food Giants Call Truce with Michelle Obama," *Politico*, September 2, 2015, https://www.politico.com/story/2015/09/michelle-obama-food-giants-school-lunch-truce-213246.

71. "Better Food, Better Communities," https://www.schwanscompany.com/social-responsibility/health-and-wellness.htm (accessed April 8, 2019).

72. School Nutrition Association, "Who We Are," https://schoolnutrition.org/AboutSchoolMeals/WhoWeAre/ (accessed October 27, 2018).

73. R. Kogan, "Rollback of Nutrition Standards Not Supported by Evidence," *Health Affairs Blog*, https://www.healthaffairs.org/do/10.1377/hblog20190312.130704/full/ (accessed November 10, 2019).

74. L. Foley, "Pizza and French Fry Lobbyists also Speak for Lunch Ladies?" *AgMag*, June 10, 2014, https://www.ewg.org/agmag/2014/06/pizza-and-french-fry-lobbyists-also-speak-lunch-ladies (accessed March 10, 2020).

75. School Nutrition Association, 2018 SNA patrons, https://schoolnutrition.org/uploadedFiles/Membership/Industry_Membership/2018-Patron-List.pdf (accessed October 27, 2018).

76. H. B. Evich, "Food Giants Call Truce with Michelle Obama," *Politico*, September 2, 2015, https://www.politico.com/story/2015/09/michelle-obama-food-giants-school-lunch-truce-213246 (accessed October 27, 2018).

77. N. Confessore, "How School Lunch Became the Latest Political Battleground," *New York Times Magazine*, October 7, 2014, https://www.nytimes.com/2014/10/12/magazine/how-school-lunch-became-the-latest-political-battleground.html.

78. School Nutrition Association, IRS Form 990 for the year ending July 31, 2016, https://pdf.guidestar.org/PDF_Images/2017/840/445/2017-840445578-0f7dd983-9O .pdf (accessed March 10, 2020).

79. B. E. Siegel, "More Strife Emerges within School Nutrition Association," *The Lunch Tray* (blog), April 2, 2015, https://www.thelunchtray.com/more-strife-emerges -within-school-nutrition-association/ (accessed October 29, 2018); "CFPB Hears Higher Ed Concerns—Muzzling Arizona Educators?—Lunchroom Spat Gets Ugly," *Politico*, March 30, 2015, https://www.politico.com/tipsheets/morning-education/ 2015/03/cfpb-hears-higher-ed-concerns-muzzling-arizona-educators-lunchroom -spat-gets-ugly-212543.

80. B. E. Siegel, "House Committee Approves Healthy School Meals Waiver; 19 Past Presidents Break with School Nutrition Association," *The Lunch Tray* (blog), May 30, 2014. https://www.thelunchtray.com/house-committee-approves-healthy-school-meals -waiver-19-past-presidents-break-school-nutrition-association/ (accessed October 29, 2018).

81. R. Nixon, "Nutrition Group Lobbies against Healthier School Meals It Sought, Citing Cost, *New York Times*, July 1, 2014, https://www.nytimes.com/2014/07/02/ us/nutrition-group-lobbies-against-healthier-school-meals-it-sought-citing-cost .html.

82. H.R. 244, *Consolidated Appropriations Act*, 2017, Section 766, https://www.congress .gov/bill/115th-congress/house-bill/244 (accessed September 15, 2019).

83. School Nutrition Association, "Model Lobbying Letter to Senators," March 3, 2015.

84. Letter from 14 trade associations to USDA Secretary Sonny Perdue, December 7, 2017.

85. US Department of Agriculture, "Child Nutrition Programs: Flexibilities for Milk, Whole Grains, and Sodium Requirements," Fed. Reg. 63775, December 12, 2018, https://thefederalregister.org/83-FR/Issue-238 (accessed February 18, 2019).

86. US Department of Agriculture, "Responding to the needs of local schools, USDA publishes school meals final rule," December 6, 2018, https://www.usda.gov/media/ press-releases/2018/12/06/responding-needs-local-schools-usda-publishes-school -meals-final (accessed December 10, 2018).

87. US Department of Agriculture, "Ag Secretary Perdue Moves to Make School Meals Great Again," press release, May 1, 2017, https://www.usda.gov/media/press -releases/2017/05/01/ag-secretary-perdue-moves-make-school-meals-great-again (accessed May 4, 2019).

88. School Nutrition Association, USDA School Meal Rule Strikes a Healthy Balance, December 6, 2018, https://schoolnutrition.org/news-publications/press-releases/2018/ usda-school-meal-rule-strikes-a-healthy-balance/ (accessed November 10, 2019).

89. Center for Science in the Public Interest, Press release, "CSPI and Healthy School Food Maryland Sue to Stop USDA's Weakening of Nutrition Standards for School Meals," April 3, 2019, https://cspinet.org/news/cspi-healthy-school-food-maryland -sue-usda-school-meals (accessed February 16, 2020).

90. US Department of Agriculture, Food and Nutrition Service, "School Nutrition and Meal Cost Study, Summary of Findings," April 2019, https://fns-prod.azureedge.net/ sites/default/files/resource-files/SNMCS_Summary-Findings.pdf (accessed May 4, 2019).

91. New York State Attorney General, "Attorney General James and Multistate Coalition Sue Trump Administration for Gutting Key Nutritional Standards for School Meals," April 3, 2019, https://ag.ny.gov/press-release/2019/attorney-general -james-and-multistate-coalition-sue-trump-administration-gutting (accessed February 25, 2020).

92. New York State Attorney General, "Attorney General James and Multistate Coalition Sue Trump Administration for Gutting Key Nutritional Standards for School Meals," press release, April 3, 2019, https://ag.ny.gov/press-release/attorney -general-james-and-multistate-coalition-sue-trump-administration-gutting-key (accessed April 6, 2019).

93. L. E. Green and S. Piccoli, "Trump Administration Sued Over Rollback of School Lunch Standards," *New York Times*, April 3, 2019, https://www.nytimes.com/2019/ 04/03/us/politics/trump-school-lunch-standards.html.

94. Center for Science in the Public Interest, "Federal Court Strikes Down Trump Administration School Nutrition Rollbacks," April 13, 2020, https://cspinet.org/ news/federal-court-strikes-down-trump-administration-school-nutrition -rollbacks-20200413 (accessed April 25, 2020); opinion, Case 8:19-cv-01004-GLS, https://cspinet.org/sites/ default/files/CSPI_v_USDA (accessed April 25, 2020).

95. C. Choi, "Court throws out Trump rollback of school nutrition rules," *Washington Post*, April 14, 2020, https://www.washingtonpost.com/health/court-vacates -trumps-rollback-of-school-nutrition-rules/2020/04/14/d3a5d794-7e78-11ea-84c2 -0792d8591911_story.html.

96. "USDA Secretary Perdue Speaks at the SNA Conference," YouTube (video), March 9, 2020, https://www.youtube.com/watch?v=Jj8n81jCZtg&feature=youtu.be (accessed March 10, 2020).

97. Campbell's Foodservice website, "K–12 Schools," https://www.campbellsfoodservice .com/solutions/solutions-by-segment/k-12-schools/ (accessed February 18, 2019).

98. T. Yarmon, telephone interview with the author, November 20, 2019.

99. P. Muntner, R. M. Carey, S. Gidding, et al., "Potential US Population Impact of the 2017 ACC/AHA High Blood Pressure Guideline," *Circulation* 137, no. 2 (January 9, 2018): 109–118.

100. City Council, City of Philadelphia, Bill 180001-A, September 12, 2018, https:// phila.legistar.com/LegislationDetail.aspx?ID=3320175&GUID=6D36BD24-B801-45D9 -8247-68408BB6AA31&FullText=1 (accessed October 11, 2019).

101. City Council, City of Philadelphia, "Councilwoman Reynolds Brown Introduces Legislation Requiring Sodium Warning Labels to Be Included on All Chain Restaurant Menus," January 25, 2018, http://phlcouncil.com/councilwoman-reynolds -brown-introduces-legislation-requiring-sodium-warning-labels-included-chain -restaurant-menus/ (accessed August 7, 2019).

102. National Restaurant Association, "Sodium Mandate Not a Done Deal...Yet," February 29, 2016, https://www.restaurant.org/News-Research/News/Sodium-mandate -not-a-done-deal-yet (accessed September 23, 2018).

103. A. Amador, National Restaurant Association, quoted in M. Shelby, "Judge Rules for Sodium Labeling in New York City," February 26, 2016, https://www.theshelbyreport .com/2016/02/26/judge-rules-for-sodium-labeling-in-new-york-city/ (accessed January 23, 2020).

104. C. Ramey, "Appeals Court Upholds NYC's Salt Warnings for Menus," *Wall Street Journal*, February 10, 2017, https://www.wsj.com/articles/appeals-court-upholds-nycs -salt-warnings-for-menus-1486767177.

105. R. Nasr, "Panera CEO: I Favor Sodium Warnings on Menus," *CNBC*, June 16, 2015, http://www.cnbc.com/2015/06/16/panera-ceo-i-favor-sodium-warnings-on -menus.html (accessed August 16, 2018).

106. Panera Bread, "Panera Responsibility Report 2015–2016," https://www .panerabread.com/panerabread/documents/press/2017/panera-bread-csr-2015-2016 .pdf (accessed April 8, 2019).

107. L. Hooper, C. Bartlett, S. G. Davey, et al., "Advice to Reduce Dietary Salt for Prevention of Cardiovascular Disease," *Cochrane Database of Systematic Reviews* 1 (2004), https://researchonline.lshtm.ac.uk/id/eprint/12704/1/Hooper_et_al-2004-The _Cochrane_library.pdf.

108. M. Zalot, "Initiative Targets Health Disparities by Reducing Salt in Takeout Food," Temple University, October 16, 2018, https://news.temple.edu/news/2018 -10-16/center-asian-health-chinese-takeout-sodium-reduce-hypertension (accessed November 21, 2018).

109. G. X. Ma, S. Shive, Y. Zhang, et al., "Evaluation of a Healthy Chinese Take-Out Sodium-Reduction Initiative in Philadelphia Low-Income Communities and Neighborhoods," *Public Health Reports* 133, no. 4 (July–August 2018): 472–480.

110. Walmart, "Our Commitments," https://corporate.walmart.com/global-responsibility/ hunger-nutrition/our-commitments (accessed November 11, 2019).

111. Walmart, "Providing Access to Affordable, Sustainable and Healthier Food," 2017, https://corporate.walmart.com/2016grr/enhancing-sustainability/providing-access -to-affordable-healthy-food (accessed November 11, 2019).

112. S. Kass, telephone interview with the author, November 11, 2019.

113. C. D. Rehm, J. L. Peñalvo, A. Afshin, et al., "Dietary Intake among US Adults, 1999–2012," *JAMA* 315, no. 23 (2016): 2542–2553.

114. J. K. C. Ahuja, Y. Li, D. B. Haytowitz, et al., "Assessing Changes in Sodium Content of Selected Popular Commercially Processed and Restaurant Foods: Results from the USDA: CDC Sentinel Foods Surveillance Program," *Nutrients* 11, no. 8 (July 30, 2019).

115. J. M. Poti, E. K. Dunford, and B. M. Popkin, "Sodium Reduction in US House-holds' Packaged Food and Beverage Purchases, 2000 to 2014," *JAMA Internal Medicine* 177, no. 7 (July 1, 2017): 986–994.

116. M. A. McCrory, A. G. Harbaugh, S. Appeadu, et al., "Fast-food Offerings in the United States in 1986, 1991, and 2016 Show Large Increases in Food Variety, Portion Size, Dietary Energy, and Selected Micronutrients," *Journal of the Academy of Nutrition and Dietetics* 119, no. 6 (June 2019): 923–933.

117. J. A. Wolfson, A. J. Moran, M. P. Jarlenski, et al., "Trends in Sodium Content of Menu Items in Large Chain Restaurants in the US," *American Journal of Preventive Medicine* 54, no.1 (January 2018): 28–36.

118. Culinary Institute of America, Harvard T.H. Chan School of Public Health, "Menus of Change: 2019 Annual Report," http://www.menusofchange.org/images/ uploads/pdf/2019MOC_AnnualReport.pdf (accessed October 8, 2019).

119. Culinary Institute of America, "Technique of the Quarter—Developing Healthy Recipes and Menus," https://www.ciachef.edu/uploadedFiles/Pages/Admissions_and _Financial_Aid/Educators/Educational_Materials/Technique_of_the_Quarter/techniques -healthy-cooking.pdf (accessed September 13, 2018).

120. Schnucks.com, November 8, 2019.

121. S. Girgis, B. Neal, and J. A. Prescott, "One-Quarter Reduction in the Salt Con-tent of Bread Can Be Made without Detection," *European Journal of Clinical Nutrition* 57 (2003): 616–620.

122. M. Mitchell, N. P. Brunton, and M. G. Wilkinson, "Current Salt Reduction Strategies and Their Effect on Sensory Acceptability: A Study with Reduced Salt Ready-Meals," *European Food Research and Technology* (2011): 1–11.

123. R. Jaenke, F. Barzi, E. McMahon, et al., "Consumer Acceptance of Reformulated Food Products: A Systematic Review and Meta-Analysis of Salt-Reduced Foods," *Critical Review of Food Science and Nutrition* 57, no 16 (2017): 3357–3372.

124. M. Breslin, interview with the author, January 3, 2019.

125. Healthy Meals R&D Collaborative, "HMC Success Stories," http://www
.ciahealthymenus.com/success-stories/ (accessed December 20, 2018).

126. E. Watson, "Cheese Trial Next after Bakers Slash Salt with 'Micro' Particles," *Food Manufacture*, August 11, 2010, https://www.foodmanufacture.co.uk/
Article/2010/08/11/Cheese-trial-next-after-bakers-slash-salt-with-micro-particles
(accessed August 20, 2018).

127. Healthy Meals R&D Collaborative, "HMC Success Stories," http://www
.ciahealthymenus.com/success-stories/ (accessed December 20, 2018).

128. L. Roberson and N. Bomm, "Partnering for Success . . . Reducing Sodium in
Hospital Settings," June 8, 2016, http://dialogue4health.org/uploads/resources/
Roberson_060816.pdf (accessed December 21, 2018).

129. Roberson and Bomm, "Partnering for Success."

130. I. Brat and M. T. Tamman, "Food Makers Quietly Cut Down on Salt," *Wall
Street Journal*, January 11, 2010, https://www.wsj.com/articles/SB1000142405274870
3585704574650562683895666.

131. T. Robinson, "Reducing Salt in Canned Foods," in *Reducing Salt in Foods: Practical Strategies*, ed. D. Kilcast and F. Angus (Boca Raton, FL: CRC Press, 2007); H.J.
Heinz Foods UK Ltd., https://www.heinz.co.uk/Products (accessed September 27,
2018).

132. P. Verduin, email to the author, November 9, 2019.

133. C. Lyles, Revolution Foods, interview with the author, December 17, 2018.

134. "Inmates Improve Health on the Inside," http://placemattersoregon.com/my
-place/ (accessed April 22, 2019).

135. "Improving Health on $2.55 a Day," Oregon Department of Corrections,
Oregon Health Authority, http://placemattersoregon.com/what-the-experts-say/
(accessed April 22, 2019).

136. L. Thorsten, interview with the author, August 14, 2019.

137. Center for Disease Control and Prevention, "Progress toward the 1990 Objec-
tives for Improved Nutrition," *Morbidity and Mortality Weekly Report* 37, no. 31
(1988): 475–479, https://www.cdc.gov/mmwr/preview/mmwrhtml/00001076.htm
(accessed August 15, 2019).

138. Campbell Soup Co., "Campbell Announces Major Step Forward in Sodium
Reduction; Adds 48 Reformulated Soups to Its Lower Sodium Portfolio," press
release, February 18, 2008, https://www.campbellsoupcompany.com/newsroom/

press-releases/campbell-announces-major-step-forward-in-sodium-reduction-adds -48-reformulated-soups-to-its-lower-sodium-portfolio/ (accessed August 20, 2018).

139. C. Scott-Thomas, "Campbell's to Add Back Sodium to Combat Soup Sales Slump," *FoodNavigator*, July 12, 2011, https://www.foodnavigator-usa.com/Article/ 2011/07/13/Campbell-s-to-add-back-sodium-to-combat-soup-sales-slump.

140. Campbell Soup Co., consumer information telephone call, April 9, 2019.

141. D. G. Liem, F. Miremadi, E. H. Zandstra, et al., "Health Labelling Can Influence Taste Perception and Use of Table Salt for Reduced-Sodium Products," *Public Health Nutrition* 15, no. 12 (December 2012): 2340–2347, https://www.cambridge.org/ core/journals/public-health-nutrition/article/health-labelling-can-influence-taste -perception-and-use-of-table-salt-for-reducedsodium-products/7F53B33A202D529FB 11F330708997CC3.

142. J. Anthony, "Progress in Sodium Reduction by the Food Industry," YouTube (video), July 19, 2018, https://www.youtube.com/watch (accessed December 27, 2018).

143. D. G. Liem, "Infants' and Children's Salt Taste Perception and Liking: A Review," *Nutrients* 9, no. 9 (2017): 1011.

144. R. D. Mattes, "The Taste for Salt in Humans," *American Journal of Clinical Nutrition* 65 (suppl.) (1997): 692S–697S.

145. S. D. Munger, "The Mechanisms of Salty and Sour Tastes," chapter 16 in *Chemosensory Transduction: The Detection of Odors, Tastes, and Other Chemostimuli* (New York: Academic Press, 2016), 287–297.

146. J. Cafasso, "The Facts about Lithium Toxicity," Healthline, https://www .healthline.com/health/lithium-toxicity (accessed November 29, 2019).

147. J. H. Tudor, *Hypertension: Community Control of High Blood Pressure*, 3rd ed. (London: CRC Press, 2004).

148. F. W. Lowenstein, "Blood-Pressure in Relation to Age and Sex in the Tropics and Subtropics," *Lancet* 277 (February 18, 1961): 389–392; B. Jansson, "Sodium: In 'NO!' Potassium: 'Yes!'" (unpublished), chapter 2 in *Human Diet before Modern Times*, 1977, https://thepaleodiet.com/wp-content/uploads/2017/05/Jansson-Chapter -2.pdf (accessed November 15, 2018).

149. NuTek Food Science, Comment to Docket No. FDA-2014-D-0055, October 17, 2016, (https://www.regulations.gov/document (accessed June 7, 2019).

150. "Soup and Steel Tariffs," Seeking Alpha$^\alpha$ (blog), March 5, 2018, https:// seekingalpha.com/article/4153129-soup-steel-tariffs (accessed January 12, 2019).

151. B. Boor, interview with the author, February 20, 2019.

152. US Food and Drug Administration, Docket ID: FDA-2016-P-1826 2016, https://www.regulations.gov/docketBrowser?rpp=50&so=DESC&sb=commentDueDate&po=0&dct=PS&D=FDA-2016-P-1826 (accessed November 10, 2018).

153. Salt Institute, Comment to US Food and Drug Administration, August 19, 2016, http://saltinstitute.org/wp-content/uploads/2016/08/Citizen-Petition-from-NuTek .pdf (accessed November 10, 2018).

154. US Food and Drug Administration, "Draft Guidance for Industry: the Use of an Alternate Name for Potassium Chloride in Food Labeling," May 2019, https://www .fda.gov/regulatory-information/search-fda-guidance-documents/draft-guidance -industry-use-alternate-name-potassium-chloride-food-labeling (accessed June 18, 2019).

155. Author's calculations based on the Label Insight database of ingredients and nutrient contents, February 2019.

156. US Food and Drug Administration 21 CFR 184.1622, https://www.accessdata. fda.gov/scripts/cdrh/cfdocs/cfcfr/CFRSearch.cfm?fr=184.1622 (accessed November 9, 2018).

157. C. Farrand, G. MacGregor, N. R. C. Campbell, et al., "Potential Use of Salt Substitutes to Reduce Blood Pressure," *Journal of Clinical Hypertension* 21, no. 3 (2019): 350–354.

158. L. D'Elia, C. Iannotta, P. Sabino, et al., "Potassium-Rich Diet and Risk of Stroke: Updated Meta-analysis," *Nutrition, Metabolism, and Cardiovascular Diseases* 24, no. 6 (2019): 585–587.

159. National Academies of Sciences, Engineering, and Medicine, *Dietary Reference Intakes for Sodium and Potassium* (Washington, DC: The National Academies Press, 2019), https://www.nap.edu/catalog/25353/dietary-reference-intakes-for-sodium-and -potassium (accessed April 11, 2019).

160. National Institute of Diabetes and Digestive and Kidney Diseases, "Nutrition for Advanced Chronic Kidney Disease in Adults," 2014, https://www.niddk.nih.gov/ health-information/kidney-disease/chronic-kidney-disease-ckd/eating-nutrition/ nutrition-advanced-chronic-kidney-disease-adults (accessed November 5, 2018); United States Renal Data System. "Chapter 1: CKD in the General Population," (download slides or data), https://www.usrds.org/2018/view/v1_01.aspx (accessed November 9, 2018).

161. M. Marklund, G. Singh, R. C. Greer, et al., "Estimated Population-wide Benefits and Risks in China of Lowering Sodium Through Potassium-enriched Salt Substitution: Modelling Study," *BMJ* 369 (2020), http://dx.doi.org/10.1136 bmj.m824.

162. Scientific Advisory Committee on Nutrition, "SACN Statement on Potassium-Based Sodium Replacers: Assessment of the Benefits of Increased Potassium Intakes

to Health," 2017, https://assets.publishing.service.gov.uk/government/uploads/system/uploads/attachment_data/file/660249/SACN_-_Potassium-based_sodium_replacers.pdf (accessed November 30, 2018).

163. Institute of Medicine, *Strategies to Reduce Sodium Intake in the United States* (Washington, DC: The National Academies Press, 2010), appendix D, https://www.ncbi.nlm.nih.gov/books/NBK50965/ (accessed December 20, 2018).

164. Senomyx, Inc., "Flavor Focus: Savory," https://web.archive.org/web/20181229073424/http://www.senomyx.com/flavor-focus/savory (accessed April 26, 2020).

165. Senomyx, Research Programs, https://web.archive.org/web/20181231103917/http://www.senomyx.com/our-expertise/research-programs/ (accessed April 26, 2020).

Chapter 10

1. F. J. He, H. C. Brinsden, and G. A. MacGregor, "Salt Reduction in the United Kingdom: A Successful Experiment in Public Health," *Journal of Human Hypertension* 28 (2014): 345–352.

2. G. A. MacGregor, interview with the author, October 15, 2019.

3. IOM (Institute of Medicine), *Strategies to Reduce Sodium Intake in the United States* (Washington, DC: The National Academies Press, 2010).

4. Public Health England, "Salt Targets 2017: Progress Report—A Report on the Food Industry's Progress towards Meeting the 2017 Salt Targets," December 2018, https://assets.publishing.service.gov.uk/government/uploads/system/uploads/attachment_data/file/765571/Salt_targets_2017_progress_report.pdf (accessed October 11, 2019).

Chapter 11

1. N. D. L. Fisher, "For the Good of Your Heart: Keep Holding the Salt," *Harvard Health Blog*, July 11, 2016, https://www.health.harvard.edu/blog/good-heart-keep-holding-salt-201607119952 (accessed November 1, 2019).

2. American Heart Association, "Heart Disease and Stroke Statistics—2019 Update," *Circulation* 139 (2019): e56–e528m, http://dx.doi.org/10.1161/CIR.0000000000000659; R. S. Vasan, A. Beiser, S. Seshadri, et al., "Residual Lifetime Risk for Developing Hypertension in Middle-Aged Women and Men: the Framingham Heart Study," *JAMA* 287 (2002): 1003–1010.

3. US Food and Drug Administration, "Sodium: Look at the Label," https://www.fda.gov/downloads/Food/IngredientsPackagingLabeling/UCM315630.pdf (accessed August 19, 2018).

4. Source for box 10.1: US Food and Drug Administration, "Sodium in Your Diet," June 2018, https://www.fda.gov/downloads/Food/IngredientsPackagingLabeling/UCM315471.pdf (accessed October 9, 2019).

5. S. Wadyka, "Must Love Pasta," *Consumer Reports* (January 2019): 20–25.

6. T. Elfassy, S. Yi, D. Eisenhower, et al., "Use of Sodium Information on the Nutrition Facts Label in New York City Adults with Hypertension," *Journal of the Academy of Nutrition and Dietetics* 115 (2015): 278–283.

7. Sources for box 11.2: "All salt is kosher": J. Feldman, "So What Exactly Is Kosher Salt, Since Salt Is Already Kosher to Begin With?" *Huffington Post*, March 21, 2016, https://www.huffpost.com/entry/what-is-kosher-salt_n_56e978a5e4b0860f99db20b5. "Drain and rinse salted canned vegetables and other foods": American Heart Association, "How to Reduce Sodium," May 23, 2018, https://www.heart.org/en/healthy-living/healthy-eating/eat-smart/sodium/how-to-reduce-sodium (accessed February 24, 2019).

8. G. K. Beauchamp, Press conference for 2010 Institute of Medicine report on lowering sodium intakes, April 20, 2010, http://www.nationalacademies.org/podcast/042110SodiumStrategies.mp3. Link no longer active.

9. Dietary Guidelines Advisory Committee, scientific report, 2005, https://health.gov/dietaryguidelines/dga2005/report/ (accessed April 14, 2019); G. K. Beauchamp, M. Bertino, and K. Engelman, "Modification of Salt Taste," *Annals of Internal Medicine* 98 (May 1983): 763–769.

10. US Department of Health and Human Services, US Department of Agriculture, "Dietary Guidelines for Americans," 2005, http://www.health.gov/dietaryguidelines/dga2005/document/html/chapter8.htm.

11. G. K. Beauchamp, M. Bertino, and K. Engelman, "Failure to Compensate Decreased Dietary Sodium with Increased Table Salt Usage," *JAMA* 258, no. 22 (1987): 3275–3278.

12. E. Heil, "Is the Best Burger at a Butcher in W. Va?," *Washington Post*, November 6, 2019.

13. A. Maloney, "For a Crunchy Crust, Cook Your Next Pizza in Blazing-Hot Cast Iron," *Washington Post*, February 12, 2020.

14. S. Nosrat, "How to Make Perfect Sweet Potatoes Every Time," *New York Times*, June 11, 2019.

15. E. F. Crown, "Cooking," *JAMA* 244 (1980): 2355.

16. C. Claiborne, "Tips from an Ex-Addict," *Time*, March 15, 1982.

17. Survey conducted from October 1–3, 2013, and sponsored by Klinge Foods Ltd., maker of LoSalt reduced-sodium salt substitute.

18. Cargill, "Sea Salts," https://www.cargill.com/food-beverage/na/cargill-sea-salts (accessed October 19, 2019); Discovery Communications produced an excellent video on how salt is obtained from underground mines and seawater and how salt is used. "How Stuff Works: Salt," YouTube (video), https://www.youtube.com/watch?v=gI5qV-kvLeg (accessed January 3, 2019); you also could visit the Kansas Underground Salt Museum in person or online: http://underkansas.org/ (accessed February 21, 2019).

19. Harvard School of Public Health, Culinary Institute of America, "Tasting Success with Cutting Salt," 2010, https://www.health.harvard.edu/PDFs/tasting-success-with-cutting-salt.pdf (accessed October 10, 2019).

20. S. Drake and M. Drake, "Comparison of Salty Taste and Time Intensity of Sea and Land Salts from Around the World," *Journal of Sensory Studies* 26 (2011): 25–34.

21. "Sorting Out Sea Salt," *Cook's Illustrated*, https://www.cooksillustrated.com/how_tos/5470-sorting-out-sea-salt?incode=MCSCD00L0&ref=new_search_experience_3 (accessed February 26, 2020).

22. Saltwell AB, "Saltwell Is a Sea Salt with Naturally Reduced Sodium," http://www.saltwellsalt.com/products (accessed September 17, 2018).

23. Alsiano, "A/S. Salona—the Low-Sodium Sea Salt," June 23, 2015, https://www.alsiano.com/News/Show/Salona-natural-sodium-reduction.aspx?Action=1&currentPage=9&M=NewsV2&PID=11945 (accessed November 9, 2019).

24. Alsiano, "Salona—Natural Sodium Reduction," June 23, 2015, http://www.alsiano.com/News/Show/Salona-natural-sodium-reduction.aspx?Action=1&currentPage=11&M=NewsV2&PID=11945 (accessed August 19, 2018).

Epilogue

1. M. Warner, "The War Over Salt, It's the Food Industry vs. an Army of Medical Experts," *New York Times*, September 13, 2008.

2. National High Blood Pressure Education Program, "Implementing Recommendations for Dietary Salt Reduction," NIH publication no. 55-728N, November 1996, https://www.nhlbi.nih.gov/files/docs/resources/heart/hbp_salt.pdf (accessed November 10, 2019).

3. L. J. Appel, interview with the author, November 25, 2019.

4. "Jeremiah Stamler," Wikipedia, https://en.wikipedia.org/wiki/Jeremiah_Stamler (accessed October 26, 2019).

5. J. Stamler and P. Elliott, "Commentary: Evidence on Salt and Blood Pressure is Consistent and Persuasive," *International Journal of Epidemiology* 31 (2002): 316–319.

6. H. Waxman, *The Waxman Report* (New York: Twelve/Hachette Book Group, 2009).

7. Waxman, *The Waxman Report*.

8. J. Morris, "Ford Spent $40 Million to Reshape Asbestos Science," February 16, 2016, https://www.publicintegrity.org/2016/02/16/19297/ford-spent-40-million-reshape-asbestos-science (accessed November 12, 2018).

9. D. Michaels, *Doubt Is Their Product* (Oxford: Cambridge University Press, 2008).

10. S. Cuozzo, "The Nanny State's War on Salt Won't Make Us Healthier," *New York Post*, December 6, 2015, https://nypost.com/2015/12/06/the-nanny-states-war-on-salt-wont-make-us-healthier/ (accessed February 19, 2020).

11. Center for Consumer Freedom website, www.consumerfreedom.com.

Index

Page numbers followed by a "b," "f," or "t" indicate boxes, figures, or tables, respectively.

About the Author

Michael F. Jacobson holds a BA in chemistry from the University of Chicago and a PhD in microbiology from the Massachusetts Institute of Technology. After graduating from MIT, Jacobson moved to Washington, DC, to volunteer with Ralph Nader. He soon met James Sullivan and Albert Fritsch, two other Nader's Raiders with doctorates, and the three created a new nonprofit organization, the Center for Science in the Public Interest. CSPI's main focus has been to educate consumers and advocate for improved government policies and corporate practices related to nutrition and health. Jacobson began his work in Washington by writing books about food additives and nutrition and has been working ever since to improve the healthfulness of the food supply. He and CSPI led efforts to ban trans fat, win passage of the that put Nutrition Facts labels on food packages and calorie counts on menus of chain restaurants, improve the nutritional quality of school foods, stop many deceptive food ads and labels, and focus public attention on health harms from sugar drinks and salt. After serving as the co-director or executive director of CSPI for more than four decades, he is now a Senior Scientist at the organization.